SNP138	91	5	96	0	94.79	5.21	0.10
SNP139	85	11	96	0	88.54	11.46	0.20
SNP140	92	3	95	1	96.84	3.16	0.06
SNP141	3	89	92	4	3.26	96.74	0.06
SNP142	24	70	94	2	25.53	74.47	0.38
SNP143	51	36	87	9	58.62	41.38	0.49
SNP144	40	47	87	9	45.98	54.02	0.50
SNP145	74	21	95	1	77.89	22.11	0.34
SNP146	73	15	88	8	82.95	17.05	0.28
SNP147	92	4	96	0	95.83	4.17	0.08
SNP148	9	86	95	1	9.47	90.53	0.17
SNP149	38	50	88	8	43.18	56.82	0.49
SNP150	65	29	94	2	69.15	30.85	0.43
SNP151	4	88	92	4	4.35	95.65	0.08
SNP152	31	61	92	4	33.70	66.30	0.45
SNP153	3	89	92	4	3.26	96.74	0.06
SNP154	29	58	87	9	33.33	66.67	0.44
SNP155	45	42	87	9	51.72	48.28	0.50
SNP156	19	71	90	6	21.11	78.89	0.33
SNP157	86	7	93	3	92.47	7.53	0.14
SNP158	66	24	90	6	73.33	26.67	0.39
SNP159	70	23	93	3	75.27	24.73	0.37
SNP160	93	3	96	0	96.88	3.13	0.06
SNP161	3	60	63	33	4.76	95.24	0.09
SNP162	74	20	94	2	78.72	21.28	0.33
SNP163	91	5	96	0	94.79	5.21	0.10
SNP164	75	17	92	4	81.52	18.48	0.30
SNP165	69	25	94	2	73.40	26.60	0.39
SNP166	56	35	91	5	61.54	38.46	0.47
SNP167	61	27	88	8	69.32	30.68	0.43
SNP168	69	24	93	3	74.19	25.81	0.38
SNP169	29	63	92	4	31.52	68.48	0.43
SNP170	30	55	85	11	35.29	64.71	0.46
SNP171	39	50	89	7	43.82	56.18	0.49
SNP172	75	17	92	4	81.52	18.48	0.30
SNP173	17	76	93	3	18.28	81.72	0.30
SNP174	41	47	88	8	46.59	53.41	0.50
SNP175	4	88	92	4	4.35	95.65	0.08
SNP176	26	65	91	5	28.57	71.43	0.41
SNP177	17	76	93	3	18.28	81.72	0.30
SNP178	9	79	88	8	10.23	89.77	0.18
SNP179	59	34	93	3	63.44	36.56	0.46
SNP180	33	59	92	4	35.87	64.13	0.46
SNP181	3	69	72	24	4.17	95.83	0.08
SNP182	25	69	94	2	26.60	73.40	0.39
SNP183	71	17	88	8	80.68	19.32	0.31
SNP184	22	69	91	5	24.18	75.82	0.37
SNP185	48	42	90	6	53.33	46.67	0.50
SNP186	81	14	95	1	85.26	14.74	0.25
SNP187	22	63	85	11	25.88	74.12	0.38
SNP188	3	92	95	1	3.16	96.84	0.06
SNP189	54	35	89	7	60.67	39.33	0.48
SNP190	13	79	92	4	14.13	85.87	0.24
SNP191	15	76	91	5	16.48	83.52	0.28
SNP192	70	21	91	5	76.92	23.08	0.36
SNP193	7	85	92	4	7.61	92.39	0.14

SNP							
SNP194	3	93	96	0	3.13	96.88	0.06
SNP195	39	49	88	8	44.32	55.68	0.49
SNP196	66	25	91	5	72.53	27.47	0.40
SNP197	7	80	87	9	8.05	91.95	0.15
SNP198	93	3	96	0	96.88	3.13	0.06
SNP199	41	50	91	5	45.05	54.95	0.50
SNP200	13	83	96	0	13.54	86.46	0.23
SNP201	53	39	92	4	57.61	42.39	0.49
SNP202	40	47	87	9	45.98	54.02	0.50
SNP203	3	93	96	0	3.13	96.88	0.06
SNP204	4	82	86	10	4.65	95.35	0.09
SNP205	92	3	95	1	96.84	3.16	0.06
SNP206	73	20	93	3	78.49	21.51	0.34
SNP207	75	18	93	3	80.65	19.35	0.31
SNP208	32	57	89	7	35.96	64.04	0.46
SNP209	60	33	93	3	64.52	35.48	0.46
SNP210	76	19	95	1	80.00	20.00	0.32
SNP211	45	46	91	5	49.45	50.55	0.50
SNP212	33	57	90	6	36.67	63.33	0.46
SNP213	19	72	91	5	20.88	79.12	0.33
SNP214	25	60	85	11	29.41	70.59	0.42

lymorphism Information Content (Totals excluding NAs).

Analysis of association between SNPs and state of collection of isolates

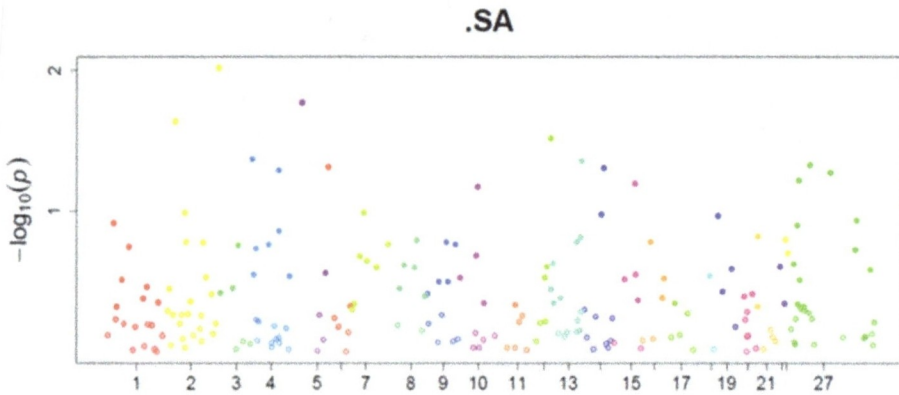

igure C1: Manhattan plot of all isolates showing association between SNPs and South Australia
xis: Supercontigs (27= SC0); y-xis $-\log_{10}$ values of association between stubble species and SNPs.

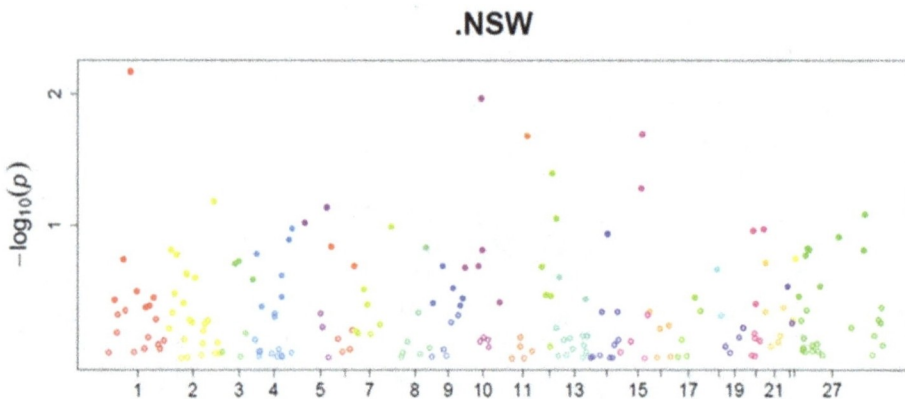

Figure C2: Manhattan plot of all isolates showing association between SNPs and New South Wales
x-axis supercontigs (27= SC0); y-xis $-\log_{10}$ values of association between stubble species and SNPs.

The Role of Hypoxia in Human Health and Disease

Editor: Ronin Wahlberg

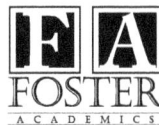

FA
FOSTER
A C A D E M I C S

www.fosteracademics.com

www.fosteracademics.com

FA
FOSTER
ACADEMICS

Cataloging-in-Publication Data

The role of hypoxia in human health and disease / edited by Ronin Wahlberg.
    p. cm.
Includes bibliographical references and index.
ISBN 978-1-63242-926-1
1. Anoxemia. 2. Oxygen in the body. 3. Hypoxia (Water). 4. Diseases--Causes and theories of causation.
5. Health. I. Wahlberg, Ronin.
RC103.A4 R65 2020
616.989 3--dc23

Foster Academics,
118-35 Queens Blvd., Suite 400,
Forest Hills, NY 11375, USA

ISBN 978-1-63242-926-1 (Hardback)

Contents

Preface

Every book is a source of knowledge and this one is no exception. The idea that led to the conceptualization of this book was the fact that the world is advancing rapidly; which makes it crucial to document the progress in every field. I am aware that a lot of data is already available, yet, there is a lot more to learn. Hence, I accepted the responsibility of editing this book and contributing my knowledge to the community.

The condition characterized by an inadequate supply of oxygen, at the level of tissues, in a region of the body is termed as hypoxia. This can arise due to decreased partial pressures of oxygen, insufficient available hemoglobin, and problems with the diffusion of oxygen in the lungs, breathing rhythm and blood flow. It may be classified as generalized or local. Generalized hypoxia can happen when people ascend to high altitudes, leading to potentially fatal consequences including high altitude cerebral edema and high altitude pulmonary edema. It can also occur when individuals breathe in a mixture of gases with low oxygen content. Hypoxia is a common complication of premature births when the lungs are not fully formed. Within minutes after the symptoms of hypoxia have set in, the brain, liver and other vital organs can be damaged. This book is a valuable compilation of topics, ranging from the basic to the most complex advancements in the understanding of the role of hypoxia in human health and disease. It includes some of the vital pieces of work being conducted across the world, on various topics related to this medical condition. Coherent flow of topics, student-friendly language and extensive use of examples make this book an invaluable source of knowledge.

While editing this book, I had multiple visions for it. Then I finally narrowed down to make every chapter a sole standing text explaining a particular topic, so that they can be used independently. However, the umbrella subject sinews them into a common theme. This makes the book a unique platform of knowledge.

I would like to give the major credit of this book to the experts from every corner of the world, who took the time to share their expertise with us. Also, I owe the completion of this book to the never-ending support of my family, who supported me throughout the project.

Editor

Hypoxia Modulates the Adenosinergic Neural Network

Susana P. Gaytán and Rosario Pasaro

Abstract

The aim of this study was to review the latest findings about the neural plasticity on the adenosinergic neural network after the exposition to hypoxia. Identification of the neuromorphology that supports the physiological adaptations underlying the response of organisms to environmental factors including injurious exposures (specifically hypoxia) has been one of the major research challenges in biomedicine. To know these responses would connect the metabolic needs and the vegetative neuronal networks in an integrated way. Hypoxia refers to a state in which oxygen supply is insufficient and several neural cardiorespiratory structures are responsible for correcting and preventing its effects. Although hypoxia is often a pathological condition, variations in arterial oxygen concentrations can be part of the normal physiological responses, for example, during hypoventilation training or strenuous physical exercise. Also, hypoxia is a serious consequence of preterm birth in the neonate. Neural plasticity is a persistent change in the morphology and/or function based on prior experiences, and it is crucial for understanding its effects. Plasticity is well evident when the triggering experience occurs early in life; but in the case of respiratory control plasticity, could also be present in adult life. The regulation of adenosinergic neural network maturation, especially in central cardiorespiratory areas, could provide new perspectives in respiratory new-born distress symptoms.

Keywords: hypoxia, purinergic network, adenosine, central respiratory control, neuronal plasticity

1. Introduction

One of the main functions of the cardiorespiratory system is to guarantee that all tissues are adequately oxygenated at all time, maintaining the normal mitochondrial oxidative process and ATP production. The most common electron acceptor is molecular oxygen (O_2), and when O_2 is present, the mitochondria will undergo aerobic respiration. To maintain O_2 levels, in healthy animals, ventilation is tightly controlled by a system that must maintain the precise constancy of alveolar and arterial blood gases and acid-base status, as well as minimizing the work and metabolic cost of breathing. Deviations from these normal values lead to hypoxic tissue environments [1–6].

In mammals, a lack of O_2 (hypoxia) induces acute reflexes including increasing ventilation and sympathetic tone in order to almost immediately improve the uptake and distribution of O_2 to all tissues of the organism. When the conditions of hypoxia were prolonged, during hours or days, as a defence mechanism it would induce the expression of different genes that, consequently, would modify the ATP metabolism. Indeed, all the homeostatic control of the animal would be affected and other changes would be induced such as increased ventilation, erythropoiesis and angiogenesis, all of that would results in improved O_2 tissue levels. In order to produce the complete response to hypoxia, a group of specialized cells are key to mediate these fast reflex responses. These cells are crucial because they are capable of sensing small variations of O_2, and this information is crucial to maintain O_2 homeostasis. Among the organs that respond acutely to hypoxia, the carotid body (CB) is currently attracting renewed medical interest, as its over-activation seems to be involved in the autonomous dysfunction that accompanies numerous highly prevalent disorders such as sleep apnoea, diabetes, hypertension and chronic heart failure [1–6].

The aim of this study was to review the latest findings about the neural plasticity of the adenosinergic neural network implicated in the central regulation of breathing after the exposition to hypoxia. Four types of hypoxia are currently known: first, the hypoxemic type, in which the blood O_2 levels fall down and they could not saturate the molecules of haemoglobin. Secondly, in the anaemic type, low concentrations of functional haemoglobin avoid the erythrocytes that could make an effective transportation of O_2. Thirdly, the stagnant type, in which hemodynamic is altered and the velocity and volume of the blood flow is diminished, as that occurs in shock or syncope. Finally, the histotoxic hypoxia was referred to a reduction due to a deficiency in the utilization of O_2 by the cells. To compensate for hypoxia, cardiovascular and respiratory functions are implemented increasing the cardiac rhythm, causing hypertension, modifying the ventilatory rhythm and increasing the activity of the accessory breathing muscles of neck and upper chest. As the hypoxia continues to worsen, these compensatory mechanisms would begin to fail [1–6].

All of these systemic responses are controlled by specific brain areas that integrate the information about the hypoxic conditions and conduct the changes during the hypoxic insult to initiate an adaptive process. As in other systems, the neural plasticity is a central cue for the cardiovascular and respiratory responses to the hypoxia functional adaptation. Neural plasticity implies a persistent change in the morphology and/or function based on prior experiences and it is crucial for understanding the changes in the central control of cardiorespiratory functions. Plasticity is well evident when the triggering experience occurs early in life; but in the case of respiratory central control, plasticity could also be present in adult life [3, 5, 7–11]. Since ATP production is compromised during exposure to hypoxia, it is interesting to try to discuss the possible role of the purinergic signalling, in general, and the neuronal adenosinergic network, among other neural structures, responsible of the defence response against hypoxia. This interplay could confer emergent properties to the central respiratory control system. Understanding these mechanisms and their interactions may enable us to optimize hypoxia-induced plasticity as a way to improve treatments for patients that suffer from different ventilatory impairments or other related pathologies [1–6]. On the other hand, the hypoxic hypometabolism differs in adults or young animals. Indeed, it would have a more evident effect in mammals when the levels of O_2 consumption are higher (i.e. in small or young animals when they are exposed to cold). It is clear that a good strategical adaptation to low O_2 levels (hypoxia) requires coordinated down-regulation of metabolic demand, as well as tissue supply, in order to prevent a mismatch in ATP utilization and production that might end in a bioenergetic collapse. In this way, substantial experimental evidence suggests that common integrative structures are probably involved in the metabolic and ventilatory responses to hypoxia [12–15]. The synthesis of adenosine is related to the cellular ratio AMP/ATP (**Figure 1**) and, obviously, to the energy metabolism of cells. In addition, in the central nervous system (CNS), an increase in neuronal activity needs a higher expense of energy and, for this reason, the extracellular levels of adenosine would be modified. The adenosinergic system acts, in CNS, to bind adenosine to one of the different adenosine receptors (A-Rs). Usually, the increased high levels of extracellular adenosine would induce a decrease in neuronal activity. Because the cells reduce its activity, its need for energy falls down too. This nucleoside usually acts via receptor-dependent mechanisms, and could also use receptor-independent mechanisms. Anyway, its complex and wide range of actions imply that adenosine could have a significant role in the defence against cell damage in areas of increased energy requirements, in tissues as well as in recovering the normal/physiological state from a pathologic one [6, 12–22].

Furthermore, the above-mentioned hypometabolism is mediated by an activation of the chemoreceptors by depletion in the arterial O_2 partial pressure (Pa_{O_2}) among other factors. The sensing of the Pa_{O_2} is the principal afferent pathway to modify the alveolar ventilation, which assure the O_2 supply. Thus, arterial chemoreceptors (aortic bodies and CBs) serve an important role in the control of alveolar ventilation, but they also exert a powerful influence on cardio-vascular function. Aortic bodies sense likewise the levels of arterial carbon dioxide partial pressure (Pa_{CO_2}) to regulate the depth and rhythm of breathing, but not changes in the blood H^+ concentration ($[H^+]$). To detect this last factor it is necessary to understand the role of the CB that detects all the previously described arterial variables, and, as its major quality, they do not desensitize. Finally, central chemoreceptors located on the ventrolateral surface of medulla oblongata detect changes in cerebrospinal fluid $[H^+]$ (**Figure 1**) [5–7, 9–11].

It is obvious then that the hypoxic response is a complex effect that must be studied at different levels, including the central areas where the respiratory rhythm and pattern is generated, as well as newly described functions of the CB, the integrative nature of central chemoreceptors and the interaction between peripheral and central chemoreception. Furthermore, it must be also taken into account the metabolic signalling influence of purinergic control, in general, and, in particular, the adenosinergic influence [1, 13, 17, 18, 23, 24].

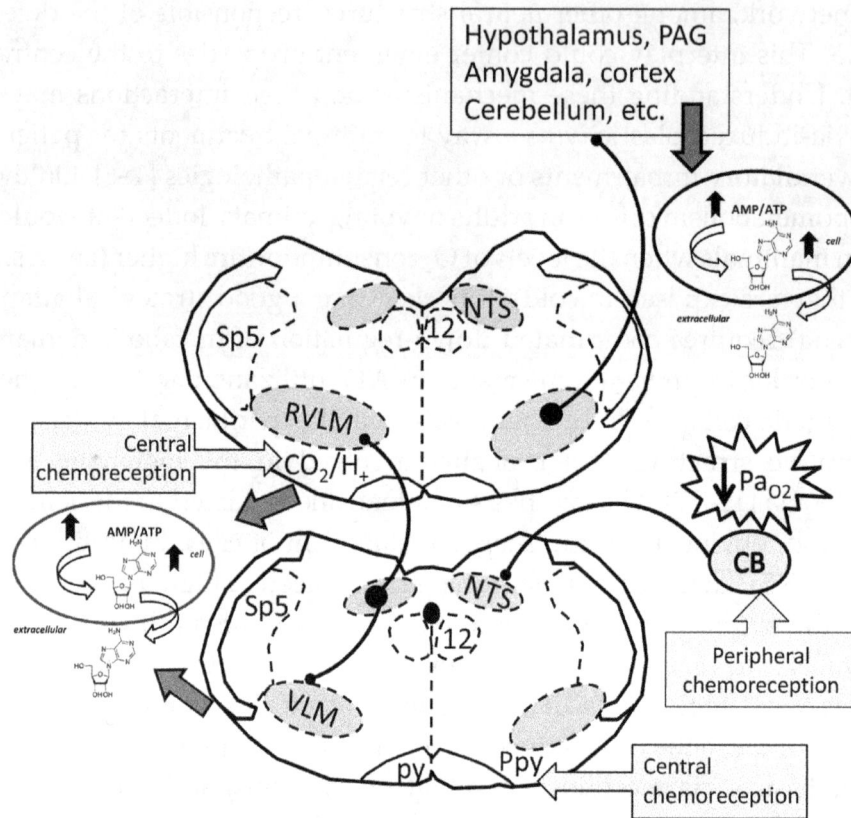

Figure 1. Schematic diagram of the hypoxic response generated at the ventrolateral medulla after the integration of peripheral and central chemoreceptors, including the role of metabolic signalling within the central neuronal network. Abbreviations: 12, hypoglossal nucleus; py, pyramidal tract; Sp5, spinal trigeminal nucleus.

2. Brain, hypoxia and pathophysiology

Normal breathing must be continuously adjusted to maintain homeostasis of arterial blood gases by means of feedback, feedforward and adaptive control strategies that depend of the brainstem respiratory network. How this process is centrally controlled is still under discussion, despite the advances (especially thanks to the development of *in vitro* preparations) that have been recently made [2, 3, 6, 7]. The precise mechanisms (cellular, synaptic and molecular) that underlie the generation and modulation of respiratory rhythm/pattern still remain largely unknown. This lack of fundamental knowledge in the field of neural control of respiration, and its relationship with other neurovegetative controls, is likely due to the complexity of the mammalian brain where synaptic connectivity between central cardiorespiratory neurons, motoneurons and their peripheral counterparts, to the present day, cannot be reliably mapped [2, 3, 7, 8].

Adaptive responses have evolved in different animal species to guarantee a sufficient supply of O_2 to tissues and to facilitate the survival of cells under transient or sustained conditions of limited O_2 availability. Although hypoxia is often related to a pathological condition, it is of great importance to recognize that variations in Pa_{O_2} can be part of normal situations that require strenuous physiological responses, for example, during hypoventilation training or intense physical exercise [4, 5, 16, 21, 25–28]. It has to be also taken into account the condition of hypercapnia that results from an excess of Pa_{CO_2}, which results in acidification of blood and tissues. The respiratory central medullary rhythm/pattern generator must respond to these chemosensory cues to maintain O_2 and carbon dioxide (CO_2) homeostasis in the blood and tissues. To do so, sensorial cells located in the periphery and CNS monitors the Pa_{O_2} and Pa_{CO_2} and initiates respiratory and autonomic reflex adjustments during hypoxic and hypercapnic. Activation of either the hypoxic or hypercapnic chemoreflex elicits both hyperventilation and sympathetic activation [4, 5, 16, 25–28]. However, the hypoxic insult is a fundamental drive to increase respiratory rate.

Traditionally, physiological research has been focused on the effect of a chronic sustained hypoxia (CH), but relatively few works were directed to the effect of periods of intermittent hypoxia that is maintained chronically. However, the different protocols resemble several pathological states that occur when patients suffer discontinuous expositions to hypoxia by malfunction of the ventilatory system. Nevertheless, these chronic intermittent hypoxia (CIH) laboratory protocols vary greatly between researches in lifespan of hypoxic exposure periods, numbers of hypoxic episodes *per day* and the total number of days of exposure. In any case, and in spite of the lack of a uniform definition, most of the recent data suggest that animals exposed to CIH would present multiple long-term pathophysiological consequences that are similar to those observed in clinic and, for that, it would be a good animal model to study different respiratory pathologies [4, 5, 16, 21, 25–28].

2.1. The role of carotid body as chemoreceptor

O_2 sensing is necessary for the activation of cardiorespiratory reflexes that permit the survival of individuals under hypoxic environments, like high altitude or pathological conditions (with reduced capacity for gas exchange between the lung alveoli and the blood). Changes are detected by the arterial chemoreceptors, in particular CB, to facilitate rapid adaptations to hypoxia including hyperventilation and sympathetic activation. The CB is located at the carotid bifurcation although its precise location varies between mammalian species. The CB is composed of functional units named glomeruli, which are clusters of cells separated by a profuse network of small capillaries and connective tissue. Each glomerulus (in close contact with blood vessels and nerve fibres) contains neuron-like glomus (or type I) cells, which can be easily identified because they are strongly dopaminergic. Glomus cells are surrounded by processes of sustentacular (type II) cells that are positive for antibodies against glial fibrillary acidic protein and other glial markers. It has been shown that type II cells, or a subpopulation of them, are quiescent stem cells that are activated under hypoxia to proliferate and differentiate into glomus and other cell types [5, 9–11]. Glomus neuron-like cells contain O_2-sensitive K^+ channels, which are inhibited by hypoxia acting through several mechanisms, including release of gaseous transmitters (NO, CO, H_2S), AMP-activated protein kinases and/or reactive oxygen species. Finally, it has been demonstrated that CBs are polymodal receptors that would respond not only to modifications in Pa_{O_2}, Pa_{CO_2} and H^+, but also to stimuli as K^+, several neurotransmitters (i.e. norepinephrine), changes in temperature and osmolarity, as well as variations in the levels of glucose or insulin. Furthermore, reductions in CB blood flow (in addition to a decrease in Pa_{O_2}) also provide powerful CB stimulation and remodelling over time [5, 9–11].

The feedback from the CB is sent to the cardiorespiratory centres in the medulla oblongata via the afferent branches of the glossopharyngeal nerve. The afferent neurons to CB have their somas in the petrosal ganglion. This ganglion is anatomically distinct in several species of mammals like cat and rabbit, but in others (i.e. rat) it is part of a structure that includes the jugular and nodose ganglia. Their afferent fibres project to the commissural or medial subnuclei of the nucleus tractus solitarius (NTS) (**Figure 1**) that convey sensory information regarding cardiorespiratory homeostasis in the form of graded action potential frequencies in fibres of the carotid sinus branch of the ninth cranial (glossopharyngeal) nerve. The efferent innervation arises primarily from the sympathetic fibres originating from the superior cervical ganglion constituting the ganglio-glomerular nerve. Efferent innervation may best be considered as a modulating influence affecting the CB chemosensitivity largely, but not solely, via a modulation of CB blood flow [5, 7–11, 29, 30].

2.2. Central integrative chemoreception process

The brainstem is the central structure that operates the integrative process of the different chemoreceptors and baroreceptors inputs and which also generates the respiratory rhythm/pattern. From these structures it should be outlined that the NTS is composed of a series of clusters of neuronal cell bodies forming a vertical column of grey matter embedded in the dorsal medulla oblongata. The NTS projects to, among other regions, the reticular formation, parasympathetic preganglionic neurons, hypothalamus and thalamus, conforming circuits that contribute to autonomic regulation (**Figure 1**). Anatomical and physiological experiments have shown that the dorsomedial part of the NTS is the primary termination site of glossopharyngeal and vagal baroreceptors, integrating the baroreceptor afferents, while the midline area, caudal to the *calamus scriptorius*, has been identified as a primary central termination site for CB afferents. The NTS neurons are stimulated by hypoxia or hypercapnia, and most profoundly by a combination of both. Under normal or pathological conditions, CB information reaches the respiratory pattern generator neuronal network via NTS glutamatergic neurons, which also target the rostral ventrolateral medulla oblongata (RVLM) presympathetic neurons, thereby raising sympathetic nerve activity (**Figure 1**). For that, NTS second-order neurons could induce chemoreceptor reflex responses that include hyperpnoea, bradycardia and a sympathetically mediated vasoconstriction for a long-term acclimatization to hypoxia [5, 7, 9–11, 29, 30].

Other group of neurons to be highlighted is the RVLM, containing several functionally distinct types of neurons, which control and orchestrate cardiovascular and respiratory responses to hypoxia and hypercapnia (**Figure 1**) [3, 7, 8, 29, 30]. At this level, chemoreceptors regulate presympathetic neurons and cardiovagal preganglionic neurons indirectly via inputs from the neurons related to the respiratory pattern generator. Secondary effects of chemoreceptors on the autonomic outflows result from changes in lung stretch afferent and baroreceptor activity [3, 7, 8, 29, 30].

On the other hand, central respiratory chemosensitivity is caused by direct effects of cerebro-spinal [H^+] on neurons and indirect effects of CO_2 via astrocytes. Central respiratory chemo-receptors are not definitively identified but several brainstem areas have been demonstrated to have a role as chemoreceptor. First, the retrotrapezoid nucleus (RTN), located at the rostral end of RVLM, is a particularly strong candidate (**Figure 1**). Indeed, the absence of RTN likely causes severe central apnoeas in congenital central hypoventilation syndrome. The RTN chemoreceptor neurons provide a CO_2/H^+-dependent drive to breathe and serve as an integrator centre of convergence of chemosensory information from other central and periph-eral sites, including the CBs. Finally, the RTN chemosensitive neurons also appear to serve as important sites of integration of several stimuli, as these neurons are significantly modulated by inputs from vagal-mediated pulmonary stretch receptors and from the hypothalamus [29, 30].

Another cluster of RVLM cells (constituted by a population of C1 catecholaminergic neurons) controls sympathetic vasomotor tone in resting and in hypoxic and hypercapnic conditions, including the peripheral chemoreflex [29, 30]. The increased sympathetic outflow elicited by peripheral chemoreceptors is mediated primarily by activation of the presympathetic neurons of the RVLM, the majority of which are C1 neurons. In fact, the cardiorespiratory effects of peripheral chemoreceptors are mediated in part by the direct glutamatergic inputs from the NTS to C1 neurons (**Figure 1**) [2, 3, 7, 8, 29, 30].

Recently, the description of the structures related to the respiratory rhythmogenesis has improved with the advent of the *in vitro* neonatal rodent brainstem preparation [31]. This recording technique has allowed for precise identification of specific medullary sites for separate but coupled rhythm generation or "oscillators". These neurons reside in the pre-Bötzinger complex and in the parafacial respiratory group (pFRG) located in the RVLM [29, 30]. The most exciting result so far was the finding that some inspiratory neurons in RVLM act as inspiratory pacemakers; they continue to produce rhythmic bursts of potentials even when the synaptic connections are blocked [2]. Although the inspiratory pacemaker neurons do not constitute a well-defined group within the medulla, this group of neurons named pre-Bötzinger complex certainly play an important role in the generation and/or modulation of the breathing rhythm [2]. Of the several models proposed for generating respiratory rhythm, the most promising appears to be a hybrid model, which combines emergent properties of networks of synaptic connections and intrinsic membrane properties of individual neurons together with independent pacemaker-type neurons [1– 3, 7, 8, 23, 29, 30].

Furthermore, several facts support that the pFRG/RTN complex is likely to be the major site of central CO_2 chemo-responsiveness. First, pFRG/RTN is characterized by glutamatergic interneurons that strongly express Phox2b (that codes for the homeodomain transcription factor expressed exclusively in the nervous system, in most neurons that control the viscera, like cardiovascular, digestive and respiratory systems). Besides, the Phox2b neurons are part of an uninterrupted chain of neurons in a circuit that includes the CBs and their afferents as well as the NTS projections to the RTN. The functional consequences of this linkage are that stimulation of the peripheral chemoreceptors enhances the slope of the central CO_2 ventilatory response,and conversely, inhibition of the CBs reduces the slope of the central CO_2 response [1–3, 7, 8, 23, 29, 30].

Another interesting central chemosensitive area is the caudal parapyramidal (Ppy), located near the ventral surface of the medulla, at the level of the pyramidal decussation and may function as well as the pFRG/RTN complex (**Figure 1**). Furthermore, medullary neurons activated in response to hypercapnia were only found in the Ppy area. Nevertheless, neurons in both regions, RTN and PPy, could belong to the same cell population based on their histochemical and physiological properties and their location, near the medullary surface that facilitates the sensing of the arterial composition [1, 23].

In any case, the brainstem cardiorespiratory control areas are connected with other areas such as periaqueductal gray (PAG), hypothalamus, amygdala, cortex and cerebellum (**Figure 1**). These areas also exert influences over the respiratory rhythm/pattern generator. In this way, it has been found, from data obtained by clinical evidences in patients submitted to deep brain stimulation (by means of stimulating electrodes that recorded field potentials during neurosurgical procedures), that the PAG and the subthalamic nucleus have a key role in activating the central command of cardiorespiratory responses to stress. The PAG is an integrative structure that maintains a wide network of connectivity with different neural systems, such as prefrontal cortex, hypothalamus and nociceptive pathways. Moreover, the PAG efferent projections also addressed to the medullary cardiorespiratory control areas. Finally, anatomical evidences support the connectivity to amygdala and cortex from RVLM and neurons of the respiratory pattern generator that supports, among others effects, the vegetative correlate of emotions or learning (**Figure 1**) [3, 7, 8, 30, 31].

All of the above described structures are part of an extended neuronal network that participates in the regulation and integration of cardiovascular and respiratory functions. From all of the neurotransmitters shared by this complex neuronal network, the purinergic network is one of the choices to regulate the physiologic responses to hypoxia. Recent evidence suggests that ATP-mediated purinergic signalling at the level of the RVLM coordinates cardiorespiratory responses triggered by hypoxia and hypercapnia by activating RTN and C1 neurons, respectively. For all of that, the role of ATP-mediated signalling in the RVLM must be critical for cardiovascular and respiratory activities (**Figure 1**) [3, 7, 8, 29, 30].

2.3. Pathophysiological responses to hypoxia

Since the condition in which the whole body (or a region) was exposed to variations in arterial O_2 concentrations can be part of the normal physiology, a mild and non-damaging intermittent hypoxia (IH) is used intentionally, for example, during altitude training to develop an athletic performance adaptation at both the systemic and cellular level [4, 5, 16, 21, 26–28]. However, hypoxia is a deprivation of adequate O_2 supply at the tissue level and, often, a pathological condition with very serious consequences of preterm birth in the neonate, for example. The main cause for this pathology is that the lungs of the human foetus are among the last organs to develop during pregnancy. The perinatal hypoxic-ischemic cerebral injuries found in the clinic are a main problem of paediatrics because of its severe consequences for the posterior development of the infants, such as the appearances of cerebral paralysis. Accumulating evidence points to an evolving process of brain injury after intrapartum hypoxia-ischemia, initiated *in utero* and extending into a recovery period. This process in the neonate originates numerous functional deficits, such as impaired resting ventilation and ventilatory response to hypoxia [17, 28, 31, 32].

On the other hand, abnormalities or mutations of the medullary neuronal breathing rhythm/pattern networks may also have a great impact on the progress of human diseases in children or adults. Failures in the breathing pattern with severe consequences are well-documented. These problems, often cause CO_2 retention in awake, and in particular, in sleeping subjects, that could be associated to neurodegenerative diseases such as Parkinson's disease, amyotrophic lateral sclerosis or post-polio syndrome. It is also been proved that these breathing alterations are often associated to medullary and multiple system atrophy of patients. These syndromes have been linked to deficits in neurons related with the respiratory control in the pre-Bötzinger complex, pontine raphe and adjacent areas. Obviously, an understanding of how the response to hypoxia is organized and when or why the system become maladapted and could induce cell damage is extremely important for knowing how to fight against the diseases in the future [4, 5, 16, 21, 26–28].

It is well known that disruption of the drive to breathe is thought to contribute to the mortality of certain pathologies, including stroke or epilepsy, and it is the cause of sudden infant death syndrome (SIDS) [1–6]. In the case of SIDS, it has generally been accepted that, in the absence of trauma, children death occurs to either respiratory or circulatory failure. The events appear to be a sequential process, first hypoxia occurs, and then there must be a failure to recover from hypoxia. The failure to recover could occur when the infant does not arouse from sleep and/or self-resuscitation mechanisms fail. For that, it has been proposed that there should be three necessary components for development of SIDS: congenital or acquired vulnerability, a critical "time-window" during maturational development and an acute stressor. The arousal response is essential for avoiding the hypoxic conditions due to certain microenvironments that could cause the loss of consciousness or the risk of dying. A failure of the neural system that would induce the arousal response from sleep, in the hypoxic condition, could be related to the progress or, in certain cases, the fatal result in diagnosed SIDS. However, these kinds of malfunctions do not explain all the process that should appear in SIDS. In fact, it seems clear that an initial respiratory failure and hypoxemia ignites the sequence of responses that, dramatically, may cause the death. Respiratory chemoreceptor studies on infants at risk for SIDS have suggested that a decreased sensitivity to CO_2 could play a causal role in these deaths [1–6, 33].

Concerning CB function, there is a significant increase in sensitivity of the peripheral chemoreceptors during the first few weeks of life and it has been frequently shown that CB denervation in animal models is followed by hypoventilation and sudden death later on. Therefore, these denervated animals for the most part are markedly symptomatic prior to death. The principal problem in translating these results to humans is that SIDS infants do not appear to have any symptoms before death. This fact implies that it could be a problem related to the central integration of CB information in SIDS, but its role is still under discussion. However,

CB must be taken into account in the pathogeny of SIDS, because a partial decrease in the sensitivity to hypercapnia or hypoxemia would be a causal role in this syndrome [2, 33].

Several studies indicate that changes in the strength and/or pattern of respiratory-sympathetic coupling may have pathological implications in the control of arterial pressure levels. Such dysfunctions can be observed in the experimental condition of CIH, and also is commonly observed in patients suffering from obstructive sleep apnoea (OSA). OSA consists of a repetitive obstruction of the upper airways during sleep. Each obstruction causes an episode of hypoxia leading to a picture of CIH causing a fall in the Pa_{O_2} and arterial haemoglobin saturation. OSA is characterized by repetitive collapse or near collapse of the upper airway during sleep, and these repetitive events impose substantial adverse effects on multiple organ systems. As a result of these mechanical changes in the airway, hypoxemia and hypercapnia develop, which further stimulate respiratory effort. Without airway opening the increased drive is ineffective at increasing ventilation. Hypoxic episodes stimulate the CB, triggering an increased motor muscles towards the inspiratory output and an arousal reaction, which together solve the obstruction [1–6]. Following even very brief periods of IH interspersed with normoxia, hyperventilation and increased sympathetic activity are sustained over an hour or more (i.e. the so-called long-term facilitation). Central adaptive responses occur following CIH in the persistent elevation of tonic hyperactivity of neurons at the level of the hypothalamus and other structures [4, 16, 21, 26–28]. As OSA progresses, it frequently generates a syndrome with associated pathologies at different systems: cardiovascular (hypertension and augmented acute vascular accidents), hepato-metabolic (insulin resistance, glucose intolerance, fatty liver disease) and neuropsychiatric (anxiety, depression and cognitive-executive deficits). Clinical and experimental studies indicate that CIH is an important event in the occurrence of OSA-associated pathologies because it causes CB sensitization [1–6]. The process probably includes increasing CB chemoreceptor input to the brainstem leading to an exaggerated sympathetic tone, which generates hypertension and subsequent cardiovascular and metabolic pathologies. In OSA patients, the repetitive respiratory events lead to IH and CO_2 retention, both of which can augment sympathetic nerve activity via stimulation of central and peripheral chemoreceptors. Conditions of hypoxia, both chronic and intermittent lack of O_2, seem to induce CNS plasticity of respiratory and sympathetic functions neuronal networks and metabolic changes that could also lead to pathological states [4, 5, 27, 28].

3. Purinergic neuronal networks and hypoxia

ATP is released in an activity-dependent manner from different cell types in the brain, fulfilling different roles as a neurotransmitter, neuromodulator, in astrocyte-to-neuron communication, propagating astrocytic responses and modulating microglia responses. So, purinergic signalling has been found to contribute at all levels of the nervous system, including enteric, autonomic and central [34–38]. The term purinergic receptor was classically introduced to name specific classes of membrane receptors that mediate the release of ATP (P2 receptors) or adenosine (P1 receptors). The group of adenosine P1 receptors (A1-R, A2a-R, A2b-R, A3-R) are expressed on presynaptic and postsynaptic neurons, on astrocytes, microglia and mature and precursor oligodendrocytes. The mechanisms of ATP signalling are equally diverse, acting by means of P2 receptors, including ionotropic (P2X-R) and metabotropic (P2Y-R) subtypes, as well as varying methods of transmission, including vesicular, volume-regulated anion channel and gap junction hemichannel release of ATP from neuronal and non-neuronal cells [34–38].

ATP is involved in central respiratory control and may mediate changes in the activity of medullary respiratory neurons during hypercapnia. The P2 receptor family comprises seven ionotropic P2X-R subunits (P2X1-7), forming both homomeric or heteromeric receptors and eight metabotropic P2Y-R subtypes (P2Y1, 2, 4, 6, 11, 12, 13, 14). The brain displays a robust mRNA expression, an intense binding, and immunoreactivity for both P2X-R and P2Y-R in neuronal and non-neuronal elements, although the role of central P2-R remains ill defined. The ATP-mediated signalling in respiratory control and central chemoreception is associated to the profile of the P2X2-R subunit. This subunit is expressed, by physiologically identified respiratory neurons, in areas of the ventral medulla, the pontine locus coeruleus, the NTS, and the raphe nuclei. There are several evidences that sustain the hypothesis that purinergic signalling could play a central role in the mechanisms underlying the chemosensitivity of RVLM (**Figure 1**). It has been demonstrated the responses evoked by ATP in neurons expressing P2X-Rs to changes in extracellular [H^+]. In that way, this evidence supports the putative mechanism of chemosensitivity of RVLM cells, and it would be necessary the tonic release of ATP. This may be the case, when P2-R blockade reduces the baseline firing of RVLM respiratory neurones. The modulation of P2X2-R function, evoked by acidification of the extracellular environment during hypercapnia, contributes to the changes in activity of the RVLM respiratory neurones that express these receptors [34–38].

Furthermore, it has been shown that several medullary areas may have chemosensitive responses mediated by ATP. In this way, experiments made in brain slices using cell-attached recordings of membrane potentials have shown that CO_2/H^+-receptive NTS neurons are activated by focal ATP applications. However, it has been evidenced that purinergic P2-R blockade did not affect their CO_2/H^+ responsiveness [38]. On the other hand, CO_2/H^+-sensitive raphe neurons were unaffected by ATP or P2-R blockade [34, 38]. When the experiments where realized *in vivo*, ATP injection into the NTS increased cardiorespiratory activity; however, injections of a P2-R antagonist into this area did not change the baseline breathing or the CO_2/H^+ responsiveness [34, 38]. Indeed, a significant proportion of respiratory neurones located in the vicinity of the Bötzinger and pre-Bötzinger areas express the P2X2-R subunit and respond with an increase in discharge during ATP application. This fact could mean that purinergic signalling plays an additional role in the generation and shaping of central respiratory output, as well as premotoneurons that are responsible for transmitting this rhythm to the spinal motoneurons controlling the diaphragm and intercostal muscles [34–38].

Finally, as above stated, RVLM contributes to peripheral chemoreceptor modulation of breathing and blood pressure, by chemosensitive RTN neurons and presympathetic C1 neurons, respectively, and these neurons are activated by purinergic agonists. In contrast, the blockade of P2-Rs in the RVLM blunted cardiorespiratory responses to peripheral chemoreceptor activation in anesthetized rats [34–38]. RTN neuronal activity was found to be independent of temperature and stimulus strength and was wholly retained when synaptic activity was blocked using high-Mg^{++}, low-Ca^{++} solution. In the RTN, mechanisms of chemoreception involved direct H^+-mediated activation of chemosensitive neurons and indirect modulation by purinergic signalling. This modulation implies a CO_2/H^+-evoked ATP release by RTN astrocytes, contributing to respiratory drive. ATP injection into the RTN increased breathing and blood pressure by a P2-R dependent mechanism, at the cellular and systems level [38]. However, because the results using antagonists of P2-R and focal injections did not elucidate the cells that were responsible, it is necessary more experimental evidence to determine the putative chemoreceptors and, if it is the case, the above observed effects could be indirect ones. Nevertheless, purinergic signalling also modulates the activity of CO_2/H^+-sensitive neurons at least in two other brainstem regions thought to contribute to central chemoreception (i.e. the caudal NTS and medullary raphe). In any case, these evidences suggest that purinergic signalling is a unique feature of RTN chemoreception and point out to a unique CO_2/H^+ sensing mechanism in the RTN [34–38].

4. Adenosine receptors, brain development and pathophysiological hypoxic response

The role of adenosine, as an extracellular signalling molecule, was defined after the observations of the ability of purines to control the functioning of the heart. Adenosine modulates the activity of the nervous system at cellular level both presynaptically by inhibiting or facilitating transmitter release, and postsynaptically by hyperpolarising or depolarising neurons, as well as exerting non-synaptic effects (i.e. on glial cells). It is usually assumed that adenosinergic signalling provides a neuroprotective role. However, several researches have shown that, under determined circumstances, changes in the levels of adenosine could have the opposite effects, contributing to neuronal damage and cell death [6, 12–15, 19–22]. These two ways of actions could be determined by the union of adenosine to different subtypes of A-Rs. Furthermore, changes in the levels of expression of the different subtypes, interactions between these receptors, differential actions on neuronal and glial cells and several "time-windows" (that are critical during development) could also provide different actions at different events, as well as adenosinergic agonist and antagonist compounds administration. Moreover, adenosine do not work isolated, and, in spite of this, it is still unclear if the role of A-R subtypes (A1-R and A2-R) in the control of neuroprotection is mostly due to the control of glutamatergic transmission. Another possible role of adenosine is that its protection is mediated by one of the homeostatic roles of its receptors, such as control of metabolism, neuroglial communication, inflammatory response, neurogenesis or mechanism of action of growth factors [6, 12–15, 19–22].

Adenosine acts in parallel as a neuromodulator and as a homeostatic modulator in the CNS [6, 12–22]. The adenosine role as a neuromodulator is especially important around the time of birth and is involved in the suppression of foetal and neonatal breathing, particularly during hypoxia when extracellular levels of this nucleoside rapidly increase. Apnoea of prematurity, defined as cessation of breathing lasting longer than 15 s and accompanied by bradycardia or hypoxia, is common occurring in 85% of infants born less than 34-week gestation. Preterm birth constitutes approximately 6–12% of all births in industrialized countries and accounts for 70% of neonatal mortality and 75% of neonatal morbidity [6, 12–21]. Depending on gestational age and birth weight, preterm infants present a wide range of abnormal physiological responses due to their immature organ systems [17, 28, 31, 32]. During development A1-Rs are especially important, being the earliest receptors expressed in the embryonic brain and heart. A1-R activation potently inhibits the development of axons and can lead to leukomalacia [18, 32].

The most common method of treatment of the apnoeas of prematurity is continuous positive airway pressure and administration of a methylxanthine. The family of methylxanthines includes caffeine (1, 3, 7-trimethylxanthine), one of the most popular human stimulants, and all of them derivate from xanthine, that is a purine present in human and other organism's tissues and fluids. This group of alkaloids has therapeutically been used for their effects stimulating respiratory function by means of its excitatory effects on the CNS, because of its capacity to suppress respiratory depression, reduce periodic breathing and enhance diaphragmatic activity. Caffeine also increases ventilatory drive and improves sensitivity and/or responsiveness to changes in the level of Pa_{O_2} [6, 12–22]. The

discovery that methylxanthines acted as antagonists of adenosine receptors represented a crucial step to establish the idea that adenosine indeed acted as an extracellular signalling molecule operating on selective receptors. Caffeine, at high doses, can also inhibit phosphodiesterases, block GABAa receptors or cause a release of intracellular Ca^{++}. Furthermore, caffeine acts on the respiratory cycle by antagonizing the actions of endogenous A1-R, A2a-R or A2b-R [6, 12–22]. Studies on A1-R have demonstrated that these receptors are found at high density in the brainstem and hypothalamus while A2a-Rs are widely distributed in the medulla [14, 17, 18]. Animal studies have shown that caffeine treatment alters A-R expression and distribution, cause transient motor impairments and could also be neurotoxic to the newborn. In rats, limited exposure to therapeutic doses of caffeine during early life (postnatal days 3–6, P3–P6) changes the distribution, density and sensitivity of A1-Rs in several regions of the CNS; these changes could persist until adulthood. Caffeine treatment at P2–P6 mimics the clinical use of caffeine in human neonates. Since the relative level of maturation of the CNS in newborn rats in the first week of life is similar to that of a premature newborn human between 20 and 40 weeks postconception, newborn rats could serve as a suitable animal model to test the potential impact of perinatal caffeine treatment on the adenosinergic system. The oral administration of caffeine in critical periods of newborn rat and immunohistological experiments showed an increase of A1-R labelling in restricted cardiorespiratory related areas. These labelled structures were the anterior hypothalamic area, ventromedial hypothalamic nucleus, parabrachial complex and ventrolateral medulla of the caffeine-treated group at P6. For the subtype A2a-R, it was found a moderate increase of immunolabelling in pontomedullary and other hypothalamic areas also related to vegetative functions. Indeed, increased A1-R and A2a-R gene expression was observed in both the brainstem and hypothalamus at P5. These results showed an up-regulation of adenosinergic maturation in central cardiorespiratory areas when the animals were caffeine treated in the neonatal period and could explain the pharmacological effects observed in caffeine treated premature infants, and it would also imply that caffeine mediated a modification of the postnatal development of the adenosinergic system during a critical period or "time-window" [6, 12–22]. To date, human data show that such caffeine treatment has no major side effects on neurodevelopmental outcome in children in the 38–42 weeks following birth and up to 2 years after the treatment. However, further research is required to determine the long-term pathologic and functional effects of caffeine and the combination of caffeine and other substances on the developing immature brain [6, 12–22].

Anyway, adenosine, is not only crucial in development, it also mediates multifactorial forms of ventilatory responses. The reduced hypoxic ventilatory response could be attributed to depressed adenosinergic peripheral excitatory mechanisms and to enhanced adenosinergic central depression mechanisms, both of which contribute to the blunted ventilatory response in different metabolic states (**Figure 1**). Several important groups of clinical studies, in which the adenosinergic network role has been demonstrated, are related to OSA, asthma and interstitial lung disease such as idiopathic pulmonary fibrosis (IPF) [1–6]. Levels of adenosine receptors are altered in the lungs of asthmatics and OSA patients and a recent study has shown that the A2b-R is increased in remodelled airway epithelial cells of rapidly progressing IPF patients [6, 12–22]. Furthermore, CIH (as an experimental OSA model) elicits phrenic long-term facilitation by an adenosine-dependent mechanism [2, 6, 12–22]. All of the above are interesting evidences about the mechanisms that support and induce inflammatory and tissue remodelling processes in these pathological states; however, it is necessary to do more research on the pathways that provoke their progressive and chronic evolution. For example, there are already implemented several models of deregulated or overactive wound healing pathways to explain how these processes contribute to an excessive remodelling response such as seen in chronic lung disease [2, 6, 12–22]. Consistent with this, adenosine levels are elevated in the lungs of patients with chronic lung disease, where it is hypothesized that adenosine regulates the balance between tissue repair and excessive airway remodelling. Furthermore, it has been demonstrated that exogenous adenosine treatment can elicit acute bronchoconstriction in patients with asthma or OSA [1–6]. In contrast, the administration of adenosine to healthy subject did not affect them, suggesting a fundamental difference with respect to adenosinergic signalling in the treated patients. The differential response could be mediated by the activation of A-Rs that would modify the activity of different cell types that play a central role in chronic lung disease. These groups of possible targets include mast cells, eosinophils, macrophages, airway epithelial cells, pulmonary fibroblasts and airway smooth muscle cells. Indeed, recent studies directly demonstrate that adenosine is involved in the regulation of pulmonary fibrosis. Lastly, there are correlations between the degree of inflammation and damage and adenosine accumulations in adenosine deaminase-deficient individuals. Furthermore, purinergic metabolism and signalling components are altered in a manner that promotes adenosine production in tissue samples from patients with OSA and IPF. These modifications were related to the very important changes found in the expression of the promoter molecules of inflammatory process that could be induced by A2b-R signalling. Finally, it was interesting to point out that it has been demonstrated that activation of A2b-Rs can influence the production of inflammatory and fibrotic mediators from macrophages isolated from these patients [6, 12–22].

All of the above findings suggest that adenosine-based therapeutics may be beneficial in the treatment of chronic lung diseases such as OSA and IPF. On the other hand, it is known that inflammation-induced release of prostaglandin E_2 changes breathing patterns and the response to CO_2 levels. This bioactive eicosanoid regulates many biologically important processes as a potent activator of several signalling pathways, through four distinct G-protein-coupled receptors. All of this alters neural network activity in the pre-Bötzinger rhythm-generating complex and in the chemosensitive brainstem respiratory regions, thereby increasing sigh frequency and the depth of inspiration with implications for inspiration and sighs throughout life, and the ability to autoresuscitate when breathing fails [2, 6, 7, 12–15, 19–22, 29, 30].

5. Conclusion

Identification of the neurophysiological mechanisms underlying the response of organisms to environmental factors, in particular, to injurious exposures like hypoxia, represents one of the most important research problems in biomedicine. Neural plasticity, as a persistent change in the morphology and/or function based on prior experiences, is crucial for understanding the effects of O_2 supply changes over neuronal networks. Plasticity is well evident when the triggering experience occurs early in life; but in the case of respiratory control plasticity, could also be present in adult life. The regulation of adenosinergic neural network maturation, especially in central cardiorespiratory areas, could provide new perspectives in respiratory newborn distress symptoms. Adenosine acts as an extracellular signalling molecule operating on selective receptors. Regulation of adenosinergic maturation in central cardiorespiratory areas in caffeine-treated neonatal mammals could explain the pharmacological effects of caffeine observed in premature infants. Anyhow, the neuroplasticity observed in the cardiorespiratory network is fundamental to maintain life in many adverse conditions.

The central and peripheral chemical drive to breathe is associated with several widespread autonomic disorders. Deficits in central chemical drive are associated with central sleep apnoea, a debilitating disease with few therapies besides constant positive airway pressure. In addition, disruption of the drive to breathe is thought to contribute to mortality of certain pathologies, including SIDS, stroke and epilepsy. Finally, in OSA, certain forms of hypertension and heart failure, it has been observed sensitization of peripheral chemoreceptor drive, particularly the sympathetic component and this over-activity is thought to contribute to the pathology.

Purinergic signalling has been proposed to be an excellent system to target for therapies of numerous pathologies, mainly due to novel pharmacological agents being developed. As more detailed understanding of the purinergic mechanisms involved in the chemical drive to breathe are uncovered, these would allow to possible pharmacological treatments of the aforementioned pathologies with the newly developed purinergic agents.

Author details

Susana P. Gaytán* and Rosario Pasaro

*Address all correspondence to: sgaytan@us.es

Department of Physiology, University of Seville, Sevilla, Spain

References

[1] Barnett WH, Abdala AP, Paton JF, Rybak IA, Zoccal DB, Molkov YI. Chemoreception and neuroplasticity in respiratory circuits. Exp Neurol. 2016;4886(16): 30156-X. DOI: 10.1016/j.expneurol.2016.05.036

[2] Guyenet PG. Regulation of breathing and autonomic outflows by chemoreceptors. Compr Physiol. 2014;4(4):1511–1562. DOI: 10.1002/cphy.c140004

[3] Molkov YI, Zoccal DB, Baekey DM, Abdala AP, Machado BH, Dick TE, Paton JF, Rybak IA. Physiological and pathophysiological interactions between the respiratory central pattern generator and the sympathetic nervous system. Prog Brain Res. 2014;212:1–23. DOI: 10.1016/B978-0-444-63488-7.00001-X

[4] Pouyssegur J, López-Barneo J. Hypoxia in health and disease. Mol Aspects Med. 2016;47–48:1–2. DOI: 10.1016/j.mam.2016.02.001

[5] Quintero M, Olea E, Conde SV, Obeso A, Gallego-Martin T, Gonzalez C, Monserrat JM, Gómez-Niño A, Yubero S, Agapito T. Age protects from harmful effects produced by chronic intermittent hypoxia. J Physiol. 2016;594(6):1773–1790. DOI: 10.1113/JP270878

[6] Ribeiro JA, Sebastião AM, de Mendonça A. Adenosine receptors in the nervous system: pathophysiological implications. Prog Neurobiol. 2002;68(6):377–392. DOI:10.1016/S0301-0082(02)00155-7

[7] Dempsey JA, Smith CA. Pathophysiology of human ventilatory control. Eur Respir J. 2014;44(2):495–512. DOI: 10.1183/09031936.00048514

[8] Gaytán SP, Pasaro R. Connections of the rostral ventral respiratory neuronal cell group: an anterograde and retrograde tracing study in the rat. Brain Res Bull. 1998;47(6):625–642. DOI: 10.1016/S0361-9230(98)00125-7

[9] Julien CA, Joseph V, Bairam A. Alteration of carotid body chemoreflexes after neonatal intermittent hypoxia and caffeine treatment in rat pups. Respir Physiol Neurobiol. 2011;177(3):301–312. DOI: 10.1016/j.resp.2011.05.006

[10] López-Barneo J, González-Rodríguez P, Gao L, Fernández-Agüera MC, Pardal R, Ortega-Sáenz P. Oxygen sensing by the carotid body: mechanisms and role in

adaptation to hypoxia. Am J Physiol Cell Physiol. 2016;310(8):629–642. DOI: 10.1152/ajpcell.00265.2015

[11] López-Barneo J, Ortega-Sáenz P, González-Rodríguez P, Fernández-Agüera MC, Macías D, Pardal R, Gao L. Oxygen-sensing by arterial chemoreceptors: mechanisms and medical translation. Mol Aspects Med. 2016;47–48:90–108. DOI: 10.1016/j.mam.2015.12.002

[12] Black AM, Pandya S, Clark D, Armstrong EA, Yager JY. Effect of caffeine and morphine on the developing pre-mature brain. Brain Res. 2008;1219:136–142. DOI: 10.1016/j.brainres.2008.04.066

[13] Borea PA, Gessi S, Merighi S, Varani K. Adenosine as a multi-signalling guardian angel in human diseases: when, where and how does it exert its protective effects? Trends Pharmacol Sci. 2016;37(6):419–434. DOI: 10.1016/j.tips.2016.02.006

[14] Gomes CV, Kaster MP, Tomé AR, Agostinho PM, Cunha RA. Adenosine receptors and brain diseases: neuroprotection and neurodegeneration. Biochim Biophys Acta. 2011;1808(5):1380–1399. DOI: 10.1016/j.bbamem.2010.12.001

[15] Wardas J. Neuroprotective role of adenosine in the CNS. Pol J Pharmacol. 2002;54:313–326 ISSN 1230-6002.PMID: 12523485

[16] Bruzzese L, Rostain JC, Née L, Condo J, Mottola G, Adjriou N, Mercier L, Berge-Lefranc JL, Fromonot J, Kipson N, Lucciano M, Durand-Gorde JM, Jammes Y, Guieu R, Ruf J, Fenouillet E. Effect of hyperoxic and hyperbaric conditions on the adenosinergic pathway and CD26 expression in rat. J Appl Physiol (1985). 2015;119(2):140–147. DOI: 10.1152/japplphysiol.00223.2015

[17] Gaytan SP, Pasaro R. Neonatal caffeine treatment up-regulates adenosine receptors in brainstem and hypothalamic cardio-respiratory related nuclei of rat pups. Exp Neurol. 2012;237(2):247–259. DOI: 10.1016/j.expneurol.2012.06.028

[18] Gaytan SP, Saadani-Makki F, Bodineau L, Frugière A, Larnicol N, Pasaro R. Effect of postnatal exposure to caffeine on the pattern of adenosine A1 receptor distribution in respiration-related nuclei of the rat brainstem. Auton Neurosci. 2006;126–127:339–346. DOI: 10.1016/j.autneu.2006.03.009

[19] Lee SD, Nakano H, Farkas GA. Adenosinergic modulation of ventilation in obese zucker rats. Obes Res. 2005;13(3):545–555. DOI: 10.1038/oby.2005.58

[20] de Mendonça A, Sebastião AM, Ribeiro JA. Adenosine: does it have a neuroprotective role after all? Brain Res Brain Res Rev. 2000;33(2–3):258–274. DOI:10.1016/S0165-0173(00)00033-3

[21] Schmidt C, Bellingham MC, Richter DW. Adenosinergic modulation of respiratory neurones and hypoxic responses in the anaesthetized cat. J Physiol. 1995;483(Pt 3):769–781. PMCID: PMC1157817

[22] Zhou Y, Murthy JN, Zeng D, Belardinelli L, Blackburn MR. Alterations in adenosine metabolism and signaling in patients with chronic obstructive pulmonary disease and idiopathic pulmonary fibrosis. PLoS One. 2010;5(2):e9224. DOI: 10.1371/journal.pone. 0009224

[23] Ribas-Salgueiro JL, Gaytán SP, Crego R, Pásaro R, Ribas J. Highly H+-sensitive neurons in the caudal ventrolateral medulla of the rat. J Physiol. 2003;549(Pt 1):181–194. DOI: 10.1113/jphysiol.2002.036624

[24] Ribas-Salgueiro JL, Gaytán SP, Ribas J, Pásaro R. Characterization of efferent projections of chemosensitive neurons in the caudal parapyramidal area of the rat brain. Brain Res Bull. 2005;66(3):235–248. DOI: 10.1016/j.brainresbull.2005.05.014

[25] Kara T, Narkiewicz K, Somers VK. Chemoreflexes-physiology and clinical implications. Acta Physiol Scand. 2003;177(3):377–384. DOI: 10.1046/j.1365-201X.2003.01083.x

[26] Nichols NL, Dale EA, Mitchell GS. Severe acute intermittent hypoxia elicits phrenic long-term facilitation by a novel adenosine-dependent mechanism. J Appl Physiol. (1985). 2012;112(10):1678–1688. DOI: 10.1152/japplphysiol.00060.2012

[27] Olea E, Gaytan SP, Obeso A, Gonzalez C, Pasaro R. Interactions between postnatal sustained hypoxia and intermittent hypoxia in the adulthood to alter brainstem structures and respiratory function. Adv Exp Med Biol. 2012;758:225–231. DOI: 10.1007/978-94-007-4584-1_31

[28] Perlman JM. Intervention strategies for neonatal hypoxic-ischemic cerebral injury. Clin Ther. 2006;28(9):1353–1365. DOI: 10.1016/j.clinthera.2006.09.005

[29] Barna BF, Takakura AC, Mulkey DK, Moreira TS. Purinergic receptor blockade in the retrotrapezoid nucleus attenuates the respiratory chemoreflexes in awake rats. Acta Physiol (Oxf). 2016;217(1):80–93. DOI: 10.1111/apha.12637

[30] Forsberg D, Horn Z, Tserga E, Smedler E, Silberberg G, Shvarev Y, Kaila K, Uhlén P, Herlenius E. CO2-evoked release of PGE2 modulates sighs and inspiration as demonstrated in brainstem organotypic culture. Elife. 2016;5(pii):e14170. DOI: 10.7554/eLife. 14170

[31] Mathew OP. Apnea of prematurity: pathogenesis and management strategies. J Perinatol. 2011;31(5):302–310. DOI: 10.1038/jp.2010.126

[32] Rivkees SA, Zhao Z, Porter G, Turner C. Influences of adenosine on the fetus and newborn. Mol Genet Metab. 2001;74(1–2):160–171. DOI:10.1006/mgme.2001.3217

[33] Thach BT. The role of respiratory control disorders in SIDS. Respir Physiol Neurobiol. 2005;149(1–3):343–353. DOI: 10.1016/j.resp.2005.06.011

[34] Gourine AV, Atkinson L, Deuchars J, Spyer KM. Purinergic signalling in the medullary mechanisms of respiratory control in the rat: respiratory neurones express the P2X2 receptor subunit. J Physiol. 2003;552(Pt 1):197–211. DOI: 10.1113/jphysiol.2003.045294

[35] Moreira TS, Wenker IC, Sobrinho CR, Barna BF, Takakura AC, Mulkey DK. Independent purinergic mechanisms of central and peripheral chemoreception in the rostral ventrolateral medulla. J Physiol. 2015;593(5):1067–1074. DOI: 10.1113/jphysiol.2014.284430

[36] Pedata F, Dettori I, Coppi E, Melani A, Fusco I, Corradetti R, Pugliese AM. Purinergic signalling in brain ischemia. Neuropharmacology. 2016;104:105–130. DOI: 10.1016/j.neuropharm.2015.11.007

[37] Rodrigues RJ, Tomé AR, Cunha RA. ATP as a multi-target danger signal in the brain. Front Neurosci. 2015;9:148. DOI: 10.3389/fnins.2015.00148

[38] Sobrinho CR, Wenker IC, Poss EM, Takakura AC, Moreira TS, Mulkey DK. Purinergic signalling contributes to chemoreception in the retrotrapezoid nucleus but not the nucleus of the solitary tract or medullary raphe. J Physiol. 2014;592(6):1309–1323.DOI: 10.1113/jphysiol.2013.268490

2

Cross-Talk Between Hypoxia and the Tumour via Exosomes

Shayna Sharma, Mona Alharbi, Andrew Lai,

Miharu Kobayashi, Richard Kline, Katrina Wade,

Gregory E. Rice and Carlos Salomon

Abstract

Cancer is one of the leading causes of death worldwide, and this is often attributed to the nonspecific symptoms. Additionally, delayed diagnosis and a lack of treatment options negatively impact prognosis. Recently, the role of extracellular vesicles in cancer progression, specifically, in metastasis and in the capacity of several tumours to invade and colonise specific organs has been established. Reduced oxygen tension due to imbalanced oxygen supply and consumption is termed hypoxia and is one of the most commonly observed features in solid tumours. This is often correlated with poor cancer prognosis. Several reports have established that low oxygen tension (i.e. hypoxia) is a common feature of the tumour microenvironment often enhancing the process of epithelial-to-mesenchymal transition (EMT) in cancer cells, thus promoting tumourigenesis and metastasis. Furthermore, hypoxia increases the number of extracellular vesicles released from cancer cells and also modifies their bioactivity and function. The aim of this chapter is to review the association between the tumour microenvironment and extracellular vesicles (EVs), focusing on a specific subpopulation of EVs of endocytic origin, termed exosomes.

Keywords: exosomes, metastasis, metastatic niche, tumourigenesis, cancer

1. Introduction

The global burden of cancer is on the rise and in 2012 around 14.1 million new cases were reported with 8.2 million deaths attributed to cancer [1]. Cancer can be subdivided into categories depending on the area that is affected, including but not limited to lung cancer, pancreatic cancer and ovarian cancer [2, 3].

Consequently, the development of targeted treatments for a large population is difficult due to the heterogeneity of the tumours. Furthermore, in cases such as ovarian cancer, current treatments, which include the use of platinum-based cytotoxic chemotherapy, antiangiogenic drugs and poly (ADP-ribose) polymerase inhibitors, are only beneficial for patients with early stage disease [2]. However, in patients with more advanced stage disease, there is often recurrence of the disease after treatment due to the development of resistance [2]. Therefore, it is essential that diagnostic procedures be explored.

This paradigm shift from focusing on treatments to focusing on early diagnosis of cancer has brought exosomes to the forefront.

Exosomes are small membranous vesicles that are released following the fusion of multive-sicular bodies (MVBs) with the cell membrane. They have multiple characteristics including a cup or spherical shape, maximum diameter of approximately 100 nm, a buoyant density of ~1.12 to ~1.19 g /mL on a sucrose gradient, endosomal origin and the enrichment of late endosomal membrane markers, including TSG101 and proteins from the tetraspanin family (e.g. CD63) [3, 4]. Exosomes are covered in a variety of cell surface receptors and contain several proteins such as cytoskeletal proteins, adhesion molecules and heat-shock proteins. Addition-ally, they encapsulate diverse miRNA and mRNA, which can impact the bioactivity and functionality of the target cells with which the exosomes interact.

While the role of exosomes during tumour progression remains to be fully established, we postulate that tumour cells release exosomes loaded with specific molecules in response to the microenvironment to prepare for and promote metastasis to specific organs.

2. Exosomes: a specific type of extracellular vesicle

Cells secrete a multitude of EVs of different origin, size, content and function. Recent reports have recognised a specific type of extracellular vesicle termed exosomes. Exosomes are believed to be tumour 'couriers', carrying signals and relocating packages of signalling molecules to initiate processes such as metastasis by preparing the metastatic niche [5, 6].

In contrast to other EVs, which are formed by an inward budding of the plasma membrane, exosomes are secreted through the intraluminal invagination of vesicles termed early endo-somes [7]. This leads to the formation of multivesicular bodies (MVBs) which contain intralu-minal vesicles (ILVs). These ILVs are then released by the cell through the fusion of the MVB with the cellular membrane. The released ILVs are termed exosomes [4, 5, 8]. Exosomes carry a common set of molecules along with cell-specific components. Therefore, exosomes contain proteins which are associated with the biogenesis of MVBs such as tetraspanins, Rab GTPases and Annexins [9]. The endosomal-sorting complex required for transport (ESCRT) pathway facilitates plasma membrane remodelling and is also believed to have a role in ILV formation

[10]. Research has also shown that other pathways independent of the ESCRT complex also exist, as an MVB is also formed when the ESCRT complexes are repressed [11, 12, 14, 15].

Whilst the biogenesis of exosomes has been well understood and defined in recent literature, a consensus on the method to extract exosomes is yet to be established. However, a detailed discussion of the current methodological approaches is beyond the scope of this chapter [16, 17]. A NanoSight Tracking Analysis (NTA) comparison between exosomes and microvesicles is shown in **Figure 1**.

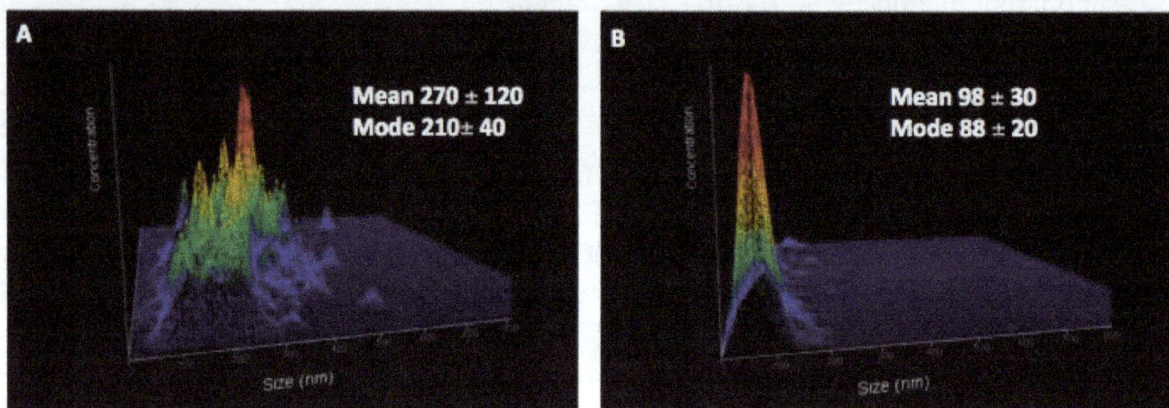

Figure 1. Nanoparticle-tracking analysis using the NanoSight. Representative image of the size distribution of 100,000 g pellet (A) and exosomes (B). The NanoSight instrument measured the rate of Brownian motion of nanoparticles and consists in a light-scattering system that provides a reproducible platform for specific and general nanoparticle characterization (NanoSight Ltd., Amesbury, UK).

Nonetheless, the requirement for a standard isolation procedure is essential as research moves towards examining exosomes as potential therapeutic agents in the context of several diseases such as cancer. Additionally, exosomes are being used to understand the characteristics of the solid tumour, circulating tumour cells and the tumour microenvironment, especially under conditions such as hypoxia.

3. The tumour microenvironment and hypoxia

Under normal conditions, the cellular microenvironment inhibits the development of cancerous cells through tumour interactions thus allowing the environment to annihilate the growth of cancerous cells. The tumour microenvironment comprises endothelial cells (ECs), fibroblasts, perivascular cells and inflammatory cells. These components tend to control the tumourigenic processes—that is, angiogenesis, desmoplasia, lymphangiogenesis and inflammation. Oxygen deficiency in tumour cells, also known as hypoxia, is among the major factors that trigger tumour development and hinder clinical diagnoses [13–15].

An imbalance between oxygen supply and demand causes hypoxic or anoxic conditions. The oxygen supply rate is equivalent to that of metabolic requirements in a normal cell or a tissue.

However, in developed solid tumours, the oxygen consumption rate may fluctuate to adjust for the insufficient oxygen supply, allowing the tissues to develop even in regions with low oxygen levels [15]. Accumulating evidence suggests that up to 60% of locally advanced tumours display hypoxic ($\leq$1% O_2 compared to 2–9% O_2 or 40 mm Hg on average in most mammalian tissues) and/or anoxic ($\leq$0.01% O_2 or undetectable oxygen) areas distributed heterogeneously throughout the tumour and that tumour hypoxia correlates with advanced stages of malignancy [16]. In cancer cells, respective mechanisms are activated to respond to changes in the availability of oxygen. The cells are subjected to lower levels of oxygen and must therefore modify their metabolism, respectively. In such conditions, the hypoxia-inducible factor-1 (HIF-1) transcription factor programme of gene expression changes. This change in expression is assumed to enable the cell to cope with the new environment [17–19].

HIF-1 is a heterodimer complex consisting of two bHLH transcription factors: HIF-1α and HIF-1β [20]. HIF-1α expression is significantly overexpressed in advanced ovarian tumours. O_2-dependent mechanisms primarily regulate HIF-1α degradation. Under normoxic conditions, the O_2-dependent hydroxylation of proline residues in HIF-1α by prolyl hydrolase-domain protein is recognised by the von Hippel-Lindau tumour-suppressor protein and ubiquitinated to be targeted for degradation. Under hypoxic conditions, HIF-1α stabilises and accumulates due to the inhibition of hydroxylation and von Hippel-Lindau protein-mediated ubiquitination, translocates to the nucleus and forms a complex with HIF-1β and a transcriptional co-activator CBP/p300 to activate the transcription of target genes by directly binding to their hypoxia-responsive elements [21].

During hypoxia, HIF-1 activates genes involved in proliferation, cell survival, angiogenesis, vascular tone, metal transport, glycolysis, mitochondrial function, cell growth and survival, and apoptosis and EMT, which all contribute to tumour progression. HIF-1-dependent expression of erythropoietin and angiogenic compounds further enhances the formation of blood vessels and thus facilitates the delivery of oxygenated blood to the hypoxic tissue through the induction of vascular endothelial growth factors (VEGFs). In vitro studies show that increasingly subjecting cancer cells to a hypoxic stimulus results in a gradual increase in VEGF mRNA levels and VEGF protein levels [22, 23].

The addition of HIF-1-induced glycolytic enzymes provides energy as a substrate for oxidative phosphorylation when mitochondria are starved of oxygen [17]. Moreover, due to lower levels of oxygen and nutrients, the ATP level decreases causing a deregulation in the actin cytoskeleton controlled by the down-regulation of Rho proteins. Rho kinase facilitates contractile force generation mediated by actin-myosin by phosphorylating a number of target proteins. Rho/Rho kinase plays a critical role in movement, penetration, cell-cell adhesion, smooth muscle contraction, cytokinesis, mitosis, multiplication, variation, apoptosis and oncogenic transformation within the cell [24–28].

Tumour hypoxia and HIF-1α overexpression have been demonstrated to induce EMT and metastatic phenotypes in cancer cells, yet the crosstalk between the HIF-signalling pathway and EMT is not completely understood [29]. Several studies propose potential molecular mechanisms, such as HIF-1-promoting EMT through the up-regulation of EMT transcriptional factors. Nonetheless, it is known that HIF-1 regulates TWIST expression by binding to their hypoxia-responsive elements. Thus, cells cultured under hypoxia or constitutive HIF-1α expression promoted EMT, whereas the repression of TWIST expression abolished the effect of HIF-1α, shifting the cells back to an epithelial phenotype from the mesenchymal phenotype [29]. HIF-1 expression induced by hypoxia represses E-cadherin-coding genes through SNAI1 and SNAI2 [30–32]. Along with transcriptional factors, hypoxia and HIF-1 activate EMT-associated signalling pathways. Hypoxia also activates the Wnt/β-catenin-signalling pathway by inhibiting GSK3β activation, preventing β-catenin phosphorylation and destruction to increase SNAI1 expression [33]. HIF-1 further interacts with the Notch intracellular domain to increase its transcriptional activity [34].

The Notch-targeted genes HES1 and HEY1 were increased under hypoxic conditions; however, a knockdown of HIF-1α abrogated the hypoxia-induced HES1 and HEY1 expression as well as the SNAI1 expression [35]. Furthermore, HIF-1α targeted lysyl oxidase and lysyl oxidase-like 2 and 3 enzymes, which promote tumour metastasis by mediating cells to matrix adhesion and stabilising SNAI1 activity to induce EMT [36, 37]. Under hypoxia, the consumption of glucose and GLUT1 expression in cancer cells increased as well [17].

It is also well established that bidirectional communication between cancer cells and their tumour microenvironment is essential for cancer progression. For example, most ovarian cancer patients present with ascites—excess fluid in the peritoneal cavity [38]. Ovarian cancer ascites contain molecular factors, including VEGF, cytokines, chemokines and TGF-β, to mediate cellular communication for effective tumourigenesis. Accumulating evidence suggests that cellular communication is not only limited to secretary molecules, but also includes EVs (such as exosomes) that mediate such communication [39]. The nomenclature of EVs is still a matter of debate due to the many terms used (e.g. microvesicles, nanovesicles, shedding vesicles and ectosomes), emphasising the range of EV populations secreted [9].

However, during tumourigenesis, hypoxia serves as a selective agent at various physiological levels. Under hypoxia, a number of transcriptional factors control the cell environment, including Nuclear Factor-kappaB (NF-κB), Activating Transcription Factors (ATFs) and p53s [40–42]. In NF-κB pathways activated by HIF during irregular hypoxia and re-oxygenation [41, 43] and ATF, anoxia drives signalling [44].

Moreover, carbonic anhydrase IX (CAIX) is among the genes in the hypoxic environment of solid tumours that increasingly express themselves. CAIX expression is perceived as causing bladder, ovarian, cervical, colorectal, oral, brain and breast cancers. It enables the balancing of intracellular pH through the extracellular hydration of CO_2 and the production of bicarbonate and protons. The bicarbonate goes back into the cell through bicarbonate transporters and balances the intracellular pH as alkaline, which is favourable for the cell's survival. The protons acidify the extracellular space, thus facilitating the tumour's migratory and invasive behaviour [45–47]. CAIX expression and activity also facilitates the production of Granulocyte-colony stimulating factor (G-CSF),which is in turn required for the transportation of granulocytic Myeloid-derived Suppressor Cells (MDSC) to the metastatic niche—an environment that promotes metastasis. CAIX expression is also required to stimulate NF-κB activity and G-CSF production mediated through hypoxia. The hypoxia-mediated NF-κB activity is triggered by a decrease in the pH level of the culture as well as hypoxia-induced glycolytic activity in the cancer cells [46, 48–50]. The hypoxic areas of tumours usually have lower levels of extracellular pH due to increased metabolic activity [45]. It has been proven that the cells are hampered from acidifying the medium due to a smaller production rate of CAIX in a hypoxic environment [51]. Therefore, hypoxia and the tumour microenvironment are essential factors in regulating disease progression and metastasis.

4. Exosomes, the tumour microenvironment and hypoxia

An evaluation of cancer cells and their microenvironment plays a critical role in hypoxia. Tumour cells under hypoxia secrete molecules that modulate their microenvironment and facilitate tumour angiogenesis and metastasis. Hypoxia is a major hallmark of the tumour environment and is caused when there is a lack of blood supply. The lowered blood supply indicates a lower number of red blood cells being able to reach the tumour cells resulting in decreased oxygen delivery [52]. Moreover, hypoxic tumours have a greater ability to resist standard treatments and the tumour cells are often in a less differentiated or more stem cell-like state [53]. Emerging evidence has shown that exosomes are key membrane vesicles secreted by most cell types under hypoxia. It has also been shown that they have an ability to modulate the tumour microenvironment to ensure adequate nutrition and oxygen supply [54]. There has been an increasing interest in the role of exosomes as a mediator of cell-to-cell communication and its role in ultimately aiding cancer progression.

There have been several processes proposed regarding the release of exosomes into the tumour microenvironment. These processes involve several molecules such as proteins involved in fusion of the multivesicular bodies as well as plasma membrane proteins. Additionally, it has been shown that exosomes present in a cell's environment also regulate exosome release. Riches and colleagues showed that when exosomes were added to the culture medium of cells, the number of exosomes released by the cells decreased evidently [55]. Other proteins that may be involved in increased exosome secretion during hypoxia include the Rab family of proteins, specifically Rab27 as they regulate exosome secretion. The Rab27 protein has two isoforms: Rab27a and Rab27b. Ostrowski and colleagues noted that inhibiting Rab9a, Rab5a, Rab27a, Rab27b and Rab2b led to an inhibition in exosome release [35]. Furthermore, it has been previously shown that the presence of calcium (Ca^{2+}) ionophores can lead to an increase in the release of exosomes [56]. Therefore, although there are several hypotheses, the exact mechanism is still unclear. Thus, the mechanisms underlying exosome release under different tumour microenvironmental conditions such as hypoxia remain to be elucidated. Nonetheless, progress is being made.

The role of exosomes in tumour progression and invasion has been highlighted in literature with a clear correlation being found between the number of hypoxic exosomes released and the aggressiveness of the tumour [57, 58]. A significant increase in the number of exosomes released under hypoxia (1% oxygen) and severe anoxia (0.1% oxygen) was found in a study conducted on three breast cancer cell lines, in which the impact of hypoxia on tumour progression and the release of exosomes was investigated [58]. King and colleagues postulated that the enhancement of exosome release might be mediated by the hypoxia-inducible factor 1 oxygen-sensing pathway (detailed above). They tested their hypothesis by using the HIF hydroxylase inhibitor, Dimethyloxalylglycine (DMOG), to treat the breast cancer cell line, MDA-MB-231 [58]. The role of the DMOG was to trigger an HIF response. This led to a minor although significant rise in the number of exosomes secreted by the cells when quantified by nanoparticle-tracking analysis (NTA). Moreover, when the HIF-1α transcription factor was silenced using siRNA, the increase in exosomes in response to hypoxia was not seen. Therefore, it was concluded that the HIF pathway may have a significant role in the release of exosomes in response to hypoxia. Similar studies were carried out on different cell lines (e.g. leukaemia cell line, K562; human microvascular endothelial cells (HMEC-1); A431 squamous carcinoma; A549 non-small-cell lung (NSCL); H1299 NSCL and HFF-1 foreskin fibroblast cells) to investigate the level of exosomes released under hypoxia and normoxia [57]. The outcome was that the number of exosomes released under hypoxic conditions increased when compared to exosomes released by cells under normoxic conditions in the same amount of time. However, the pathways underlying the hypoxic enhancement of exosome release were unclear [15].

In addition, oncogenic miR-21 was identified at a significant level in exosome fractions [59, 64]. miR-21 is known to down-regulate programmed cell death 4 (PDCD4) expression by directly targeting its 3′-untranslated region. Moreover, it was found that exosomes isolated from peritoneal effusions (ovarian cancer) contained low PDCD4 expression, whereas oncogenic miR-21 was highly expressed compared to exosomes isolated from non-neoplastic peritoneal effusions [59]. The use of exosomal miR-21 as a biomarker for cancer diagnosis has been suggested in several studies as it exists in almost all bodily fluids, is stable and is protected from degradation [60]. Exosomal miR-21 has an effect on a number of signalling pathways which promote metastatic capacity and proliferation. It has been found that miR-21 suppresses phosphatase and tensin homolog expression and promotes the growth and migration of tumour cells [61]. miR-21 also regulates cellular functions by influencing signal transduction, proliferation, carcinogenesis, differentiation and immune response [62–64]. These observations provide key evidence that elevated exosome release under hypoxia is a critical factor affecting tumour proliferation.

Tumour-derived exosomes have the ability to transfer oncogenic activity among tumour cells. Human glioma cells can horizontally transfer an oncogenic form of epidermal growth factor variant III (EGFRvIII) to glioma cells lacking EGFRvIII [65]. The transfer results in an increased expression of the pro-survival gene and a reduction in the cell cycle inhibitor, increasing anchorage-independent growth capacity [65]. An interesting possibility that exosomes are key factors that affect the neighbouring cells is provided by these studies.

Exosomes facilitate communication among tumour cells and contribute to the development of a favourable microenvironment for tumour progression by enhancing processes such as angiogenesis. Angiogenesis is promoted by the activation of endothelial cells through tumour-derived exosomes, and is followed up by the activation of myofibroblasts, a source of matrix-remodelling protein [66, 67]. Tumour-derived exosomes trigger fibroblast to myofibroblast differentiation [68]. In addition to fibroblasts, exosomes can trigger conversion of mesenchymal stem cells from the tumour stroma and adipose tissue to myofibroblasts [69]. The exosomes also contribute to the formation of pre-metastatic niches by educating the bone marrow-derived cells (BMDC). BMDCs when combined with exosomes derived from highly and poorly metastatic melanoma cells accelerated primary tumour growth and also increased the magnitude and number of metastases [6]. Additionally, evidence has shown that exosomes interact with immune cells to suppress antitumour responses and skew them towards the pro-tumourigenic phenotype [70]. Exosomes from hypoxic endothelial cells (EC) show up-regulation of collagen crosslinking activity by activation of lysyl oxidase-like 2 [71]. Lysyl oxidase-like 2 (LOXL2) has been linked to extracellular matrix (ECM) remodelling, angiogenesis, cell proliferation, migration, transcription regulation, fibroblast activation, EMT and metastatic niche formation through a number of processes [36, 72, 73]. The tumour cells can communicate with multiple different cell types via exosomes. Therefore, it is highly likely that this leads to a complex network of interactions.

The reaction of the target cells upon treatment with exosomes depends on the exosomal composition, which has been previously described as being diverse, and the transfer of encapsulated molecules [4, 67]. This ability of exosomes to protect and transfer molecules has led to the hypothesis that they could be used as potential tumour biomarkers or as a non-invasive tumour biopsy.

5. *In vivo* biodistribution of exosomes

Functional characterisation of exosomes often involves the use of an *in vivo* mouse model. Such experiments can give the biodistribution and pharmacokinetic parameters of the exosomes tested, which is important for understanding exosome trafficking and their physiological roles [74].

The starting point at which exosomes are to be isolated varies based on the experimental goals. In studies investigating the role of tumour-derived exosomes in cancer progression, exosomes were isolated from various cancer cell lines such as breast cancer, pancreatic cancer, gastric cancer and colorectal cancer [75]. Another area of interest is the potential use of exosomes as therapeutic carriers of antitumour microRNA or chemotherapy agents [76, 77]. This may allow for improved tissue targeting, increasing the potency of the delivered drug [78]. Exosomes are often isolated from cell-conditioned media with differential centrifugation being the most common method of enriching exosomes [75–77, 79, 80]. Most of the exosome isolation protocols involved low-speed centrifugation steps to remove cells and cell debris followed by high-speed centrifugation at 100,000 g and a washing step of the pellet with a final centrifugation. In a study by Alvarez-Erviti et al. [77], exosomes were derived from cultured dendritic cells, which was chosen based on data demonstrating that dendritic cell-derived exosomes contained immune-stimulating components such as major histocompatibility complex (MHC) class I and class II molecules in addition to T-cell-stimulating molecule, CD86 [81]. Studies also showed that isolated exosomes can be loaded with exogenous RNA or chemotherapy drugs by different methods, including electroporation and sonication [77, 78].

To enable the *in vivo* tracking of exosomes, they can be labelled post isolation with a lipophilic membrane dye such as Paul Karl Horan (PKH), DiOC18 (DIR) or DiIC18 (DiI) [75, 80, 82]. An alternative method of generating labelled exosomes is by transfecting donor cells with a construct encoding for a fluorescence-membrane fusion protein. In this approach, a membrane-bound variant of bioluminescence reporter, Gaussia luciferase, is transfected into the donor cells, producing luciferase-labelled exosomes [82, 83]. A major difference between the two labelling approaches is the time and expertise required. The post-isolation membrane dye labelling is quick (~1 h), whereas the transfection of cells requires additional time (~2 weeks) and expertise in vector and viral cloning and transfection [79, 84]. Additionally, a study by Lai et al [83] reported quicker rates of clearance of transfected luciferase-labelled exosomes compared to the dye-labelled exosomes. The authors attributed this difference to the possibility of the highly stable dyes being an artefact instead of indicating intact exosomal presence.

Exosomes injected into mice are commonly quantified using the Coomassie dye (Bradford)-based method, or copper-based chemistry such as the Bicinchoninic Acid Assay (BCA) [75–77, 82–85]. The yield of exosomes obtained often ranges from 6 to 12 μg/10^6-cultured dendritic cells, 69.2 μg/2–5 × 10^7 of HEK293 and 2–4 ug/10^6 HEK cells [76, 77, 79]. There is some ambiguity in the quantification of exosomal protein concentration in these studies. Presumably, the exosomes were first lysed pre-quantification as without lysing the exosomes, only the membrane-bound proteins would be quantified. Another method of determining the required number of exosomes is to use the number of exosomes per gram of animal weight. Techniques such as NTA are used to quantify the number of exosomal particles and their size distribution [85, 90]. Importantly, in order to translate the use of exosomes into a clinical setting, standardising the dose of exosomes injected is critical. Given that isolated exosomes from current techniques such as ultracentrifugation are heterogeneous in size when observed using NTA [85], it is likely that the difference in size translates to differences in total protein concentration. Therefore, methods that quantify the total protein content within exosomes such as the Bradford/BCA assays are a better means of measuring the protein content and thus exosomal dose.

For biodistribution and tissue-uptake studies, the dose of injected exosomes ranged from 4 to 10 μg per mouse [75, 82]. Alternatively, a dosing range of 1.5 × 10^{10} particles/gram body weight (p/g), 1.0 × 10^{10} p/g and 0.25 × 10^{10} p/g was used [85]. In studies where exosomes were used as a potential therapeutic siRNA carrier, the dose of exosomes chosen was much higher, at 150 μg/mouse [77]. An explanation of a higher dose employed could be that systemically administered exosomes are rapidly cleared from the bloodstream, with evidence to suggest that macrophages play a role in exosome clearance [80]. Therefore, the higher dose was chosen to induce a measurable response.

Once the labelled exosomes are administered, the duration of monitoring ranged from 10 min to 6 h for biodistribution studies, which met the goal of tracking the localisation of exosomes over time [82, 83]. It was demonstrated that injected exosomes localised primarily in the liver and lungs [82, 85]. Moreover, it was shown recently that particular integrin expression on tumour-derived exosomes could be used to predict organ-specific metastasis [75]. In particular, exosomes expressing $\alpha6\beta4$ and $\alpha6\beta1$ were linked with lung metastasis, while exosomal integrin $\alpha v\beta5$ was associated with liver metastasis. For exosomes which carried modified cargo, such as siRNA targeting the abundant GAPDH, the effect induced by the cargo was measured 3 days post injection [77]. This study showed the possibility of using exosome-mediated delivery of potentially therapeutic siRNA to induce a gene-specific knockdown.

In summary, *in vivo* characterisation is an important step in gaining an understanding of the physiological pathways that exosomes are involved in. Further research will strengthen the proposal of using exosomes as a therapeutic carrier and potential diagnostic tool.

6. New approaches to elucidate the role of exosomes in cancer

Identification of biomarkers to detect cancer during its early stages has the potential to improve patient outcomes significantly with exosomes currently being considered. As exosomes are released and circulate in the peripheral circulation, they can be collected from diverse bio-fluids through minimally invasive procedures from the blood and non-invasive procedures from saliva and urine. Through the isolation and purification process, exosomes are separated from highly abundant proteins present in bodily fluids [56]. Furthermore, cancer-derived exosomes can be specifically distinguished from exosomes originating from other cells by the expression of markers such as CD24 and EpCAM [86]. Storage of exosomes does not significantly affect their protein and miRNA contents thus highlighting their high stability [87]. Most importantly, the release and content of exosomes reflect the tumour state and their microenvironment [88].

Encapsulation of cellular proteins and RNA molecules into exosomes makes exosomes an enriched source of tumour markers, which provides an insight into the originating tumour cells. miRNAs are evolutionarily conserved regulating several cellular processes such as cell differentiation, proliferation and apoptosis [89]. These cellular processes are often altered in cancer-enhancing cellular transformation and tumourigenesis by impaired miRNA biogenesis; therefore, miRNA profiles can differentiate cancer tissues from benign tissues [90]. A complete miRNA-profiling study in epithelial ovarian cancer (EOC) has identified aberrantly expressed miRNA in different subtypes of EOC compared to normal ovaries [91]. Ovarian tumour-derived exosomes isolated from patient sera exhibited similar miRNA profiles to originating tumour cells and the exosome concentration was positively correlated with the progression of disease, highlighting the diagnostic potential of exosomal miRNA [92]. High exosomal miR-21, miR-23b and miR-29a expression of ovarian cancer patient effusion correlated with poor progression-free survival and poor overall survival was related to high expression of miR-21 suggesting their use as prognostic markers [93].

A recent study established the role of EOC-derived exosomes in mediating the activation of macrophages to a tumour-associated macrophage (TAM) state [94]. They also demonstrated that SKOV-3 cells when grown with conditioned media from the transformed macrophages were more likely to migrate and proliferate.

Additional studies have proposed the use of exosomes as both diagnostic biomarkers and therapeutic agents [95]. It has been proposed that exosomes be used to transport antitumour complexes such as drugs to the tumour cells, thus providing a form of targeted therapy.

Furthermore, it has been shown that decreasing exosome production by blocking Rab27a (responsible for exosome release) can also reduce primary tumour growth [96].

Compared to the currently available detection methods, the use of exosomes as biomarkers will involve minimally invasive procedures and as the exosomal content reflects the originating cancer cells and their microenvironment, they will have greater specificity. This will decrease the need for surgical interventions and deaths from surgical complications as a result of false-positive results [97].

Author details

Shayna Sharma[1], Mona Alharbi[1], Andrew Lai[1], Miharu Kobayashi[1], Richard Kline[2], Katrina Wade[2], Gregory E. Rice[1,2] and Carlos Salomon[1,2*]

*Address all correspondence to: c.salomongallo@uq.edu.au

1 Exosome Biology Laboratory, Centre for Clinical Diagnostics, University of Queensland Centre for Clinical Research, Royal Brisbane and Women's Hospital, The University of Queensland, Brisbane, QLD, Australia

2 Department of Obstetrics and Gynecology, Maternal-Fetal Medicine, Ochsner Clinic Foundation, New Orleans, LA, USA

References

[1] Ferlay, J., et al., Cancer incidence and mortality worldwide: sources, methods and major patterns in GLOBOCAN 2012. Int J Cancer, 2015. 136(5): p. E359–86.

[2] Jayson, G.C., et al., Ovarian cancer. The Lancet, 2014. 384(9951): p. 1376-1388.

[3] Salomon, C., et al., Exosomal signaling during hypoxia mediates microvascular endothelial cell migration and vasculogenesis. PLoS One, 2013. 8(7): p. e68451.

[4] Rice, G.E., et al., The effect of glucose on the release and bioactivity of exosomes from first trimester trophoblast cells. J Clin Endocrinol Metab, 2015. 100(10): p. E1280–8.

[5] Brinton, L.T., et al., Formation and role of exosomes in cancer. Cell Mol Life Sci, 2014. 72(4): p. 659-671.

[6] Peinado, H., et al., Melanoma exosomes educate bone marrow progenitor cells toward a pro-metastatic phenotype through MET. Nature Med, 2012. 18(6): p. 883–91.

[7] Salomon, C., et al., Exosomes are fingerprints of originating cells: potential biomarkers for ovarian cancer. Research and Reports in Biochemistry, 2015. 5(15): p. 101-109.

[8] Johnstone, R.M., et al., Vesicle formation during reticulocyte maturation. Association of plasma membrane activities with released vesicles (exosomes). J Biol Chem, 1987. 262(19): p. 9412–20.

[9] Théry, C., Zitvogel, L. and Amigorena, S., Exosomes: composition, biogenesis and function. Nat Rev Immunol, 2002. 2(8): p. 569–79.

[10] Colombo, M., et al., Analysis of ESCRT functions in exosome biogenesis, composition and secretion highlights the heterogeneity of extracellular vesicles. J Cell Sci, 2013. 126(Pt 24): p. 5553–65.

[11] Stuffers, S., et al., Multivesicular endosome biogenesis in the absence of ESCRTs. Traffic, 2009. 10(7): p. 925–37.

[12] Trajkovic, K., et al., Ceramide triggers budding of exosome vesicles into multivesicular endosomes. Science, 2008. 319(5867): p. 1244–7.

[13] Finger, E.C. and Giaccia, A.J., Hypoxia, inflammation, and the tumor microenvironment in metastatic disease. Cancer Metastasis Rev, 2010. 29(2): p. 285–93.

[14] Chan, D.A. and Giaccia, A.J., Hypoxia, gene expression, and metastasis. Cancer Metastasis Rev, 2007. 26(2): p. 333–9.

[15] Vaupel, P. and Mayer, A., Hypoxia in cancer: significance and impact on clinical outcome. Cancer Metastasis Rev, 2007. 26(2): p. 225–39.

[16] Favaro, E., et al., Gene expression and hypoxia in breast cancer. Genome Medicine, 2011. 3(8): p. 55.

[17] Papandreou, I., et al., HIF-1 mediates adaptation to hypoxia by actively downregulating mitochondrial oxygen consumption. Cell Metabolism, 2006. 3(3): p. 187–97.

[18] Ke, Q. and Costa, M., Hypoxia-inducible factor-1 (HIF-1). Mol Pharmacol, 2006. 70(5): p. 1469–80.

[19] Zhou, J., et al., Tumor hypoxia and cancer progression. Cancer Lett, 2006. 237(1): p. 10–21.

[20] Semenza, G.L., Targeting HIF-1 for cancer therapy. Nat Rev Cancer, 2003. 3(10): p. 721–32.

[21] Harris, A.L., Hypoxia – A key regulatory factor in tumour growth. Nat Rev Cancer, 2002. 2(1): p. 38–47.

[22] Zhu, P., et al., The proliferation, apoptosis, invasion of endothelial-like epithelial ovarian cancer cells induced by hypoxia. Journal of Experimental and Clinical Cancer Research, 2010. 29(1): p. 124.

[23] Ziello, J.E., Jovin, I.S. and Huang, Y., Hypoxia-Inducible factor (HIF)-1 regulatory pathway and its potential for therapeutic intervention in malignancy and ischemia. Yale J Biol Med, 2007. 80(2): p. 51–60.

[24] Rĕdowicz, M.J., Rho-associated kinase: involvement in the cytoskeleton regulation. Arch Biochem Biophys, 1999. 364(1): p. 122–24.

[25] Leong, H.S. and Chambers, A.F., Hypoxia promotes tumor cell motility via RhoA and ROCK1 signaling pathways. Proc Natl Acad Sci, 2014. 111(3): p. 887–8.

[26] Street, C.A. and Bryan, B.A., Rho kinase proteins—pleiotropic modulators of cell, survival and apoptosis. Anticancer Res, 2011. 31(11): p. 3645–57.

[27] Gilkes, D.M., et al., Hypoxia-inducible factors mediate coordinated RhoA-ROCK1 expression and signaling in breast cancer cells. Proc Natl Acad Sci, 2014. 111(3): p. E384–93.

[28] Horiuchi, A., et al., Up-regulation of small GTPases, RhoA and RhoC, is associated with tumor progression in ovarian carcinoma. Lab Investig, 2003. 83(6): p. 861–70.

[29] Yang, M.H., et al., Direct regulation of TWIST by HIF-1alpha promotes metastasis. Nat Cell Biol, 2008. 10(3): p. 295–305.

[30] Kurrey, N.K., et al., Snail and slug mediate radioresistance and chemoresistance by antagonizing p53-mediated apoptosis and acquiring a stem-like phenotype in ovarian cancer cells. Stem Cells, 2009. 27(9): p. 2059–68.

[31] Imai, T., et al., Hypoxia attenuates the expression of E-cadherin via up-regulation of SNAIL in ovarian carcinoma cells. Am J Pathol, 2003. 163(4): p. 1437–47.

[32] Zhang, Y., Fan, N. and Yang, J., Expression and clinical significance of hypoxia-inducible factor 1alpha, Snail and E-cadherin in human ovarian cancer cell lines. Mol Med Rep, 2015. 12(3): p. 3393–9.

[33] Cannito, S., et al., Redox mechanisms switch on hypoxia-dependent epithelial-mesenchymal transition in cancer cells. Carcinogenesis, 2008. 29(12): p. 2267–78.

[34] Haase, V.H., Oxygen regulates epithelial-to-mesenchymal transition: insights into molecular mechanisms and relevance to disease. Kidney Int, 2009. 76(5): p. 492–9.

[35] Ostrowski, M., et al., Rab27a and Rab27b control different steps of the exosome secretion pathway. Nat Cell Biol, 2010. 12(1): p. 19–30; sup pp 1–13.

[36] Peinado, H., et al., A molecular role for lysyl oxidase-like 2 enzyme in Snail regulation and tumor progression. EMBO J, 2005. 24(19): p. 3446–58.

[37] Erler, J.T., et al., Lysyl oxidase is essential for hypoxia-induced metastasis. Nature, 2006. 440(7088): p. 1222–6.

[38] Kipps, E., Tan, D.S. and Kaye, S.B., Meeting the challenge of ascites in ovarian cancer: new avenues for therapy and research. Nat Rev Cancer, 2013. 13(4): p. 273–82.

[39] Kahlert, C. and Kalluri, R., Exosomes in tumor microenvironment influence cancer progression and metastasis. J Mol Med (Berl), 2013. 91(4): p. 431–7.

[40] Graeber, T.G., et al., Hypoxia induces accumulation of p53 protein, but activation of a G1-phase checkpoint by low-oxygen conditions is independent of p53 status. Mol Cell Biol, 1994. 14(9): p. 6264–77.

[41] Cummins, E.P., et al., Hypoxic regulation of NF-kappaB signaling. Methods Enzymol, 2007. 435: p. 479–92.

[42] Köditz, J., et al., Oxygen-dependent ATF-4 stability is mediated by the PHD3 oxygen sensor. Blood, 2007. 110(10): p. 3610–17.

[43] Ameri, K., et al., Induction of activating transcription factor 3 by anoxia is independent of p53 and the hypoxic HIF signalling pathway. Oncogene, 2007. 26(2): p. 284–9.

[44] Ameri, K., et al., Anoxic induction of ATF-4 through HIF-1–independent pathways of protein stabilization in human cancer cells. Blood, 2004. 103(5): p. 1876–82.

[45] Gatenby, R.A. and Gillies, R.J., Why do cancers have high aerobic glycolysis? Nat Rev Cancer, 2004. 4(11): p. 891–9.

[46] Chafe, S.C., et al., Carbonic anhydrase IX promotes myeloid-derived suppressor cell mobilization and establishment of a metastatic niche by stimulating G-CSF production. Cancer Res, 2015. 75(6): p. 996–1008.

[47] McDonald, P.C., et al., Recent developments in targeting carbonic anhydrase IX for cancer therapeutics. Oncotarget, 2012. 3(1): p. 84–97.

[48] Perkins, N.D., The diverse and complex roles of NF-κB subunits in cancer. Nat Rev Cancer, 2012. 12(2): p. 121–32.

[49] Xu, L. and Fidler, I.J., Acidic pH-induced elevation in interleukin 8 expression by human ovarian carcinoma cells. Cancer Res, 2000. 60(16): p. 4610–6.

[50] Fukumura, D., et al., Hypoxia and acidosis independently up-regulate vascular endothelial growth factor transcription in brain tumors in vivo. Cancer Res, 2001. 61(16): p. 6020–4.

[51] Lou, Y., et al., Targeting tumor hypoxia: suppression of breast tumor growth and metastasis by novel carbonic anhydrase IX inhibitors. Cancer Res, 2011. 71(9): p. 3364–76.

[52] Kumar, V. and Gabrilovich, D.I., Hypoxia-inducible factors in regulation of immune responses in tumour microenvironment. Immunology, 2014. 143(4): p. 512–9.

[53] Kim, Y., et al., Hypoxic tumor microenvironment and cancer cell differentiation. Curr Mol Med, 2009. 9(4): p. 425–34.

[54] Dorayappan, K.D.P., et al., The biological significance and clinical applications of exosomes in ovarian cancer. Gynecologic oncology, 2016. 142(1): p. 199-205.

[55] Riches, A., et al., Regulation of exosome release from mammary epithelial and breast cancer cells – A new regulatory pathway. Eur J Cancer, 2014. 50(5): p. 1025–34.

[56] Colombo, M., Raposo, G. and Théry, C., Biogenesis, secretion, and intercellular interactions of exosomes and other extracellular vesicles. Annu Rev Cell Dev Biol, 2014. 30: p. 255–89.

[57] Park, J.E., et al., Hypoxic tumor cell modulates its microenvironment to enhance angiogenic and metastatic potential by secretion of proteins and exosomes. Mol Cell Proteomics: MCP, 2010. 9(6): p. 1085–99.

[58] King, H.W., Michael, M.Z. and Gleadle, J.M., Hypoxic enhancement of exosome release by breast cancer cells. BMC Cancer, 2012. 12(1): p. 1–10.

[59] Cappellesso, R., et al., Programmed cell death 4 and microRNA 21 inverse expression is maintained in cells and exosomes from ovarian serous carcinoma effusions. Cancer Cytopathol, 2014. 122(9): p. 685–93.

[60] Shi, J., Considering exosomal miR-21 as a biomarker for cancer. J Clin Med, 2016. 5(4): p. 42.

[61] Meng, F., et al., MicroRNA-21 regulates expression of the PTEN tumor suppressor gene in human hepatocellular cancer. Gastroenterology, 2007. 133(2): p. 647–58.

[62] Taylor, D.D. and Gercel-Taylor, C., MicroRNA signatures of tumor-derived exosomes as diagnostic biomarkers of ovarian cancer. Gynecol Oncol, 2008. 110(1): p. 13–21.

[63] Ratner, E.S., et al., MicroRNA signatures differentiate uterine cancer tumor subtypes. Gynecol Oncol, 2010. 118(3): p. 251–7.

[64] Bartel, D.P., MicroRNAs: target recognition and regulatory functions. Cell, 2009. 136(2): p. 215–33.

[65] Kucharzewska, P., et al., Exosomes reflect the hypoxic status of glioma cells and mediate hypoxia-dependent activation of vascular cells during tumor development. Proc Natl Acad Sci, 2013. 110(18): p. 7312–7.

[66] Vong, S. and Kalluri, R., The role of stromal myofibroblast and extracellular matrix in tumor angiogenesis. Genes Cancer, 2011. 2(12): p. 1139–45.

[67] Zhuang, G., et al., Tumour-secreted miR-9 promotes endothelial cell migration and angiogenesis by activating the JAK-STAT pathway. EMBO J, 2012. 31(17): p. 3513–23.

[68] Webber, J., et al., Cancer exosomes trigger fibroblast to myofibroblast differentiation. Cancer Res, 2010. 70(23): p. 9621–30.

[69] Cho, J.A., et al., Exosomes from breast cancer cells can convert adipose tissue-derived mesenchymal stem cells into myofibroblast-like cells. Int J Oncol, 2012. 40(1): p. 130–8.

[70] Filipazzi, P., et al. Recent advances on the role of tumor exosomes in immunosuppression and disease progression. in Seminars in cancer biology. 2012. 22(4): p. 342-349.

[71] Jong, O.G., et al., Exosomes from hypoxic endothelial cells have increased collagen crosslinking activity through up-regulation of lysyl oxidase-like 2. Journal of cellular and molecular medicine, 2016. 20(2): p. 342-350.

[72] Hollosi, P., et al., Lysyl oxidase-like 2 promotes migration in noninvasive breast cancer cells but not in normal breast epithelial cells. Int J Cancer, 2009. 125(2): p. 318–27.

[73] Barker, H.E., et al., Tumor-secreted LOXL2 activates fibroblasts through FAK signaling. Mol Cancer Res, 2013. 11(11): p. 1425–36.

[74] Choi, H. and Lee, D.S., Illuminating the physiology of extracellular vesicles. Stem Cell Res Ther, 2016. 7: p. 55.

[75] Hoshino, A., et al., Tumour exosome integrins determine organotropic metastasis. Nature, 2015. 527(7578): p. 329–35.

[76] Ohno, S.-I., et al., Systemically injected exosomes targeted to EGFR deliver antitumor microRNA to breast cancer cells. Mol Ther, 2013. 21(1): p. 185–91.

[77] Alvarez-Erviti, L., et al., Delivery of siRNA to the mouse brain by systemic injection of targeted exosomes. Nat Biotech, 2011. 29(4): p. 341–5.

[78] Kim, M.S., et al., Development of exosome-encapsulated paclitaxel to overcome MDR in cancer cells. Nanomed: Nanotechnol Biol Med, 2016. 12(3): p. 655–64.

[79] El-Andaloussi, S., et al., Exosome-mediated delivery of siRNA in vitro and in vivo. Nat Protocols, 2012. 7(12): p. 2112–26.

[80] Imai, T., et al., Macrophage-dependent clearance of systemically administered B16BL6-derived exosomes from the blood circulation in mice. J Extracell Ves, 2015. 4: p. 10.3402/jev.v4.26238.

[81] Zitvogel, L., et al., Eradication of established murine tumors using a novel cell-free vaccine: dendritic cell derived exosomes. Nat Med, 1998. 4(5): p. 594–600.

[82] Takahashi, Y., et al., Visualization and in vivo tracking of the exosomes of murine melanoma B16-BL6 cells in mice after intravenous injection. J Biotechnol, 2013. 165(2): p. 77–84.

[83] Lai, C.P., et al., Dynamic biodistribution of extracellular vesicles in vivo using a multimodal imaging reporter. ACS Nano, 2014. 8(1): p. 483–94.

[84] Tian, T., et al., Dynamics of exosome internalization and trafficking. J Cell Physiol, 2013. 228(7): p. 1487–95.

[85] Wiklander, O.P.B., et al., Extracellular vesicle in vivo biodistribution is determined by cell source, route of administration and targeting. Journal of Extracellular Vesicles, 2015. 4: p. 26316.

[86] Im, H., et al., Label-free detection and molecular profiling of exosomes with a nano-plasmonic sensor. Nat Biotechnol, 2014. 32(5): p. 490–5.

[87] Sarker, S., et al., Placenta-derived exosomes continuously increase in maternal circulation over the first trimester of pregnancy. J Transl Med, 2014. 12: p. 204.

[88] Kobayashi, M., et al., Ovarian cancer cell invasiveness is associated with discordant exosomal sequestration of Let-7 miRNA and miR-200. J Transl Med, 2014. 12: p. 4.

[89] Paranjape, T., Slack, F.J. and Weidhaas, J.B., MicroRNAs: tools for cancer diagnostics. Gut, 2009. 58(11): p. 1546–54.

[90] Kumar, M.S., et al., Impaired microRNA processing enhances cellular transformation and tumorigenesis. Nat Genet, 2007. 39(5): p. 673–7.

[91] Iorio, M.V., et al., MicroRNA signatures in human ovarian cancer. Cancer Res, 2007. 67(18): p. 8699–707.

[92] Taylor, D.D. and Gercel-Taylor, C., MicroRNA signatures of tumor-derived exosomes as diagnostic biomarkers of ovarian cancer. Gynecol Oncol, 2008. 110(1): p. 13–21.

[93] Vaksman, O., et al., Exosome-derived miRNAs and ovarian carcinoma progression. Carcinogenesis, 2014. 35(9): p. 2113–20.

[94] Ying, X., et al., Epithelial ovarian cancer-secreted exosomal miR-222-3p induces polarization of tumor-associated macrophages. Oncotarget, 2016. 7(28): p. 43076-43087.

[95] Tickner, J.A., et al., Functions and therapeutic roles of exosomes in cancer. Front Oncol, 2014. 4: p. 127.

[96] Bobrie, A., et al., Rab27a supports exosome-dependent and -independent mechanisms that modify the tumor microenvironment and can promote tumor progression. Cancer Res, 2012. 72(19): p. 4920–30.

[97] Moyer, V.A., Screening for ovarian cancer: U.S. Preventive Services Task Force reaffirmation recommendation statement. Ann Intern Med, 2012. 157(12): p. 900–4.

3

The Multifaceted Role of Hypoxia-Inducible Factor 1 (HIF1) in Lipid Metabolism

Guomin Shen and Xiaobo Li

Abstract

Hypoxia-inducible factor 1 (HIF1) is a master transcription factor and regulates expression of a large number of genes involving many aspects of biology. In addition to HIF1's roles in glucose metabolism and angiogenesis, numerous studies have revealed an emerging role of HIF1 in controlling lipid homeostasis. In this chapter, we discuss that lipid accumulation is related to HIF1's activity in several diseases and the growing evidence demonstrating the functional importance of HIF1 in controlling lipid metabolism. The functions include lipid uptake and trafficking, fatty acid metabolism, sterol metabolism, triacylglycerol synthesis, phospholipid metabolism, lipid droplet biogenesis, and lipid signaling. Defining the role of HIF1 in lipid metabolism is crucial to understand the pathophysiology of lipid in disease and may help us to identify additional target sites for drug development. This review would shed light on our understanding of the critical role of HIF1 in lipid metabolism.

Keywords: hypoxia-inducible factor 1, lipid accumulation, lipid metabolism

1. Introduction

Hypoxia has been identified as a common symptom in many diseases, such as cancer [1, 2], obesity [3], atherosclerosis [4], and ischemic heart disease (IHD) [5]. Adaptation to hypoxia involves hypoxia-inducible factor 1 (HIF1) and requires reprogramming of essential elements of cellular metabolism [6]. HIF1 was described about 20 years ago [7]. It is a heterodimeric transcription factor that is composed of an oxygen-regulated HIF1α subunit and a constitutively expressed HIF1β subunit [7, 8]. HIF1α is mainly regulated by protein degradation. Under normoxic conditions, HIF1α is subjected to oxygen-dependent hydroxylation by three prolyl hydroxylase domain proteins (PHD1–3) on two proline residues in the oxygen-dependent degradation (ODD) domain [9]. The prolyl-hydroxylated HIF1α is targeted for degradation by the tumor suppressor protein von Hippel-Lindau (VHL), an E3 ubiquitin-protein ligase [10, 11]. HIF1α is also regulated in an oxygen-dependent manner by factor inhibiting HIF1 (FIH1) [12, 13]. In this case, FIH1 mediates the hydroxylation of an asparagine residue in the C-terminal trans-activation domain, which prevents the binding of HIF1α with coactivators p300 and CBP [13–15]. Hydroxylation of proline and asparagine is inhibited under hypoxic conditions causing HIF1α to rapidly accumulate [12, 13]. HIF1α subsequently heterodimerizes with HIF1β, and the complex binds to hypoxic responsive elements (HREs) within the promoter regions of target genes, and allows for recruitment of coactivators and activation of transcription [16]. In addition to hypoxia, HIF1 accumulation can also be induced by growth-factor stimulation, gene mutations, and intermediate metabolites [17] (**Figure 1**).

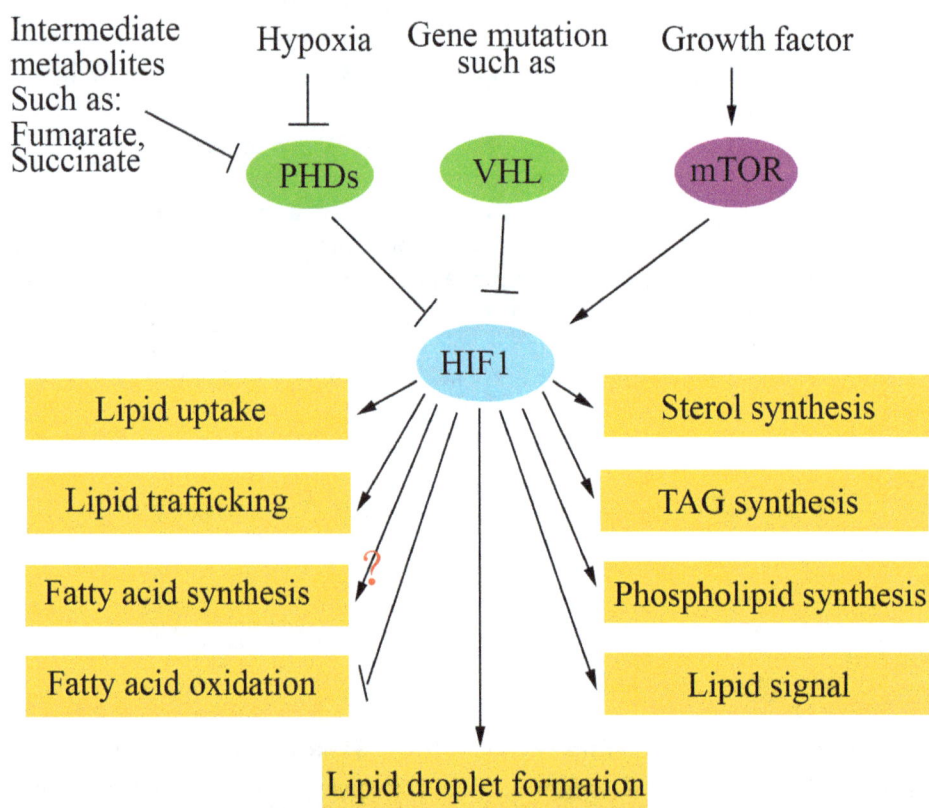

Figure 1. Regulation of HIF1 and its downstream roles related to lipid metabolism. HIF1 accumulation can be induced by hypoxia, gene mutations, intermediate metabolites, and growth factors. HIF1 plays a pivotal role in lipid metabolism. It can increase lipid uptake and trafficking, fatty acid synthesis, sterol synthesis, TAG synthesis, lipid droplet biogenesis, and lipid signal production, and suppress fatty acid β-oxidation. Lipid droplet accumulation may be the final result of HIF1 in lipid metabolism. It is unclear about its role in phospholipids metabolism.

It has been reported that HIF1 regulates the transcription of hundreds of genes involving many aspect of biology, especially energy metabolism and vascularization [16]. The role of HIF1 in glucose metabolism had been well established [17]. Most of genes involving glucose uptake and glycolysis are directly regulated by HIF1 [17]. Recent studies demonstrated that HIF1 also plays an important role in lipid metabolism [1, 2, 18–21]. Currently, our understanding of HIF1 in regulating lipid metabolism has lagged behind that of glucose metabolism. Lipids, structurally and functionally important in all organisms, are not only one of the major components of cellular membrane systems, but also the source of energy storage. Moreover, signal molecules, such as prostaglandin E2 (PGE2), hydroxyeicosatetraenoic acid (HETE), and steroid hormones, are derived from lipids. This review would focus on the HIF1's activity related to dysregulation of lipid metabolism in several diseases, including atherosclerosis [4], fatty liver disease (FLD) [19], heart failure diseases [5], obesity [3], and cancer [1, 2] as well as the involvement of HIF1 in lipid metabolism, including lipid uptake and trafficking, fatty acid metabolism, sterol metabolism, triacylglycerol (TAG) synthesis, phospholipid metabolism, lipid droplet (LD) biogenesis, and lipid signaling.

2. Lipid accumulation is associated with HIF1's activity in diseases

Most of the studies have demonstrated that HIF1's activity is associated with lipid accumulation positively [3, 18, 20–27], while few researches have indicated the opposite effect [28–31]. PHD2 inhibition or deletion, increasing HIF1's activity (**Figure 1**), decreased lipid accumulation in different animal models [28, 30, 31]. It indicated that the role of HIF1 in lipid metabolism may be different in different animal models. Details were described and discussed in the following sections.

2.1. Atherosclerosis

Hypoxia has been demonstrated in atherosclerotic plaques [4]. Arterial wall hypoxia exists in a rabbit atherosclerosis injury model [32–34], confirmed in rabbit atherosclerotic plaques [35, 36] as well as in several mouse models [23, 37, 38]. Recently, in vivo studies have demonstrated hypoxia in human atherosclerotic plaques [39]. Macrophages are the major cell types in human plaques that display signs of hypoxia. TAG-loaded foam cells derived from macrophages are characteristic of both early and late atherosclerotic plaques [40, 41]. Exposure of human macrophages to hypoxia causes an accumulation of TAG-containing lipid droplets [42]. HIF1α is expressed in various cell types of atherosclerotic lesions and is associated with lesional inflammation [43]. Knockdown of HIF1α with small interfering RNAs inhibits TAG-loaded foam cell formation in the human monoblastic cell line U937 [22]. Dyslipidemia are regarded as the key risk factors for the development of atherosclerosis, and HIF1 has been suggested to have both detrimental and beneficial roles in atherosclerosis [28, 44, 45]. In murine atherosclerosis, the hypoxia-induced accumulation of cholesterol was substantially reversed in vitro by reducing the expression of the HIF1α [23]. While in another model, PHD2 inhibition stabilized HIF1α and reduced serum cholesterol levels in low-density lipoprotein receptor-deficient mice that were fed a high-fat diet (HFD) [28]. So the role of HIF1 should be further studied in atherosclerosis lipid metabolism.

2.2. Heart failure diseases

Ischemic heart disease, systemic hypertension, and pathological cardiac hypertrophy eventually result in heart failure. Myocardial hypoxia has been associated with these clinical conditions [25, 46]. Several studies showed a correlation between TAG accumulation and heart failure [26, 47–49]. Hypoxia promotes TAG accumulation in cardiomyocytes [48, 50]. Overexpression of the constitutive active form of HIF1α in cardiomyocytes promotes intracellular lipid accumulation under normoxia [24]. The specific deletion of VHL in mice cardiac myocytes results in lipid accumulation [25, 26]. In a pathological cardiac hypertrophy mouse model, cardiac TAG accumulation in ventricles was abolished in HIF1α knockout mice [26].

2.3. Fatty liver disease (FLD)

Lipid accumulation is a common feature of fatty liver disease, whether it is alcoholic (AFLD) or nonalcoholic (NAFLD) [19]. FLD initially begins with simple hepatic steatosis, but can irreversibly progress to steatohepatitis, fibrosis, cirrhosis, or hepatocellular carcinoma [19]. Hypoxia in liver has been documented in vivo in rats on a continuous ethanol diet at a constant rate for prolonged periods [51–54]. Recent studies have demonstrated that hypoxia is also observed in NAFLD [55]. Indeed, HIF1 expression is increased in fatty liver diseases [19]. Nath and his colleagues found that ethanol feeding resulted in liver steatosis in wild-type mice compared with isocaloric diet-fed controls [27]. Constitutive activation of HIF1α in hepatocytes accelerates lipid accumulation with chronic ethanol feeding compared with wild-type mice [27]. In contrast, hepatocyte-specific deletion of HIF1α protected mice from alcohol-induced liver lipid accumulation [27]. However, another group reported that hepatocyte-specific HIF1α-null mice developed severe hyper-triglyceridemia with enhanced lipid accumulation in the liver of mice after 4 weeks of exposure to a 6% ethanol-containing liquid diet [29]. Different genetic techniques used to create specific gene expression or knockout mice in each of these studies may offer some explanation of the different results each described. The other possible explanation is that the presence of inflammation may rewire the HIF-1 pathway, which leads to a different gene expression profile compared to that observed in simple steatosis [19].

2.4. Obesity

Hypoxia has been directly demonstrated in adipose tissue of several obese mouse models, such as ob/ob mice [56, 57], KKAy obese mice [58], and high-fat diet-induced obese mice [56–58]. In HFD-induced obese mice, HIF1 activation in visceral white adipocytes is critical to maintain dietary obesity [3] and adipocyte-specific HIF1β or HIF1α knockout mice exhibit reduced fat formation compared with wild-type controls [59]. Conversely, another group, using transgenic mice with adipose tissue selective expression of a dominant negative version of HIF1, found that mice with inhibition of HIF1's activity developed a more severe obesity in HFD-induced obese mice [60]. Inactivation of PHD2 resulted in the activation of HIF1. Transgenic mice with PHD2-specific deletion in adipocyte were resistant to HFD-induced obesity and decreased lipid accumulation [30]. In another PHD2-deficient mice model, they also had improved glucose tolerance and insulin sensitivity. Whether fed normal chow or HFD, PHD2 inhibition had less adipose tissue, smaller adipocytes, and less adipose tissue inflammation than their littermates. In addition, serum cholesterol level and de novo lipid synthesis were decreased, and the mice were protected against hepatic steatosis in PHD2-deficient mice [31]. It seems that HIF1 in adipocyte of obesity had different effect on lipid metabolism compared with other models. Thus, the effect of HIF1 in lipid metabolism of obesity has yet to be defined.

2.5. Cancer

Hypoxia in the tumor microenvironment leads to the metabolic changes in cancer cells. Over 50% cellular energy is produced by glycolysis and HIF1 plays a central role in the changes [16, 61]. Recently disorders of lipid metabolism had been demonstrated in solid tumors [62, 63], such as pancreatic cancer [64], liver cancer [1], breast cancer [65], colon cancer [66], and ovarian cancer [67]. Lipid accumulation is observed in human tumor tissue [66, 68]. Accumulation of cholesterol also has been reported in prostate cancer [69]. Indeed, recent researches had demonstrated that HIF1's activity is really involved abnormal lipid metabolism of cancer cells. Hypoxia-induced lipid accumulation depends on HIF1's activity in cancer cells [18, 20, 21]. Under hypoxic condition, the flux from glutamine into fatty acid is mediated by reductive carboxylation, and HIF1α plays an important role in this metabolic shift in tumor cells [70]. HIF1α also inhibits fatty acid β-oxidation to promote lipid accumulation in human hepatocellular carcinoma [1]. Valli and his colleagues revealed that hypoxia induced many changes in lipid metabolites. Enzymatic steps in fatty acid synthesis and the Kennedy pathway were modified in an HIF1α-dependent fashion in HCT116 cell line [2]. However, the role of HIF1 in cancer lipid metabolism has not been well addressed, so more researches should be further studied.

3. The role of HIF1 in lipid metabolism

Lipid metabolism is more complicated than glucose metabolism. Besides as major components of membrane, lipids are also a source of energy storage and signal molecules. HIF1-induced genes involving lipid metabolism are listed in **Table 1**. We would discuss the role of HIF1 in lipid metabolism from the following linked aspects: lipid uptake and trafficking, fatty acid metabolism, sterol metabolism, TAG synthesis, phospholipids metabolism, lipid droplets biogenesis, and lipid signaling (**Figure 1**).

3.1. Lipid uptake and trafficking

3.1.1. Free fatty acid (FFA) uptake

At the plasma membrane, uptake of fatty acid is mainly regulated by the fatty acid transport protein family, such as CD36 [89–91], and plasma membrane-associated fatty-acid-binding proteins (FABPs). Fatty acid transporter CD36 transports long chain fatty acid (LCFA) across plasma membrane. In cardiac myocytes, acute hypoxia (15 min) induced the redistribution of CD36 from an intracellular pool to the plasma membrane [92]. Similarly, in intact Langendorff-perfused heart, a similar effect was demonstrated [92]. Thus, indicating the increased intracellular lipid accumulation in hypoxic hearts is attributable to accumulation of fatty acid in the heart [92]. CD36 also can be regulated at the transcriptional level. In neonatal mouse cardiac myocytes, phenyl-epinephrine (PE) induced free fatty acid uptake in an HIF1α -dependent fashion while inhibition of CD36 led to decreased TAG accumulation upon PE stimulation [26]. In this model, CD36 was induced through HIF1-PPARγ axis [26]. In human retinal pigment epithelial cells, CD36 is mediated by HIF1 binding on its promoter region [71]. Hypoxia also markedly induced CD36 mRNA in corneal and retinal tissue in in vivo [71].

Products of HIF1's target genes	Functions in lipid metabolism	References
CD36, PPARγ, FABP3, FABP7	Fatty acid uptake	[21, 26, 71]
VLDLR, LRP1	LDL and VLDL uptake	[18, 48, 72, 73]
CAV1, RAB20	Endocytosis and lipid trafficking	[74, 75]
PPARα*, TWIST1, Sirt2*	Fatty acid β-oxidation	[3, 76, 77]
DEC1	Fatty acid synthesis	[30, 78]
ABCA1*	Cholesterol efflux	[79]
PPARγ, Lipin1	TAG synthesis	[20, 26]
CHKA	Phospholipids synthesis	[80, 81]
ADRP, HIG2, CAV1	Lipid droplet biogenesis	[42, 74, 82–85]
COX2, PTGES1	Lipid signaling	[86–88]

PPARγ, peroxisome proliferator-activated receptor gamma; VLDLR, very-low-density lipoprotein receptor; LRP1, low-density lipoprotein receptor-related protein 1; CAV1, caveolin 1; PPARα, peroxisome proliferator-activated receptor alpha; TWIST1, twist family bHLH transcription factor 1; SIRT2, sirtuin 2; DEC1, deleted in esophageal cancer 1; ABCA1, ATP-binding cassette subfamily A member 1; LPIN1, lipin 1; HIG2, hypoxia inducible gene 2; CHKA, choline kinase alpha; COX2, cyclooxygenase 2; PTGES, prostaglandin E synthase 1.

"*" genes suppressed by HIF1.

Table 1. HIF1 targets genes that regulate lipid metabolism.

FABPs are part of a larger family of cytoplasmic proteins comprising nine members (FABP1–FABP9) [93], and are involved in reversibly binding intracellular hydrophobic ligands and trafficking them throughout cellular compartments [89]. Some evidence suggested that FABPs could interact directly with CD36 [94]. In *in vitro*, FABP3 and FABP7 were induced by hypoxia in a HIF1-dependent manner, and both are involved in fatty acid uptake [21]. Knockdown of endogenous expression of FABP3 or FABP7 significantly impaired lipids droplets formation under hypoxia [21]. More specifically, the role of FABP3 is evident from the phenotype of FABP3 knockout mice, which show a rate of palmitate uptake reduced by 50% in cardiac myocytes [95, 96]. FABP7 binds long-chain polyunsaturated FA (PUFA), allowing uptake and intracellular trafficking [97], and is involved in proliferation and invasion of melanoma cells [98] and glioblastoma cells [21]. High expression of FABP7 in glioblastomas is associated with poor prognosis and more invasive tumors [99].

3.1.2. LDL and VLDL uptake

LDL and VLDL are major source of extracellular lipid, and HIF1 has been implicated in the transport of LDL and VLDL into cells. LDL receptor (LDLR) and VLDL receptor (VLDLR) are major receptors that are responsible for LDL and VLDL uptake. It had been reported that hypoxia significantly increased LDL uptake and enhances lipid accumulation in arterial smooth muscle cells (SMCs), exclusive LDLR activity [100]. In addition, hypoxia increased VLDL uptake in cardiac myocytes, which might be partially dependent on up-regulating VLDLR expression [101]. Some studies had also reported that VLDLR could be induced under hypoxia [102]. In human cancer cell lines, we had demonstrated that HIF1-mediated VLDLR induction influenced intracellular lipid accumulation through regulating LDL and VLDL uptake under hypoxia [18]. In hepatocellular carcinoma, expression of VLDR was associated positively with HIF1 [18]. In mice, hypoxia-induced VLDLR expression in HL-1 cells was dependent on HIF1α through its interaction with an HRE in the *VLDLR* promoter. VLDLR promoted the endocytosis of lipoproteins, and causes lipid accumulation in cardiomyocytes [48].

Low-density lipoprotein receptor related protein 1 (LRP1) belongs to LDL receptor superfamily, and is a key receptor for selective cholesterol uptake in human vascular smooth muscle cells (VSMCs). Hypoxia increased LRP1 expression through HIF1α, and overexpression of LRP1 mediated hypoxia-induced aggregated LDL (agLDL) uptake in human VSMCs [72] as well as VLDL-cholesteryl ester (VLDL-CE) uptake in neonatal rat ventricular myocytes (NRVMs) [73]. In contrast to the strong impact of LRP1 inhibition on VLDL-CE uptake in hypoxic cardiomyocytes, LRP1 deficiency did not exert any significant effect on VLDL-TG uptake or VLDL-TG accumulation [73]. This indicated that VLDLR might be a key receptor for VLDL-TG uptake. Therefore, more experiments should be done to value the precise contribution of VLDLR and LRP1 in myocardial VLDL-CE and VLDL-TG uptake in pathophysiological situation in the heart.

LDL and VLDL uptake are through vesicular transport pathways [103]. The LDL receptor superfamily has NPXY motif in cytoplasmic domain that interacts with the endocytotic machinery to mediate rapid clathrin-dependent endocytosis of the receptor-ligand complex [104, 105]. Caveolaes are formed in the process of receptor-mediated endocytosis. Numerous proteins are involved in caveolae formation, including caveolins, Rabs, VAT-1, SNAP, and VAMP [106]. Caveolin-1 (CAV1) is an essential structural constituent of caveolae that is involved in constitutive endocytic vesicular trafficking. Loss of VHL function, an E3 ligase involving HIF1α degradation, was associated with increased caveolae formation [74]. CAV1, as a direct target of HIF1, accentuated the formation of caveolae [74]. Knockdown expression of CAV1 inhibited uptake of oxidized LDL (oxLDL) without changing its binding to the plasma membrane [107]. These results indicated that CAV1 was part of the pathway that allowed cells to take up oxLDL [107]. Rab20, a member of the Rab family of small GTP-binding proteins, regulating intracellular trafficking and vesicle formation, had also been characterized as an HIF-1 target [75]. Although there was no direct evidence of the involvement of CAV1 and Rab20 in hypoxia-induced LDL and VLDL uptake, we hypothesized that they might play role in hypoxia-induced LDL and VLDL uptake and/or intracellular lipid trafficking.

Taken together, HIF1 promoting lipid accumulation may increase lipid uptake and intracellular lipid trafficking by inducing related genes directly. It should be further studied if there are more genes targeted by HIF1 in the process.

3.2. Fatty acid metabolism

3.2.1. Fatty acid β-oxidation

Hypoxia increased intracellular lipid accumulation through suppression of fatty acid β-oxidation (FAO) in several models, and the molecular mechanism involvement of HIF1 in the process had been demonstrated (**Figure 2**). Under hypoxic condition, human macrophages showed in an increased TAG accumulation that was associated with a decreasing rate of FAO. The decreasing rate of FAO was shown to be partly dependent on the reduced expression of enzymes involved in FAO [42]. Peroxisome proliferator-activated receptors (PPARs), including α, γ, and β/δ, belong to the nuclear receptor family of ligand-activated transcription factors that were originally described as gene regulators of various metabolic pathways. PPARα and PPARβ/δ control expression of genes implicated in FAO. PPARγ, in contrast, is a key regulator of glucose homeostasis and adipogenesis [108].

Muscle carnitine palmitoyltransferase 1 (M-CPT1), a known PPARα target gene, catalyzes the rate-limiting step in the mitochondrial import of fatty acids for the FAO cycle [109]. In cardiomyocytes, hypoxia and adenovirus-mediated expression of a constitutively active form of HIF1α reduced the mRNA and protein levels of PPARα and M-CPT1 [24, 50, 110] as well as the DNA binding activity of PPARα [24, 50]. CoCl$_2$ treatment also decreased PPARα and M-CPT1 mRNA levels [110]. In intestinal epithelial cells, hypoxia rapidly down-regulated PPARα mRNA and protein in an HIF1-dependent manner in vitro and in vivo [76]. HIF1 could down-regulate PPARα directly through binding a functional HRE in the promoter region [76]. These results suggested that the mechanism of HIF-1 suppression of FAO involved the partial reduction of the expression of PPARα and M-CPT1.

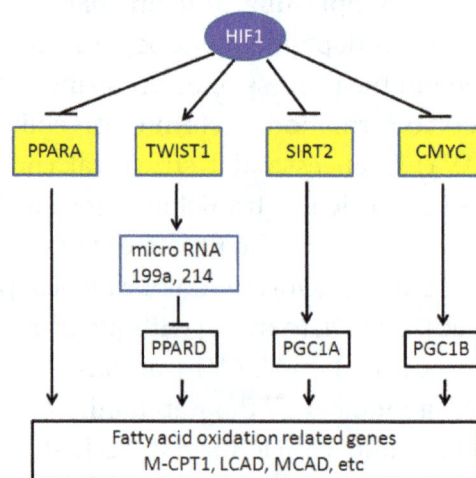

Figure 2. The molecular mechanism involving HIF1 repression of fatty acid β-oxidation. HIF1 targets PPARα, PPARδ, and Sirt2 directly and thereby suppresses the genetic expression of fatty acid β-oxidation.

HIF1 also suppressed FAO by inhibition of PPARδ's activity. In a pathological cardiac hypertrophy mouse model, myocardial hypoxia provoked Dnm3os activation and concomitantly mir-199a and mir-214 expression through the HIF1-TWIST1 axis [49]. TWIST1 is a direct target gene of HIF1 [77]. DNM3os is a noncoding RNA transcript that harbors the mi-RNA cluster mir-199a~214, for which PPARδ is a target. Increased expression of mir-199a and mir-214 decreased cardiac PPARδ expression and mitochondrial fatty acid oxidative capacity. Reduced expression of enzymes involved in FAO, for example long-chain acyl-CoA dehydrogenase (LCAD) and medium-chain acyl-CoA dehydrogenase (MCAD), was also observed. Conversely, antagomir-based silencing of miR-199a~214 in mice subjected to pressure overload de-repressed cardiac PPARδ, LCAD and MCAD levels, and restored mitochondrial FAO [49].

PPARγ coactivator 1α (PGC-1α) has been prominently associated with the expression of the genes involving FAO and energy expenditure [111]. In obese mouse model, HIF1α suppressed FAO in visceral white adipocytes, in part, through transcriptional repression of sirtuin 2 (Sirt2), an NAD$^+$-dependent deacetylase [3]. Reduced Sirt2 function directly translated into diminished deacetylation of PGC1α and the expression of FAO genes. HIF1α negated adipocyte-intrinsic pathway of fatty acid catabolism by negatively regulating the Sirt2-PGC1α regulatory axis [3].

PPARγ coactivator 1β (PGC-1β) is a transcription factor that also plays critical roles in regulating mitochondrial function and lipid metabolism [112, 113]. PGC-1β could regulate FAO through activating medium-chain acyl-CoA dehydrogenase (MCAD) and long-chain acyl-CoA dehydrogenase (LCAD), which catalyzes the first step of FAO in mitochondria [1, 112]. It had been documented previously that hypoxia inhibited PGC-1β activity through HIF1-dependent c-Myc suppression in VHL-null RCC4 renal carcinoma cells [114]. Under hypoxic condition in Hep3B and HepG2 cells, and also in PC3 prostate cancer cells, Huang and his colleagues revealed a role of the HIF1/C-MYC/PGC-1β regulatory axis in hypoxia-mediated regulation of MCAD and LCAD by which HIF1 suppressed FAO [1]. This study confirmed that hypoxia inhibited FAO in an HIF1-dependent mechanism in cancer cells [1].

In summary, it had been confirmed by different models that hypoxia inhibits FAO depending on HIF1's activity (**Figure 2**). However, HIF1 did not target FAO-related genes directly, and it was always cross-talk with other pathway to suppress FAO indirectly. It should be further studied if HIF1 could involve cross-talk with more pathways to suppress FAO.

3.2.2. Fatty acid synthesis

De novo fatty acid synthesis begins with acetyl coenzyme A (Ac-CoA). Ac-CoA is primarily generated from glucose through tri-carboxylic acid (TCA) cycle in the mitochondrion, the citrate shuttle and ATP citrate lyase in the cytosol. Under hypoxic condition, cells converted glucose to lactate and the TCA cycle is largely disconnected from glycolysis [70, 115–117], thereby directing glucose carbon away from fatty acid synthesis. Recently, several groups had found that hypoxic tumor cells maintain proliferation by running the TCA cycle in reverse [70, 115–117]. In these cells, the source of carbon for Ac-CoA and fatty acid switched from glucose to glutamine. This hypoxic flux from glutamine to fatty acid was mediated by the reductive carboxylation of glutamine-derived α-ketoglutarate.

The reductive carboxylation of glutamine was part of the metabolic reprogramming associated with HIF1. Glutamine-derived α-ketoglutarate is reductively carboxylated by the cytosolic isocitrate dehydrogenase 1 (IDH1) [70, 115] and the mitochondrial isocitrate dehydrogenase 2 (IDH2) to form isocitrate [70, 115, 116], which could then be isomerized to citrate. The combined action of IDH1 and IDH2 was necessary and sufficient to affect the reverse TCA flux [115]. Citrate was converted into Ac-CoA by ATP citrate lyase in the cytosol. Renal cell lines deficient in the VHL preferentially used reductive glutamine metabolism for lipid biosynthesis even at normal oxygen levels [70]. Constitutive activation of HIF1 recapitulated the preferential reductive metabolism of glutamine-derived α-ketoglutarate even in normoxic condition [116]. This regulation by HIF1 of the reverse TCA cycle occurred partly through HIF1-inducing PDK1. Knocking down PDK1 suppressed reductive carboxylation [70, 118]. However, more details should be studied about the role of HIF1 in TCA cycle reverse.

The first step of fatty acid synthesis is catalyzed by AcCoA carboxylase (ACC) which converts Ac-CoA to malonyl-CoA. Then fatty-acid synthase (FASN) catalyzes acetyl-CoA and malonyl-CoA to palmitate. Further elongation and de-saturation of newly synthesized fatty acid takes place at the cytoplasmic face of the endoplasmic reticulum membrane. It had been reported that hypoxia regulated FASN expression [78, 119, 120]. However, different conclusions on hypoxia regulation of FASN had been reported. One group using human breast cancer cell lines found that FASN was significantly up-regulated by hypoxia via activation of the Akt and HIF1 followed by the induction of the SREBP1 gene [119]. Another group, using several cell lines other than breast cancer cell lines, found that hypoxia suppressed FASN expression through HIF1-DEC1 and/or DEC2-SREBP1 axis. They found that HIF1 repressed the SREBP1 gene by inducing DEC1 and DEC2, and further repressing FASN expression [78]. These results might indicate that HIF1 regulated FASN in a cell-type specific manner. In addition, it had been reported that hypoxia could induce the expression of SCD1 which introduces a double bond in the $\Delta 9$ position of palmitic acid and stearic acid to produce mono-unsaturated fatty acid [42, 121]. It is unknown if HIF1 is involved in hypoxic-induced SCD1.

Taken together, the role of HIF1 in de novo fatty acid synthesis may depend on different models and conditions, and more researches should be done in the direction.

3.3. Cholesterol metabolism

Cholesterol is an essential structural component of membrane. It modulates membrane permeability and fluidity and also forms microdomains named lipid rafts that integrate the activation of some signal transduction pathways [14]. Intermediates generated by the cholesterol biosynthesis pathway were required for the posttranslational modification of small GTPases, such as the farnesylation of Ras and the geranyl-geranylation of Rho [15]. Finally, cholesterol also serves as a precursor for the biosynthesis of steroid hormones, bile acids, and vitamin D.

Cellular cholesterol level can be modulated by three processes: cholesterol uptake, synthesis, and efflux [122]. In the preceding paragraph, we had discussed the role of HIF1 in LDL and VLDL uptake that are main source of extracellular cholesterol. Here, we discuss the cholesterol synthesis and efflux. Cholesterol biosynthesis begins with the condensation of AcCoA with acetoacetyl-CoA to form 3-hydroxy-3-methylglutaryl (HMG)-CoA. Then HMG-CoA reductase (HMGCR) reduces of HMG-CoA to mevalonate. Early research found that Hypoxia also suppressed cholesterol synthesis in cultured rabbit skin fibroblasts [123]. However, recently research indicated that hypoxia increased sterol synthesis depending on HIF1's activity [23, 124]. In hypoxic macrophages, the increase of intracellular cholesterol content was correlated with elevated HMGCR's activity and mRNA levels [23]. In HepG2 cells, HIF1α accumulation was able to increase the level and activity of HMGCR by stimulating its transcription [124]. But it was unclear if HIF1 regulated HMGCR directly.

Hypoxia suppressed the efflux of cholesterol, and this efflux was substantially reversed in vitro by reducing the expression of HIF1 [23, 123]. ATP-binding cassette transporter A1 (ABCA1) plays a major role in cholesterol efflux. Hypoxia severely reduced ABCA1-mediated cholesterol efflux, which could be explained by subcellular redistribution of ABCA1 protein under acute hypoxia and decreased protein level under prolonged hypoxia [23]. One group reported that HIF1 could repress the transcription of ABCA1 directly [79]. Hypoxia, partly mediated by HIF1α, increased intracellular cholesterol content due to the induction of cholesterol synthesis and the suppression of cholesterol efflux [23]. In addition, accumulation of cholesterol in hypoxic cells was in esterified form [23, 100]. At 2% O_2 tension, twice the total cholesteryl ester was observed compared with that at 21% O_2. At the same time, no significant difference was found in the concentration of cellular-free cholesterol [100]. Accumulation of cholesteryl ester in hypoxic cells might depend on the increased activity of AcCoA:cholesterol acyltransferases (ACATs) [123], which are important enzymes for the esterification of cholesterol. Therefore, more studies should be done to define the role of HIF1 involving the cholesterol metabolism in detail.

3.4. TAG synthesis and phospholipids metabolism

3.4.1. TAG synthesis

TAG is formed by the addition of three molecules of fatty acid to glycerol. There are two major pathways for TAG biosynthesis in mammalian cell: the glycerol phosphate pathway and the mono-acylglycerol (MG) pathway. In the glycerol phosphate pathway, two molecules of fatty acyl-CoA are esterified to glycerol-3-phosphate to yield 1,2-diacylglycerol (DAG) phosphate (commonly identified as phosphatidic acid). The phosphate is then removed to yield 1,2-diacylglycerol, which is followed by addition of the third fatty acid to form TAG. TAG accumulation under hypoxia could be mediated by HIF1-inducing Lipin1 [20], a phosphatidate phosphatase isoform that catalyzes the penultimate step in TAG biosynthesis, the removal of phosphate from diacylglycerol phosphate to yield DAG. It also had been reported that hypoxia produced a marked intracellular accumulation of diacylglycerol in different cell types [125]. DAG may also serve a feedback role regulating HIF1's activity [125]. In a mouse model of pathological hypertrophy, HIF1α promoted TAG accumulation in cardiomyocytes via the regulation of PPARγ expression. PPARγ was the principal mediator of TAG anabolism through its transcriptional regulation glycerol-3-phosphate generation (via GPD1), and downstream esterification processes (via GPAT) [26].

3.4.2. Phospholipids metabolism

Phospholipids are indispensable for cell growth. Phospholipids synthesis and TAG synthesis share similar steps. DAG is a precursor for phosphatidylcholine and phosphatidylethanolamine. Phosphatidic acid utilizes cytidine triphosphate (CTP) as an energy source to produce a CDP-DAG intermediate followed by conversion to phosphatidylcholine. It had been reported that the intracellular level of phosphatidic acid (PA) and DAG rose in response to hypoxia [125, 126]. However, PA accumulation in response to hypoxia was both HIF1 and VHL-independent [127]. Choline kinase α (ChKα) catalyzes the phosphorylation of choline, the first step of phosphatidylcholine synthesis. In cancer cells, one group had shown that hypoxia increased ChKα expression and this was driven by HIF1 [80]. Conversely, another group had shown that choline kinase activity and choline phosphorylation were decreased, that might be mediated via HIF1α binding to the promoter of ChKα gene [81]. Thus, further studies should be done to address the role of HIF1 in phospholipids metabolism.

3.5. Lipid droplet (LD) biogenesis and lipid signaling

Lipid droplet, also named lipid body, has been largely associated with neutral lipid storage and transport in cells [106]. The internal core of the LD is rich in neutral lipids, predominantly TAGs or cholesteryl esters, that are surrounded by an outer monolayer of phospholipids and associated proteins [128]. LD was considered to be highly regulated, dynamic and functionally active organelle [106]. Proteins on the surface of lipid droplets are crucial to the droplet structure and dynamics. Currently, the complete protein composition of LD has not been defined. The best characterized LD' proteins are the perilipin/ADRP/TIP47 (PAT) domain family. Apart from the PAT domain proteins, there are other lipid droplets associated proteins which involve the catabolism of lipids, vesicular transport, eicosanoid-forming enzymes, protein kinases, etc. [106]. Hypoxia increased LD number and size [42, 129]. Several LD-associated proteins were induced by HIF1 and might also involve HIF1-induced LD biogenesis and lipid signaling (**Figure 3**).

3.5.1. Lipid droplet biogenesis

Adipose differentiation-related protein (ADRP), a PAT domain protein, is a structural component of LD and had been reported by several groups to be inducible by HIF1 [42, 82–84]. Lipid accumulation was associated with high expression level of ADRP in solid tumors [68, 130], especially in clear cell lesions [131]. During the process of carcinogenesis, the ADRP expression was increased during early tumorigenesis and was associated with the proliferation rate [68]. The expression of ADRP was also correlated with atherosclerosis [132]. In mouse macrophages in vitro, ADRP expression facilitated foam cell formation induced by modified lipoproteins [132]. In apolipoprotein E-deficient mice, ADRP inactivation reduced the number of LD in foam cells in atherosclerotic lesions [132]. Under hypoxia, knockdown of ADRP in U87 and T98G or in MCF-7 and MDA-MB-231 cells significantly decreased the formation of LD, and resulted in decreased fatty acid uptake [21]. It indicated that ADRP promoted LD formation mainly through increasing FA uptake under hypoxic condition. It had been reported that ADRP can also stimulate LCFA uptake [133]. While another research reported that ADRP did not involve LDL- and VLDL-induced LD formation under hypoxia [84].

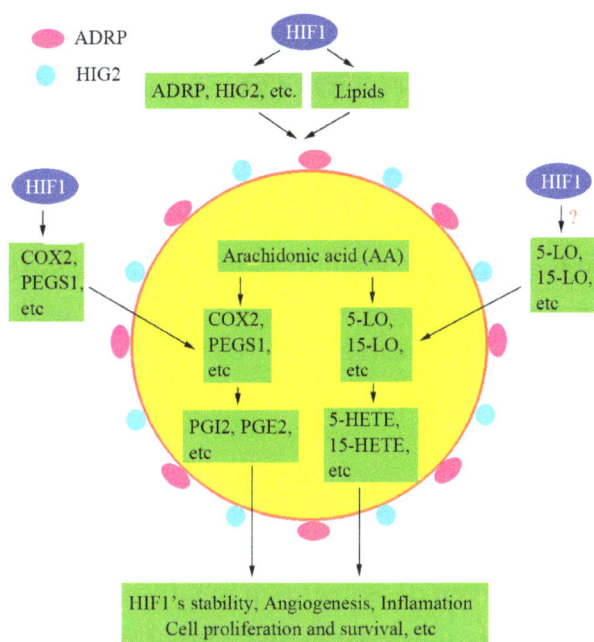

Figure 3. A hypothetical representation of molecular mechanism involving hypoxia-induced lipid droplet biogenesis and function. HIF1-induced structural proteins of the LD, such as ADRP, HIG2, combine with HIF1-increased lipids to form the LD. Enzymes involving eicosanoid production are also induced by HIF1, and are recruited to the LD. These proteins can increase lipid signaling that can involve many aspects of biology, such as HIF1α's stability, angiogenesis, inflammation, cell proliferation and survival.

Hypoxia-inducible protein 2 (HIG2), a newly identified protein associated with LD, was up-regulated by hypoxia and was a direct and specific target gene of HIF1 [85]. Overexpression of HIG2 under normoxic condition was sufficient to increase LD in HeLa cells. HIG2-driven LD might contribute to an inflammatory response. Overexpression of HIG2 stimulated cytokine expression of vascular endothelial growth factor-A (VEGFA), macrophage migration inhibitory factor (MIF), and interleukin-6 (IL-6). Increasing expression of HIG2 was also detected under several conditions of pathological lipid accumulation, such as atherosclerotic arteries and fatty liver disease [85]. We had mentioned that CAV1 was a target of HIF1. CAV1 could distribute to LD under several conditions [134–137] and the association with LD was reversible [134]. However, It is unknown if hypoxia can redistribute CAV1 to LD and CAV1 involves LD biogenesis under hypoxia.

3.5.2. Lipid signaling

Eicosanoids are signaling molecules made by oxidation of 20-carbon fatty acids, mainly from arachidonic acid. Cyclooxygenases and Lipoxygenases are two families of enzymes catalyzing fatty acid oxygenation to produce the eicosanoids. There are multiple subfamilies of eicosanoids, including prostaglandins, prostacyclins, thromboxanes, lipoxins, and leukotrienes. Prostaglandins, such as PGI_2 and PGE_2, are synthesized via cyclooxygenase (COX) by oxidation of arachidonic acid. PGE_2 is synthesized in three steps catalyzed by phospholipase (PL) A2, COX, and terminal prostaglandin E synthase (PTGES), where each catalytic activity is represented by multiple enzymes and/or isoenzymes. It had been reported that hypoxia could increase prostaglandins (PGI_2 and PGE_2) synthesis [138]. Hypoxia-induced synthesis of PGE_2 was accompanied by up-regulation of COX2, which is a direct target gene of HIF1 [86]. Several studies had indicated that LD was reservoirs of COX2 and sites of PGE_2 synthesis [66, 139, 140]. PTGES1 could also be regulated by HIF1 directly [87, 88]; however, it is unknown if PTGES1 localizes to hypoxia-induced LD.

Lipoxygenases are a family of nonheme iron-containing enzymes which dioxygenate polyunsaturated fatty acid to hydroperoxyl metabolite, and mainly include 5-lipoxygenase (5-LO), 12-lipoxygenase (12-LO), and 15-lipoxygenase (15-LO). 5-LO and 15-LO were shown by immuno-cytochemistry, immuno-fluorescence, ultrastructural postembedding immuno-gold EM and/or western blotting from subcellular fractions to localize within lipid droplets stimulated in vitro [141–144]. Increasing level of 5-LO was detected in lung tissue of rodent model of hypoxia-induced pulmonary hypertension [145]. Hypoxia increased 12-LO in rat lung and in in vitro cultured rat pulmonary artery smooth muscle cell (PASMC) and may contribute to the production of 12(S)-hydroxyeicosatetraenoic acid (12(S)-HETE) [146]. Increasing 12(S)-HETE had also been demonstrated in hypoxic macrophage cells [147]. Under hypoxia, increased levels of 15-LO had been demonstrated by different groups [147, 148] and its product, 15-hydroperoxyeicosatetraenoic acid (15-HETE), was up-regulated [147]. Up-regulation of 15-LO/15-HETE in response to hypoxia might be partially mediated by HIF1α [149]. In addition, HIF1α was shown to be regulated by 15-HETE in a positive feedback manner [149]. However, it is unknown if lipoxygenases are regulated by HIF1 directly.

4. Conclusions and perspectives

HIF1 plays an important role in lipid metabolism and a number of studies support the findings that HIF1 promotes lipid accumulation. Nevertheless, many questions remain. HIF1, as a master transcriptional factor, may target many genes directly or indirectly involved in lipid metabolism. HIF1 plays a pivotal role in glucose metabolism. Inhibition of GULT3, an HIF1 target gene, could significantly reduce both glucose uptake and hypoxia-induced de novo lipid synthesis in human monocyte-derived macrophages [150]. PGAM1, induced by hypoxia [151], catalyzes the reversible reaction of 3-phosphoglycerate (3-PGA) to 2-phosphoglycerate (2-PGA) in the glycolytic pathway. Inhibition of PGAM1 led to significantly decreased glycolysis and de novo lipid synthesis in cancer cells [152]. Thus, it is possible that glucose metabolism might couple with lipid metabolism under hypoxia. The source of carbon for fatty acid switched from glucose to glutamine under hypoxia [70]. The question thus arises. Does HIF1 induce lipid accumulation through targeting genes involving glucose metabolism, and how does glucose metabolism affect lipid metabolism under hypoxia?

HIF1 could interact with other pathways to regulate lipid metabolism besides PPARα, PPARγ, PPARδ, PGC1α, and SREBP1. There might be a pivotal role for mTOR in controlling lipid homeostasis in many settings, both physiological and pathological [153]. AMPK is a cellular energy sensor that normalizes lipid, glucose, and energy imbalances [154]. Inhibition of cMYC was accompanied by accumulation of intracellular LD in tumor cells as a direct consequence of mitochondrial dysfunction [155]. Recently, p53 had also been shown to regulate lipid metabolism [156]. The role of HIF1 in these pathways and the molecular mechanism will require further investigation.

Lipid accumulation in diseases, including obesity, atherosclerosis, ALD, heart failure disease and cancer, had been associated with HIF1's activity. There may be additional pathologies with lipid metabolism disorder associated with HIF1. HIF1 is an attractive target candidate for therapeutic intervention in diseases with disorder of lipid metabolism including cancer. Its involvement in the etiology of a number of diseases and its interaction with a number of regulatory genes make it an important area for further study.

Acknowledgements

This review is supported by a National Natural Science Foundation of China (Grant No. 31301076 to G. S; Grant No. 81401961 to X. L.), We thank Gerard Moskowitz, Ph. D. (Washington University in St. Louis, St. Louis, MO) for critical reading of the manuscript. We sincerely apologize to the colleagues whose works are not covered in this review due to limitations of time and space.

Author details

Guomin Shen[1*] and Xiaobo Li[2]

*Address all correspondence to: shenba433@163.com

1 Department of Medical Genetics, Medical College, Henan University of Science and Technology, Luoyang, Henan Province, China

2 Department of Pathology & Translational Medicine Center, Harbin Medical University, Harbin, Heilongjiang Province, China

References

[1]   D. Huang, T. Li, X. Li, L. Zhang, L. Sun, X. He, X. Zhong, D. Jia, L. Song, G.L. Semenza, P. Gao, H. Zhang, HIF-1-mediated suppression of acyl-CoA dehydrogenases and fatty acid oxidation is critical for cancer progression, Cell Rep 8 (2014) 1930–1942.

[2] A. Valli, M. Rodriguez, L. Moutsianas, R. Fischer, V. Fedele, H.L. Huang, R. Van Stiphout, D. Jones, M. McCarthy, M. Vinaxia, K. Igarashi, M. Sato, T. Soga, F. Buffa, J. McCullagh, O. Yanes, A. Harris, B. Kessler, Hypoxia induces a lipogenic cancer cell phenotype via HIF1alpha-dependent and -independent pathways, Oncotarget 6 (2015) 1920–1941.

[3] J. Krishnan, C. Danzer, T. Simka, J. Ukropec, K.M. Walter, S. Kumpf, P. Mirtschink, B. Ukropcova, D. Gasperikova, T. Pedrazzini, W. Krek, Dietary obesity-associated Hif1alpha activation in adipocytes restricts fatty acid oxidation and energy expenditure via suppression of the Sirt2-NAD+ system, Genes Dev 26 (2012) 259–270.

[4] E. Marsch, J.C. Sluimer, M.J. Daemen, Hypoxia in atherosclerosis and inflammation, Curr Opin Lipidol 24 (2013) 393–400.

[5] G.L. Semenza, Hypoxia-inducible factor 1 and cardiovascular disease, Annu Rev Physiol 76 (2013) 39–56.

[6] G.L. Semenza, Hypoxia-inducible factors in physiology and medicine, Cell 148 (2012) 399–408.

[7] G.L. Wang, B.H. Jiang, E.A. Rue, G.L. Semenza, Hypoxia-inducible factor 1 is a basic-helix-loop-helix-PAS heterodimer regulated by cellular O2 tension, Proc Natl Acad Sci U S A 92 (1995) 5510–5514.

[8] G.L. Wang, G.L. Semenza, Purification and characterization of hypoxia-inducible factor 1, J Biol Chem 270 (1995) 1230–1237.

[9] A.C. Epstein, J.M. Gleadle, L.A. McNeill, K.S. Hewitson, J. O'Rourke, D.R. Mole, M. Mukherji, E. Metzen, M.I. Wilson, A. Dhanda, Y.M. Tian, N. Masson, D.L. Hamilton, P. Jaakkola, R. Barstead, J. Hodgkin, P.H. Maxwell, C.W. Pugh, C.J. Schofield, P.J. Ratcliffe, C. elegans EGL-9 and mammalian homologs define a family of dioxygenases that regulate HIF by prolyl hydroxylation, Cell 107 (2001) 43–54.

[10] P.H. Maxwell, M.S. Wiesener, G.W. Chang, S.C. Clifford, E.C. Vaux, M.E. Cockman, C.C. Wykoff, C.W. Pugh, E.R. Maher, P.J. Ratcliffe, The tumour suppressor protein VHL targets hypoxia-inducible factors for oxygen-dependent proteolysis, Nature 399 (1999) 271–275.

[11] M. Ohh, C.W. Park, M. Ivan, M.A. Hoffman, T.Y. Kim, L.E. Huang, N. Pavletich, V. Chau, W.G. Kaelin, Ubiquitination of hypoxia-inducible factor requires direct binding to the beta-domain of the von Hippel-Lindau protein, Nat Cell Biol 2 (2000) 423–427.

[12] P.C. Mahon, K. Hirota, G.L. Semenza, FIH-1: a novel protein that interacts with HIF-1alpha and VHL to mediate repression of HIF-1 transcriptional activity, Genes Dev 15 (2001) 2675–2686.

[13] K.S. Hewitson, L.A. McNeill, M.V. Riordan, Y.M. Tian, A.N. Bullock, R.W. Welford, J.M. Elkins, N.J. Oldham, S. Bhattacharya, J.M. Gleadle, P.J. Ratcliffe, C.W. Pugh, C.J. Schofield, Hypoxia-inducible factor (HIF) asparagine hydroxylase is identical to factor

inhibiting HIF (FIH) and is related to the cupin structural family, J Biol Chem 277 (2002) 26351–26355.

[14] D. Lando, D.J. Peet, J.J. Gorman, D.A. Whelan, M.L. Whitelaw, R.K. Bruick, FIH-1 is an asparaginyl hydroxylase enzyme that regulates the transcriptional activity of hypoxia-inducible factor, Genes Dev 16 (2002) 1466–1471.

[15] D. Lando, D.J. Peet, D.A. Whelan, J.J. Gorman, M.L. Whitelaw, Asparagine hydroxylation of the HIF transactivation domain a hypoxic switch, Science 295 (2002) 858–861.

[16] G.L. Semenza, Defining the role of hypoxia-inducible factor 1 in cancer biology and therapeutics, Oncogene 29 (2010) 625–634.

[17] N.C. Denko, Hypoxia, HIF1 and glucose metabolism in the solid tumour, Nat Rev Cancer 8 (2008) 705–713.

[18] G.M. Shen, Y.Z. Zhao, M.T. Chen, F.L. Zhang, X.L. Liu, Y. Wang, C.Z. Liu, J. Yu, J.W. Zhang, Hypoxia-inducible factor-1 (HIF-1) promotes LDL and VLDL uptake through inducing VLDLR under hypoxia, Biochem J 441 (2012) 675–683.

[19] T. Suzuki, S. Shinjo, T. Arai, M. Kanai, N. Goda, Hypoxia and fatty liver, World J Gastroenterol 20 (2014) 15087–15097.

[20] I. Mylonis, H. Sembongi, C. Befani, P. Liakos, S. Siniossoglou, G. Simos, Hypoxia causes triglyceride accumulation by HIF-1-mediated stimulation of lipin 1 expression, J Cell Sci 125 (2012) 3485–3493.

[21] K. Bensaad, E. Favaro, C.A. Lewis, B. Peck, S. Lord, J.M. Collins, K.E. Pinnick, S. Wigfield, F.M. Buffa, J.L. Li, Q. Zhang, M.J. Wakelam, F. Karpe, A. Schulze, A.L. Harris, Fatty acid uptake and lipid storage induced by HIF-1alpha contribute to cell growth and survival after hypoxia-reoxygenation, Cell Rep 9 (2014) 349–365.

[22] G. Jiang, T. Li, Y. Qiu, Y. Rui, W. Chen, Y. Lou, RNA interference for HIF-1alpha inhibits foam cells formation in vitro, Eur J Pharmacol 562 (2007) 183–190.

[23] S. Parathath, S.L. Mick, J.E. Feig, V. Joaquin, L. Grauer, D.M. Habiel, M. Gassmann, L.B. Gardner, E.A. Fisher, Hypoxia is present in murine atherosclerotic plaques and has multiple adverse effects on macrophage lipid metabolism, Circ Res 109 (2011) 1141–1152.

[24] A.J. Belanger, Z. Luo, K.A. Vincent, G.Y. Akita, S.H. Cheng, R.J. Gregory, C. Jiang, Hypoxia-inducible factor 1 mediates hypoxia-induced cardiomyocyte lipid accumulation by reducing the DNA binding activity of peroxisome proliferator-activated receptor alpha/retinoid X receptor, Biochem Biophys Res Commun 364 (2007) 567–572.

[25] L. Lei, S. Mason, D. Liu, Y. Huang, C. Marks, R. Hickey, I.S. Jovin, M. Pypaert, R.S. Johnson, F.J. Giordano, Hypoxia-inducible factor-dependent degeneration, failure, and malignant transformation of the heart in the absence of the von Hippel-Lindau protein, Mol Cell Biol 28 (2008) 3790–3803.

[26] J. Krishnan, M. Suter, R. Windak, T. Krebs, A. Felley, C. Montessuit, M. Tokarska-Schlattner, E. Aasum, A. Bogdanova, E. Perriard, J.C. Perriard, T. Larsen, T. Pedrazzini,

W. Krek, Activation of a HIF1alpha-PPARgamma axis underlies the integration of glycolytic and lipid anabolic pathways in pathologic cardiac hypertrophy, Cell Metab 9 (2009) 512–524.

[27] B. Nath, I. Levin, T. Csak, J. Petrasek, C. Mueller, K. Kodys, D. Catalano, P. Mandrekar, G. Szabo, Hepatocyte-specific hypoxia-inducible factor-1alpha is a determinant of lipid accumulation and liver injury in alcohol-induced steatosis in mice, Hepatology 53 (2011) 1526–1537.

[28] L. Rahtu-Korpela, J. Maatta, E.Y. Dimova, S. Horkko, H. Gylling, G. Walkinshaw, J. Hakkola, K.I. Kivirikko, J. Myllyharju, R. Serpi, P. Koivunen, Hypoxia-inducible factor prolyl 4-hydroxylase-2 inhibition protects against development of atherosclerosis, Arterioscler Thromb Vasc Biol 36 (2016) 608–617.

[29] Y. Nishiyama, N. Goda, M. Kanai, D. Niwa, K. Osanai, Y. Yamamoto, N. Senoo-Matsuda, R.S. Johnson, S. Miura, Y. Kabe, M. Suematsu, HIF-1alpha induction suppresses excessive lipid accumulation in alcoholic fatty liver in mice, J Hepatol 56 (2012) 441–447.

[30] H. Matsuura, T. Ichiki, E. Inoue, M. Nomura, R. Miyazaki, T. Hashimoto, J. Ikeda, R. Takayanagi, G.H. Fong, K. Sunagawa, Prolyl hydroxylase domain protein 2 plays a critical role in diet-induced obesity and glucose intolerance, Circulation 127 (2013) 2078–2087.

[31] L. Rahtu-Korpela, S. Karsikas, S. Horkko, R. Blanco Sequeiros, E. Lammentausta, K.A. Makela, K.H. Herzig, G. Walkinshaw, K.I. Kivirikko, J. Myllyharju, R. Serpi, P. Koivunen, HIF prolyl 4-hydroxylase-2 inhibition improves glucose and lipid metabolism and protects against obesity and metabolic dysfunction, Diabetes 63 (2014) 3324–3333.

[32] J. Niinikoski, C. Heughan, T.K. Hunt, Oxygen tensions in the aortic wall of normal rabbits, Atherosclerosis 17 (1973) 353–359.

[33] C. Heughan, J. Niinikoski, T.K. Hunt, Oxygen tensions in lesions of experimental atherosclerosis of rabbits, Atherosclerosis 17 (1973) 361–367.

[34] J.F. Martin, R.F. Booth, S. Moncada, Arterial wall hypoxia following hyperfusion through the vasa vasorum is an initial lesion in atherosclerosis, Eur J Clin Invest 20 (1990) 588–592.

[35] T. Bjornheden, M. Evaldsson, O. Wiklund, A method for the assessment of hypoxia in the arterial wall, with potential application in vivo, Arterioscler Thromb Vasc Biol 16 (1996) 178–185.

[36] T. Bjornheden, M. Levin, M. Evaldsson, O. Wiklund, Evidence of hypoxic areas within the arterial wall in vivo, Arterioscler Thromb Vasc Biol 19 (1999) 870–876.

[37] J.M. Silvola, A. Saraste, S. Forsback, V.J. Laine, P. Saukko, S.E. Heinonen, S. Yla-Herttuala, A. Roivainen, J. Knuuti, Detection of hypoxia by [18F]EF5 in atherosclerotic plaques in mice, Arterioscler Thromb Vasc Biol 31 (2011) 1011–1015.

[38] B. Ramkhelawon, Y. Yang, J.M. van Gils, B. Hewing, K.J. Rayner, S. Parathath, L. Guo, S. Oldebeken, J.L. Feig, E.A. Fisher, K.J. Moore, Hypoxia induces netrin-1 and Unc5b in atherosclerotic plaques: mechanism for macrophage retention and survival, Arterioscler Thromb Vasc Biol 33 (2013) 1180–1188.

[39] J.C. Sluimer, J.M. Gasc, J.L. van Wanroij, N. Kisters, M. Groeneweg, M.D. Sollewijn Gelpke, J.P. Cleutjens, L.H. van den Akker, P. Corvol, B.G. Wouters, M.J. Daemen, A.P. Bijnens, Hypoxia, hypoxia-inducible transcription factor, and macrophages in human atherosclerotic plaques are correlated with intraplaque angiogenesis, J Am Coll Cardiol 51 (2008) 1258–1265.

[40] S. Parathath, Y. Yang, S. Mick, E.A. Fisher, Hypoxia in murine atherosclerotic plaques and its adverse effects on macrophages, Trends Cardiovasc Med 23 (2013) 80–84.

[41] L.M. Hulten, M. Levin, The role of hypoxia in atherosclerosis, Curr Opin Lipidol 20 (2009) 409–414.

[42] P. Bostrom, B. Magnusson, P.A. Svensson, O. Wiklund, J. Boren, L.M. Carlsson, M. Stahlman, S.O. Olofsson, L.M. Hulten, Hypoxia converts human macrophages into triglyceride-loaded foam cells, Arterioscler Thromb Vasc Biol 26 (2006) 1871–1876.

[43] S. Akhtar, P. Hartmann, E. Karshovska, F.A. Rinderknecht, P. Subramanian, F. Gremse, J. Grommes, M. Jacobs, F. Kiessling, C. Weber, S. Steffens, A. Schober, Endothelial hypoxia-inducible factor-1alpha promotes atherosclerosis and monocyte recruitment by upregulating MicroRNA-19a, Hypertension 66 (2015) 1220–1226.

[44] J. Ben-Shoshan, A. Afek, S. Maysel-Auslender, A. Barzelay, A. Rubinstein, G. Keren, J. George, HIF-1alpha overexpression and experimental murine atherosclerosis, Arterioscler Thromb Vasc Biol 29 (2009) 665–670.

[45] L. Gao, Q. Chen, X. Zhou, L. Fan, The role of hypoxia-inducible factor 1 in atherosclerosis, J Clin Pathol 65 (2012) 872–876.

[46] G.L. Semenza, Hypoxia-inducible Factor 1 and cardiovascular disease, Annu Rev Physiol 76 (2014) 39–56.

[47] T.S. Park, I.J. Goldberg, Sphingolipids, lipotoxic cardiomyopathy, and cardiac failure, Heart Fail Clin 8 (2012) 633–641.

[48] J.C. Perman, P. Bostrom, M. Lindbom, U. Lidberg, M. StAhlman, D. Hagg, H. Lindskog, M. Scharin Tang, E. Omerovic, L. Mattsson Hulten, A. Jeppsson, P. Petursson, J. Herlitz, G. Olivecrona, D.K. Strickland, K. Ekroos, S.O. Olofsson, J. Boren, The VLDL receptor promotes lipotoxicity and increases mortality in mice following an acute myocardial infarction, J Clin Invest 121 (2011) 2625–2640.

[49] H. El Azzouzi, S. Leptidis, E. Dirkx, J. Hoeks, B. van Bree, K. Brand, E.A. McClellan, E. Poels, J.C. Sluimer, M.M. van den Hoogenhof, A.S. Armand, X. Yin, S. Langley, M. Bourajjaj, S. Olieslagers, J. Krishnan, M. Vooijs, H. Kurihara, A. Stubbs, Y.M. Pinto, W. Krek, M. Mayr, P.A. da Costa Martins, P. Schrauwen, L.J. De Windt, The hypoxia-

inducible MicroRNA cluster miR-199a approximately 214 targets myocardial PPAR-delta and impairs mitochondrial fatty acid oxidation, Cell Metab 18 (2013) 341–354.

[50] J.M. Huss, F.H. Levy, D.P. Kelly, Hypoxia inhibits the peroxisome proliferator-activated receptor alpha/retinoid X receptor gene regulatory pathway in cardiac myocytes: a mechanism for O2-dependent modulation of mitochondrial fatty acid oxidation, J Biol Chem 56–84 (2001) 27605–27612.

[51] G.E. Arteel, Y. Iimuro, M. Yin, J.A. Raleigh, R.G. Thurman, Chronic enteral ethanol treatment causes hypoxia in rat liver tissue in vivo, Hepatology 25 (1997) 920–926.

[52] G.E. Arteel, J.A. Raleigh, B.U. Bradford, R.G. Thurman, Acute alcohol produces hypoxia directly in rat liver tissue in vivo: role of Kupffer cells, Am J Physiol 271 (1996) G494–G500.

[53] S.W. French, The role of hypoxia in the pathogenesis of alcoholic liver disease, Hepatol Res 29 (2004) 69–74.

[54] F. Bardag-Gorce, B.A. French, J. Li, N.E. Riley, Q.X. Yuan, V. Valinluck, P. Fu, M. Ingelman-Sundberg, S. Yoon, S.W. French, The importance of cycling of blood alcohol levels in the pathogenesis of experimental alcoholic liver disease in rats, Gastroenterology 123 (2002) 325–335.

[55] S.K. Mantena, D.P. Vaughn, K.K. Andringa, H.B. Eccleston, A.L. King, G.A. Abrams, J.E. Doeller, D.W. Kraus, V.M. Darley-Usmar, S.M. Bailey, High fat diet induces dysregulation of hepatic oxygen gradients and mitochondrial function in vivo, Biochem J 417 (2009) 183–193.

[56] M.E. Rausch, S. Weisberg, P. Vardhana, D.V. Tortoriello, Obesity in C57BL/6J mice is characterized by adipose tissue hypoxia and cytotoxic T-cell infiltration, Int J Obes (Lond) 32 (2008) 451–463.

[57] J. Ye, Z. Gao, J. Yin, Q. He, Hypoxia is a potential risk factor for chronic inflammation and adiponectin reduction in adipose tissue of ob/ob and dietary obese mice, Am J Physiol Endocrinol Metab 293 (2007) E1118–E1128.

[58] N. Hosogai, A. Fukuhara, K. Oshima, Y. Miyata, S. Tanaka, K. Segawa, S. Furukawa, Y. Tochino, R. Komuro, M. Matsuda, I. Shimomura, Adipose tissue hypoxia in obesity and its impact on adipocytokine dysregulation, Diabetes 56 (2007) 901–911.

[59] C. Jiang, A. Qu, T. Matsubara, T. Chanturiya, W. Jou, O. Gavrilova, Y.M. Shah, F.J. Gonzalez, Disruption of hypoxia-inducible factor 1 in adipocytes improves insulin sensitivity and decreases adiposity in high-fat diet-fed mice, Diabetes 60 (2011) 2484–2495.

[60] X. Zhang, K.S. Lam, H. Ye, S.K. Chung, M. Zhou, Y. Wang, A. Xu, Adipose tissue-specific inhibition of hypoxia-inducible factor 1{alpha} induces obesity and glucose intolerance by impeding energy expenditure in mice, J Biol Chem 285 (2010) 32869–32877.

[61] O. Warburg, On respiratory impairment in cancer cells, Science 124 (1956) 269–270.

[62] J.A. Menendez, R. Lupu, Fatty acid synthase and the lipogenic phenotype in cancer pathogenesis, Nat Rev Cancer 7 (2007) 763–777.

[63] C.R. Santos, A. Schulze, Lipid metabolism in cancer, FEBS J 279 (2012) 2610–2623.

[64] J. Swierczynski, A. Hebanowska, T. Sledzinski, Role of abnormal lipid metabolism in development, progression, diagnosis and therapy of pancreatic cancer, World J Gastroenterol 20 (2014) 2279–2303.

[65] P.L. Alo, P. Visca, G. Trombetta, A. Mangoni, L. Lenti, S. Monaco, C. Botti, D.E. Serpieri, U. Di Tondo, Fatty acid synthase (FAS) predictive strength in poorly differentiated early breast carcinomas, Tumori 85 (1999) 35–40.

[66] M.T. Accioly, P. Pacheco, C.M. Maya-Monteiro, N. Carrossini, B.K. Robbs, S.S. Oliveira, C. Kaufmann, J.A. Morgado-Diaz, P.T. Bozza, J.P. Viola, Lipid bodies are reservoirs of cyclooxygenase-2 and sites of prostaglandin-E2 synthesis in colon cancer cells, Cancer Res 68 (2008) 1732–1740.

[67] D.K. Nomura, J.Z. Long, S. Niessen, H.S. Hoover, S.W. Ng, B.F. Cravatt, Monoacylgly-cerol lipase regulates a fatty acid network that promotes cancer pathogenesis, Cell 140 (2010) 49–61.

[68] B.K. Straub, E. Herpel, S. Singer, R. Zimbelmann, K. Breuhahn, S. Macher-Goeppinger, A. Warth, J. Lehmann-Koch, T. Longerich, H. Heid, P. Schirmacher, Lipid droplet-associated PAT-proteins show frequent and differential expression in neoplastic steatogenesis, Mod Pathol 23 (2010) 480–492.

[69] M.H. Hager, K.R. Solomon, M.R. Freeman, The role of cholesterol in prostate cancer, Curr Opin Clin Nutr Metab Care 9 (2006) 379–385.

[70] C.M. Metallo, P.A. Gameiro, E.L. Bell, K.R. Mattaini, J. Yang, K. Hiller, C.M. Jewell, Z.R. Johnson, D.J. Irvine, L. Guarente, J.K. Kelleher, M.G. Vander Heiden, O. Iliopoulos, G. Stephanopoulos, Reductive glutamine metabolism by IDH1 mediates lipogenesis under hypoxia, Nature 481 (2011) 380–384.

[71] B.R. Mwaikambo, C. Yang, S. Chemtob, P. Hardy, Hypoxia up-regulates CD36 expression and function via hypoxia-inducible factor-1- and phosphatidylinositol 3-kinase-dependent mechanisms, J Biol Chem 284 (2009) 26695–26707.

[72] J. Castellano, R. Aledo, J. Sendra, P. Costales, O. Juan-Babot, L. Badimon, V. Llorente-Cortes, Hypoxia stimulates low-density lipoprotein receptor-related protein-1 expression through hypoxia-inducible factor-1alpha in human vascular smooth muscle cells, Arterioscler Thromb Vasc Biol 31 (2011) 1411–1420.

[73] R. Cal, J. Castellano, E. Revuelta-Lopez, R. Aledo, M. Barriga, J. Farre, G. Vilahur, L. Nasarre, L. Hove-Madsen, L. Badimon, V. Llorente-Cortes, Low-density lipoprotein receptor-related protein 1 mediates hypoxia-induced very low density lipoprotein-

cholesteryl ester uptake and accumulation in cardiomyocytes, Cardiovasc Res 94 (2012) 469–479.

[74] Y. Wang, O. Roche, C. Xu, E.H. Moriyama, P. Heir, J. Chung, F.C. Roos, Y. Chen, G. Finak, M. Milosevic, B.C. Wilson, B.T. Teh, M. Park, M.S. Irwin, M. Ohh, Hypoxia promotes ligand-independent EGF receptor signaling via hypoxia-inducible factor-mediated upregulation of caveolin-1, Proc Natl Acad Sci U S A 109 (2012) 4892–4897.

[75] T. Hackenbeck, R. Huber, R. Schietke, K.X. Knaup, J. Monti, X. Wu, B. Klanke, B. Frey, U. Gaipl, B. Wullich, D. Ferbus, G. Goubin, C. Warnecke, K.U. Eckardt, M.S. Wiesener, The GTPase RAB20 is a HIF target with mitochondrial localization mediating apoptosis in hypoxia, Biochim Biophys Acta 1813 (2011) 1–13.

[76] S. Narravula, S.P. Colgan, Hypoxia-inducible factor 1-mediated inhibition of peroxisome proliferator-activated receptor alpha expression during hypoxia, J Immunol 166 (2001) 7543–7548.

[77] M.H. Yang, M.Z. Wu, S.H. Chiou, P.M. Chen, S.Y. Chang, C.J. Liu, S.C. Teng, K.J. Wu, Direct regulation of TWIST by HIF-1alpha promotes metastasis, Nat Cell Biol 10 (2008) 295–305.

[78] S.M. Choi, H.J. Cho, H. Cho, K.H. Kim, J.B. Kim, H. Park, Stra13/DEC1 and DEC2 inhibit sterol regulatory element binding protein-1c in a hypoxia-inducible factor-dependent mechanism, Nucleic Acids Res 36 (2008) 6372–6385.

[79] P. Ugocsai, A. Hohenstatt, G. Paragh, G. Liebisch, T. Langmann, Z. Wolf, T. Weiss, P. Groitl, T. Dobner, P. Kasprzak, L. Gobolos, A. Falkert, B. Seelbach-Goebel, A. Gellhaus, E. Winterhager, M. Schmidt, G.L. Semenza, G. Schmitz, HIF-1beta determines ABCA1 expression under hypoxia in human macrophages, Int J Biochem Cell Biol 42 (2010) 241–252.

[80] K. Glunde, T. Shah, P.T. Winnard, Jr., V. Raman, T. Takagi, F. Vesuna, D. Artemov, Z.M. Bhujwalla, Hypoxia regulates choline kinase expression through hypoxia-inducible factor-1 alpha signaling in a human prostate cancer model, Cancer Res 68 (2008) 172–180.

[81] A. Bansal, R.A. Harris, T.R. DeGrado, Choline phosphorylation and regulation of transcription of choline kinase alpha in hypoxia, J Lipid Res 53 (2012) 149–157.

[82] S.T. Saarikoski, S.P. Rivera, O. Hankinson, Mitogen-inducible gene 6 (MIG-6), adipophilin and tuftelin are inducible by hypoxia, FEBS Lett 530 (2002) 186–190.

[83] X. Xia, M.E. Lemieux, W. Li, J.S. Carroll, M. Brown, X.S. Liu, A.L. Kung, Integrative analysis of HIF binding and transactivation reveals its role in maintaining histone methylation homeostasis, Proc Natl Acad Sci U S A 106 (2009) 4260–4265.

[84] G. Shen, N. Ning, X. Zhao, X. Liu, G. Wang, T. Wang, R. Zhao, C. Yang, D. Wang, P. Gong, Y. Shen, Y. Sun, Y. Jin, W. Yang, Y. He, L. Zhang, X. Jin, X. Li, Adipose differen-

tiation-related protein is not involved in hypoxia inducible factor-1-induced lipid accumulation under hypoxia, Mol Med Rep 12 (2015) 8055–8061.

[85] T. Gimm, M. Wiese, B. Teschemacher, A. Deggerich, J. Schodel, K.X. Knaup, T. Hackenbeck, C. Hellerbrand, K. Amann, M.S. Wiesener, S. Honing, K.U. Eckardt, C. Warnecke, Hypoxia-inducible protein 2 is a novel lipid droplet protein and a specific target gene of hypoxia-inducible factor-1, FASEB J 24 (2010) 4443–4458.

[86] A. Kaidi, D. Qualtrough, A.C. Williams, C. Paraskeva, Direct transcriptional up-regulation of cyclooxygenase-2 by hypoxia-inducible factor (HIF)-1 promotes colorectal tumor cell survival and enhances HIF-1 transcriptional activity during hypoxia, Cancer Res 66 (2006) 6683–6691.

[87] J.J. Lee, M. Natsuizaka, S. Ohashi, G.S. Wong, M. Takaoka, C.Z. Michaylira, D. Budo, J.W. Tobias, M. Kanai, Y. Shirakawa, Y. Naomoto, A.J. Klein-Szanto, V.H. Haase, H. Nakagawa, Hypoxia activates the cyclooxygenase-2-prostaglandin E synthase axis, Carcinogenesis 31 (2010) 427–434.

[88] C. Grimmer, D. Pfander, B. Swoboda, T. Aigner, L. Mueller, F.F. Hennig, K. Gelse, Hypoxia-inducible factor 1alpha is involved in the prostaglandin metabolism of osteoarthritic cartilage through up-regulation of microsomal prostaglandin E synthase 1 in articular chondrocytes, Arthritis Rheum 56 (2007) 4084–4094.

[89] G.S. Hotamisligil, D.A. Bernlohr, Metabolic functions of FABPs—mechanisms and therapeutic implications, Nat Rev Endocrinol 11 (2015) 592–605.

[90] A. Chabowski, J. Gorski, J.J. Luiken, J.F. Glatz, A. Bonen, Evidence for concerted action of FAT/CD36 and FABPpm to increase fatty acid transport across the plasma membrane, Prostaglandins Leukot Essent Fatty Acids 77 (2007) 345–353.

[91] R.W. Schwenk, G.P. Holloway, J.J. Luiken, A. Bonen, J.F. Glatz, Fatty acid transport across the cell membrane: regulation by fatty acid transporters, Prostaglandins Leukot Essent Fatty Acids 82 (2010) 149–154.

[92] A. Chabowski, J.C. Chatham, N.N. Tandon, J. Calles-Escandon, J.F. Glatz, J.J. Luiken, A. Bonen, Fatty acid transport and FAT/CD36 are increased in red but not in white skeletal muscle of ZDF rats, Am J Physiol Endocrinol Metab 291 (2006) E675–E682.

[93] R.L. Smathers, D.R. Petersen, The human fatty acid-binding protein family: evolutionary divergences and functions, Hum Genomics 5 (2011) 170–191.

[94] V.L. Spitsberg, E. Matitashvili, R.C. Gorewit, Association and coexpression of fatty-acid-binding protein and glycoprotein CD36 in the bovine mammary gland, Eur J Biochem 230 (1995) 872–878.

[95] F.G. Schaap, B. Binas, H. Danneberg, G.J. van der Vusse, J.F. Glatz, Impaired long-chain fatty acid utilization by cardiac myocytes isolated from mice lacking the heart-type fatty acid binding protein gene, Circ Res 85 (1999) 329–337.

[96]   B. Binas, H. Danneberg, J. McWhir, L. Mullins, A.J. Clark, Requirement for the heart-type fatty acid binding protein in cardiac fatty acid utilization, FASEB J 13 (1999) 805–812.

[97]   L.Z. Xu, R. Sanchez, A. Sali, N. Heintz, Ligand specificity of brain lipid-binding protein, J Biol Chem 271 (1996) 24711–24719.

[98]   A. Slipicevic, K. Jorgensen, M. Skrede, A.K. Rosnes, G. Troen, B. Davidson, V.A. Florenes, The fatty acid binding protein 7 (FABP7) is involved in proliferation and invasion of melanoma cells, BMC Cancer 8 (2008) 276.

[99]   G. Kaloshi, K. Mokhtari, C. Carpentier, S. Taillibert, J. Lejeune, Y. Marie, J.Y. Delattre, R. Godbout, M. Sanson, FABP7 expression in glioblastomas: relation to prognosis, invasion and EGFR status, J Neurooncol 84 (2007) 245–248.

[100] Y. Wada, A. Sugiyama, T. Yamamoto, M. Naito, N. Noguchi, S. Yokoyama, M. Tsujita, Y. Kawabe, M. Kobayashi, A. Izumi, T. Kohro, T. Tanaka, H. Taniguchi, H. Koyama, K. Hirano, S. Yamashita, Y. Matsuzawa, E. Niki, T. Hamakubo, T. Kodama, Lipid accumulation in smooth muscle cells under LDL loading is independent of LDL receptor pathway and enhanced by hypoxic conditions, Arterioscler Thromb Vasc Biol 22 (2002) 1712–1719.

[101] J. Castellano, J. Farre, J. Fernandes, A. Bayes-Genis, J. Cinca, L. Badimon, L. Hove-Madsen, V. Llorente-Cortes, Hypoxia exacerbates Ca(2+)-handling disturbances induced by very low density lipoproteins (VLDL) in neonatal rat cardiomyocytes, J Mol Cell Cardiol 50 (2011) 894–902.

[102] N. Loewen, J. Chen, V.J. Dudley, V.P. Sarthy, J.R. Mathura, Jr., Genomic response of hypoxic Muller cells involves the very low density lipoprotein receptor as part of an angiogenic network, Exp Eye Res 88 (2009) 928–937.

[103] W.A. Prinz, Lipid trafficking sans vesicles: where, why, how?, Cell 143 (2010) 870–874.

[104] Y. Li, M.P. Marzolo, P. van Kerkhof, G.J. Strous, G. Bu, The YXXL motif, but not the two NPXY motifs, serves as the dominant endocytosis signal for low density lipoprotein receptor-related protein, J Biol Chem 275 (2000) 17187–17194.

[105] L. Auderset, L.M. Landowski, L. Foa, K.M. Young, Low density lipoprotein receptor related proteins as regulators of neural stem and progenitor cell function, Stem Cells Int 2016 (2016) 1–16.

[106] P.T. Bozza, K.G. Magalhaes, P.F. Weller, Leukocyte lipid bodies – biogenesis and functions in inflammation, Biochim Biophys Acta 1791 (2009) 540–551.

[107] P.G. Frank, F. Galbiati, D. Volonte, B. Razani, D.E. Cohen, Y.L. Marcel, M.P. Lisanti, Influence of caveolin-1 on cellular cholesterol efflux mediated by high-density lipo-proteins, Am J Physiol Cell Physiol 280 (2001) C1204–1214.

[108] N. Marx, H. Duez, J.C. Fruchart, B. Staels, Peroxisome proliferator-activated receptors and atherogenesis: regulators of gene expression in vascular cells, Circ Res 94 (2004) 1168–1178.

[109] J.M. Brandt, F. Djouadi, D.P. Kelly, Fatty acids activate transcription of the muscle carnitine palmitoyltransferase I gene in cardiac myocytes via the peroxisome proliferator-activated receptor alpha, J Biol Chem 273 (1998) 23786–23792.

[110] P. Razeghi, M.E. Young, S. Abbasi, H. Taegtmeyer, Hypoxia in vivo decreases peroxisome proliferator-activated receptor alpha-regulated gene expression in rat heart, Biochem Biophys Res Commun 287 (2001) 5–10.

[111] C. Handschin, B.M. Spiegelman, Peroxisome proliferator-activated receptor gamma coactivator 1 coactivators, energy homeostasis, and metabolism, Endocr Rev 27 (2006) 728–735.

[112] D.O. Espinoza, L.G. Boros, S. Crunkhorn, H. Gami, M.E. Patti, Dual modulation of both lipid oxidation and synthesis by peroxisome proliferator-activated receptor-gamma coactivator-1alpha and -1beta in cultured myotubes, FASEB J 24 (2010) 1003–1014.

[113] J. Lin, R. Yang, P.T. Tarr, P.H. Wu, C. Handschin, S. Li, W. Yang, L. Pei, M. Uldry, P. Tontonoz, C.B. Newgard, B.M. Spiegelman, Hyperlipidemic effects of dietary saturated fats mediated through PGC-1beta coactivation of SREBP, Cell 120 (2005) 261–273.

[114] H. Zhang, P. Gao, R. Fukuda, G. Kumar, B. Krishnamachary, K.I. Zeller, C.V. Dang, G.L. Semenza, HIF-1 inhibits mitochondrial biogenesis and cellular respiration in VHL-deficient renal cell carcinoma by repression of C-MYC activity, Cancer Cell 11 (2007) 407–420.

[115] F.V. Filipp, D.A. Scott, Z.A. Ronai, A.L. Osterman, J.W. Smith, Reverse TCA cycle flux through isocitrate dehydrogenases 1 and 2 is required for lipogenesis in hypoxic melanoma cells, Pigment Cell Melanoma Res 25 (2012) 375–383.

[116] D.R. Wise, P.S. Ward, J.E. Shay, J.R. Cross, J.J. Gruber, U.M. Sachdeva, J.M. Platt, R.G. DeMatteo, M.C. Simon, C.B. Thompson, Hypoxia promotes isocitrate dehydrogenase-dependent carboxylation of alpha-ketoglutarate to citrate to support cell growth and viability, Proc Natl Acad Sci U S A 108 (2011) 19611–19616.

[117] A. Le, A.N. Lane, M. Hamaker, S. Bose, A. Gouw, J. Barbi, T. Tsukamoto, C.J. Rojas, B.S. Slusher, H. Zhang, L.J. Zimmerman, D.C. Liebler, R.J. Slebos, P.K. Lorkiewicz, R.M. Higashi, T.W. Fan, C.V. Dang, Glucose-independent glutamine metabolism via TCA cycling for proliferation and survival in B cells, Cell Metab 15 (2012) 110–121.

[118] P.A. Gameiro, J. Yang, A.M. Metelo, R. Perez-Carro, R. Baker, Z. Wang, A. Arreola, W.K. Rathmell, A. Olumi, P. Lopez-Larrubia, G. Stephanopoulos, O. Iliopoulos, In vivo HIF-mediated reductive carboxylation is regulated by citrate levels and sensitizes VHL-deficient cells to glutamine deprivation, Cell Metab 17 (2013) 372–385.

[119] E. Furuta, S.K. Pai, R. Zhan, S. Bandyopadhyay, M. Watabe, Y.Y. Mo, S. Hirota, S. Hosobe, T. Tsukada, K. Miura, S. Kamada, K. Saito, M. Iiizumi, W. Liu, J. Ericsson, K.

Watabe, Fatty acid synthase gene is up-regulated by hypoxia via activation of Akt and sterol regulatory element binding protein-1, Cancer Res 68 (2008) 1003–1011.

[120] S.Y. Jung, H.K. Jeon, J.S. Choi, Y.J. Kim, Reduced expression of FASN through SREBP-1 down-regulation is responsible for hypoxic cell death in HepG2 cells, J Cell Biochem 113 (2012) 3730–3739.

[121] R.M. Young, D. Ackerman, Z.L. Quinn, A. Mancuso, M. Gruber, L. Liu, D.N. Giannoukos, E. Bobrovnikova-Marjon, J.A. Diehl, B. Keith, M.C. Simon, Dysregulated mTORC1 renders cells critically dependent on desaturated lipids for survival under tumor-like stress, Genes Dev 27 (2013) 1115–1131.

[122] J.R. Krycer, A.J. Brown, Cholesterol accumulation in prostate cancer: a classic observation from a modern perspective, Biochim Biophys Acta 1835 (2013) 219–229.

[123] J. Mukodani, Y. Ishikawa, H. Fukuzaki, Effects of hypoxia on sterol synthesis, acyl-CoA: cholesterol acyltransferase activity, and efflux of cholesterol in cultured rabbit skin fibroblasts, Arteriosclerosis 10 (1990) 106–110.

[124] V. Pallottini, B. Guantario, C. Martini, P. Totta, I. Filippi, F. Carraro, A. Trentalance, Regulation of HMG-CoA reductase expression by hypoxia, J Cell Biochem 104 (2008) 701–709.

[125] E. Temes, S. Martin-Puig, J. Aragones, D.R. Jones, G. Olmos, I. Merida, M.O. Landazuri, Role of diacylglycerol induced by hypoxia in the regulation of HIF-1alpha activity, Biochem Biophys Res Commun 315 (2004) 44–50.

[126] J. Aragones, D.R. Jones, S. Martin, M.A. San Juan, A. Alfranca, F. Vidal, A. Vara, I. Merida, M.O. Landazuri, Evidence for the involvement of diacylglycerol kinase in the activation of hypoxia-inducible transcription factor 1 by low oxygen tension, J Biol Chem 276 (2001) 10548–10555.

[127] S. Martin-Puig, E. Temes, G. Olmos, D.R. Jones, J. Aragones, M.O. Landazuri, Role of iron (II)-2-oxoglutarate-dependent dioxygenases in the generation of hypoxia-induced phosphatidic acid through HIF-1/2 and von Hippel-Lindau-independent mechanisms, J Biol Chem 279 (2004) 9504–9511.

[128] S. Martin, R.G. Parton, Lipid droplets: a unified view of a dynamic organelle, Nat Rev Mol Cell Biol 7 (2006) 373–378.

[129] L.M. Scarfo, P.F. Weller, H.W. Farber, Induction of endothelial cell cytoplasmic lipid bodies during hypoxia, Am J Physiol Heart Circ Physiol 280 (2001) H294–H301.

[130] L.M. Pawella, M. Hashani, P. Schirmacher, B.K. Straub, Lipid droplet-associated proteins in steatosis. Effects of induction and siRNA-mediated downregulation of PAT proteins in cell culture models of hepatocyte steatosis, Pathologe 31 Suppl 2 (2010) 126–131.

[131] D.A. Ostler, V.G. Prieto, J.A. Reed, M.T. Deavers, A.J. Lazar, D. Ivan, Adipophilin expression in sebaceous tumors and other cutaneous lesions with clear cell histology: an immunohistochemical study of 117 cases, Mod Pathol 23 (2010) 567–573.

[132] A. Paul, B.H. Chang, L. Li, V.K. Yechoor, L. Chan, Deficiency of adipose differentiation-related protein impairs foam cell formation and protects against atherosclerosis, Circ Res 102 (2008) 1492–1501.

[133] J. Gao, G. Serrero, Adipose differentiation related protein (ADRP) expressed in transfected COS-7 cells selectively stimulates long chain fatty acid uptake, J Biol Chem 274 (1999) 16825–16830.

[134] A. Pol, S. Martin, M.A. Fernandez, C. Ferguson, A. Carozzi, R. Luetterforst, C. Enrich, R.G. Parton, Dynamic and regulated association of caveolin with lipid bodies: modulation of lipid body motility and function by a dominant negative mutant, Mol Biol Cell 15 (2004) 99–110.

[135] A. Pol, R. Luetterforst, M. Lindsay, S. Heino, E. Ikonen, R.G. Parton, A caveolin dominant negative mutant associates with lipid bodies and induces intracellular cholesterol imbalance, J Cell Biol 152 (2001) 1057–1070.

[136] D.L. Brasaemle, G. Dolios, L. Shapiro, R. Wang, Proteomic analysis of proteins associated with lipid droplets of basal and lipolytically stimulated 3T3-L1 adipocytes, J Biol Chem 279 (2004) 46835–46842.

[137] D. Marchesan, M. Rutberg, L. Andersson, L. Asp, T. Larsson, J. Boren, B.R. Johansson, S.O. Olofsson, A phospholipase D-dependent process forms lipid droplets containing caveolin, adipocyte differentiation-related protein, and vimentin in a cell-free system, J Biol Chem 278 (2003) 27293–27300.

[138] A.J. North, T.S. Brannon, L.B. Wells, W.B. Campbell, P.W. Shaul, Hypoxia stimulates prostacyclin synthesis in newborn pulmonary artery endothelium by increasing cyclooxygenase-1 protein, Circ Res 75 (1994) 33–40.

[139] A.M. Dvorak, P.F. Weller, V.S. Harvey, E.S. Morgan, H.F. Dvorak, Ultrastructural localization of prostaglandin endoperoxide synthase (cyclooxygenase) to isolated, purified fractions of guinea pig peritoneal macrophage and line 10 hepatocarcinoma cell lipid bodies, Int Arch Allergy Immunol 101 (1993) 136–142.

[140] A. Arend, R. Masso, M. Masso, G. Selstam, Electron microscope immunocytochemical localization of cyclooxygenase-1 and -2 in pseudopregnant rat corpus luteum during luteolysis, Prostaglandins Other Lipid Mediat 74 (2004) 1–10.

[141] P.T. Bozza, W. Yu, J.F. Penrose, E.S. Morgan, A.M. Dvorak, P.F. Weller, Eosinophil lipid bodies: specific, inducible intracellular sites for enhanced eicosanoid formation, J Exp Med 186 1997 909–920.

[142] P.T. Bozza, W. Yu, J. Cassara, P.F. Weller, Pathways for eosinophil lipid body induction: differing signal transduction in cells from normal and hypereosinophilic subjects, J Leukoc Biol 64 (1998) 563–569.

[143] P. Pacheco, F.A. Bozza, R.N. Gomes, M. Bozza, P.F. Weller, H.C. Castro-Faria-Neto, P.T. Bozza, Lipopolysaccharide-induced leukocyte lipid body formation in vivo: innate immunity elicited intracellular Loci involved in eicosanoid metabolism, J Immunol 169 (2002) 6498–6506.

[144] A. Vieira-de-Abreu, E.F. Assis, G.S. Gomes, H.C. Castro-Faria-Neto, P.F. Weller, C. Bandeira-Melo, P.T. Bozza, Allergic challenge-elicited lipid bodies compartmentalize in vivo leukotriene C4 synthesis within eosinophils, Am J Respir Cell Mol Biol 33 (2005) 254–261.

[145] N.F. Voelkel, R.M. Tuder, K. Wade, M. Hoper, R.A. Lepley, J.L. Goulet, B.H. Koller, F. Fitzpatrick, Inhibition of 5-lipoxygenase-activating protein (FLAP) reduces pulmonary vascular reactivity and pulmonary hypertension in hypoxic rats, J Clin Invest 97 (1996) 2491–2498.

[146] I.R. Preston, N.S. Hill, R.R. Warburton, B.L. Fanburg, Role of 12-lipoxygenase in hypoxia-induced rat pulmonary artery smooth muscle cell proliferation, Am J Physiol Lung Cell Mol Physiol 290 (2006) L367–L374.

[147] E.K. Rydberg, A. Krettek, C. Ullstrom, K. Ekstrom, P.A. Svensson, L.M. Carlsson, A.C. Jonsson-Rylander, G.I. Hansson, W. McPheat, O. Wiklund, B.G. Ohlsson, L.M. Hulten, Hypoxia increases LDL oxidation and expression of 15-lipoxygenase-2 in human macrophages, Arterioscler Thromb Vasc Biol 24 (2004) 2040–2045.

[148] Y. Liu, X. Tang, C. Lu, W. Han, S. Guo, D. Zhu, Expression of 15-lipoxygenases in pulmonary arteries after hypoxia, Pathology 41 (2009) 476–483.

[149] L. Yao, X. Nie, S. Shi, S. Song, X. Hao, S. Li, D. Zhu, Reciprocal regulation of HIF-1alpha and 15-LO/15-HETE promotes anti-apoptosis process in pulmonary artery smooth muscle cells during hypoxia, Prostaglandins Other Lipid Mediat 99 (2012) 96–106.

[150] L. Li, B. Liu, L. Haversen, E. Lu, L.U. Magnusson, M. Stahlman, J. Boren, G. Bergstrom, M.C. Levin, L.M. Hulten, The importance of GLUT3 for de novo lipogenesis in hypoxia-induced lipid loading of human macrophages, PLoS One 7 (2012) e42360.

[151] D.R. Mole, C. Blancher, R.R. Copley, P.J. Pollard, J.M. Gleadle, J. Ragoussis, P.J. Ratcliffe, Genome-wide association of hypoxia-inducible factor (HIF)-1alpha and HIF-2alpha DNA binding with expression profiling of hypoxia-inducible transcripts, J Biol Chem 284 (2009) 16767–16775.

[152] T. Hitosugi, L. Zhou, S. Elf, J. Fan, H.B. Kang, J.H. Seo, C. Shan, Q. Dai, L. Zhang, J. Xie, T.L. Gu, P. Jin, M. Aleckovic, G. LeRoy, Y. Kang, J.A. Sudderth, R.J. DeBerardinis, C.H. Luan, G.Z. Chen, S. Muller, D.M. Shin, T.K. Owonikoko, S. Lonial, M.L. Arellano, H.J. Khoury, F.R. Khuri, B.H. Lee, K. Ye, T.J. Boggon, S. Kang, C. He, J. Chen, Phosphogly-

cerate mutase 1 coordinates glycolysis and biosynthesis to promote tumor growth, Cancer Cell 22 (2012) 585–600.

[153] S.J. Ricoult, B.D. Manning, The multifaceted role of mTORC1 in the control of lipid metabolism, EMBO Rep 14 (2013) 242–251.

[154] R.A. Srivastava, S.L. Pinkosky, S. Filippov, J.C. Hanselman, C.T. Cramer, R.S. Newton, AMP-activated protein kinase: an emerging drug target to regulate imbalances in lipid and carbohydrate metabolism to treat cardio-metabolic diseases, J Lipid Res 53 (2012) 2490–2514.

[155] H. Zirath, A. Frenzel, G. Oliynyk, L. Segerstrom, U.K. Westermark, K. Larsson, M. Munksgaard Persson, K. Hultenby, J. Lehtio, C. Einvik, S. Pahlman, P. Kogner, P.J. Jakobsson, M.A. Henriksson, MYC inhibition induces metabolic changes leading to accumulation of lipid droplets in tumor cells, Proc Natl Acad Sci U S A 110 (2013) 10258–10263.

[156] X. Wang, X. Zhao, X. Gao, Y. Mei, M. Wu, A new role of p53 in regulating lipid metabolism, J Mol Cell Biol 5 (2013) 147–150.

4

A Novel Hypoxia Imaging Endoscopy System

Kazuhiro Kaneko, Hiroshi Yamaguchi and

Tomonori Yano

Abstract

Measurement of tumor hypoxia is required for the diagnosis of tumor and the evaluation of therapeutic outcome. Currently, invasive and noninvasive techniques being exploited for tumor hypoxia measurement include polarographic needle electrodes, immunohistochemical (IHC) staining, magnetic resonance imaging (MRI), radionuclide imaging (positron emission tomography [PET] and single-photon emission computed tomography [SPECT]), optical imaging (bioluminescence and fluorescence), and hypoxia imaging endoscopy. This review provides a summary of the modalities available for assessment of tissue oxygenation as well as a discussion of current arguments for and against each modality, with a particular focus on noninvasive hypoxia imaging with emerging agents and new imaging technologies intended to detect molecular events associated with tumor hypoxia.

Keywords: Hypoxia imaging endoscopy, innovation of endoscopy

1. Introduction

In the 1950s, hypoxia research began, and many clinical trials have been reported. Hypoxia of tumor affects outcomes after radiotherapy. But hypoxia has also been shown to be a poor prognostic factor after chemotherapy and surgery. These findings are attributed to chronic hypoxia. Hypoxic tumors are more likely to recur loco-regionally than well-oxygenated tumors regardless of whether surgery or radiation therapy is the primary local treatment. However, the common oxygen measurement used in these reports was polarographic needle electrodes inserted directly into specific sections of tumor tissue. In this method, hypoxia was measured in only pinpointed area for the tumor. In other words, there was no modality used in which the hypoxia imaging results were visible in real time and which reflected the hypoxic state in the whole tumor. Therefore, hypoxia imaging is expected to allow direct visualization of the biological and functional changes in cancer.

Hypoxia is a histopathological condition in which cells in tissues suffer from lack of oxygen for their normal metabolism. An oxygen saturation (StO_2) of arterial blood is almost 100% and that of venous blood is approximately 70%. In contrast, the StO_2 in half of cancers is 50–60% at the highest. Hypoxia takes hold as a tumor becomes large enough to disrupt the balance of oxygen supply and consumption in the area. Approximately, 50–60% of advanced cancer forming solid tumor may show hypoxic and/or anoxic conditions exhibiting heterogeneous distribution in the inside of tumor [1]. Hypoxia proliferates rapidly in solid tumors, and their intratumoral vessels with significantly structural abnormalities are distributed spatially with dilated, tortuous, saccular, and heterogeneous figures. As a result, this distribution leads to perfusion-limited delivery of O_2 [2]. There are mainly two types of hypoxia regarding solid tumor and tissue around tumor. One is perfusion-limited O_2 delivery type, the so-called acute hypoxia, which leads to ischemic condition, however, it is often transient. Another type is diffusion-limited hypoxia, the so-called chronic hypoxia, which can also be caused by an increase in diffusion distances, so that cells far away (>70 μm) from a nutritive blood vessel receive less oxygen (and nutrients) than needed [1]. Regarding hypoxia-induced proteome and/or genome changes, cell cycle arrest, differentiation, apoptosis, and necrosis are found in solid tumor. In contrast, hypoxia-induced changes of proteome may progress tumor growth because of mechanisms enabling cells to overcome nutritive deprivation, to escape from the hostile environment and to favor unrestricted growth. Furthermore, continuous hypoxia can also bring cellular changes as a more aggressive phenotype [3]. Since the presence of hypoxic status in solid tumors was first reported in 1953 to be among the factors associated with treatment failure following radiation therapy [4], tumor hypoxia has drawn attention as a pivotal event in tumor invasion, angiogenesis, apoptosis, metastasis [1], resistance to chemotherapy [5], surgery, and resistance to radiotherapy [6]. In tumor diagnosis and treatment planning, it is crucial to have a grasp of the degree and extent of tumor hypoxia involved prior to the start of treatment.

2. Clinical importance for measurement of tumor hypoxic state

A variety of techniques are being proposed to assess tumor hypoxia, which can be broadly categorized into direct measurements and indirect measurements according to different principles and the ability to quantify tissue oxygenation. Direct measurements, including polarographic needle electrode, phosphorescence imaging, near-infrared spectroscopy (NIRS), blood oxygen level dependent (BOLD) and ^{19}F magnetic resonance imaging (MRI) and electron paramagnetic resonance (EPR) imaging, can detect oxygen partial pressure (pO_2), oxygen concentration, or oxygen percentage. Recently, a hypoxia imaging endoscopy that can derive the oxygen saturation (StO_2) was developed in endoscopic fields. Indirect measurements, including measuring exogenous and endogenous hypoxia markers, can provide parameters related to oxygenation.

Many clinical trials have been performed using direct and indirect measurement methods. It is now known that hypoxia affects outcome after radiotherapy, with poor prognosis in hypoxic cancers. Next, hypoxia has also been shown to be a poor prognostic factor after chemotherapy and surgery. Furthermore, hypoxic tumors are more likely to recur loco-regionally than well-oxygenated tumors regardless of whether surgery or radiation therapy was the primary local treatment.

3. Direct measurements for hypoxia

3.1. Polarographic needle electrodes for direct tumor tissue

The invasive polarographic needle electrodes have been widely employed since the 1990s to assess tumor oxygen status and to measure pO_2 in both human and animal studies [7, 8]. As the gold standard modality, their use has been extended not only to lymph node metastases but to more accessible tumors, which include head and neck cancer, cervical cancer, soft tissue sarcomas of the extremities, astrocytic brain tumors, lung cancer, pancreatic cancer, prostate cancer, and lymph node metastases [8–12]. With the average median pO_2 before treatment of 11.2 mmHg (range 0.4–60 mmHg) [7], these measured values help prediction of the tumor response to treatment [13] and tumor metastatic potential [14]. The polarographic needle electrode is currently available under CT guidance for evaluating tumor pO_2 in deep-seated organs as well as for assessing overall tumor oxygen status [15] with the caveat, however, that insertion of an electrode into the tumor leads to disruption of tissues, thus rendering it difficult to distinguish the necrotic areas and to establish the patterns of hypoxia involved. Furthermore, the use of the modality not only calls for great expertise but is associated with large interobserver variability.

4. Noninvasive imaging of hypoxia

While the polarographic needle electrode and immunohistochemical (IHC) staining can provide a relatively accurate estimation of tumor oxygenation, being subject to selection bias, provide only a partial, but not complete, picture of the entire tumor site [16]. This has led to an increasing interest in the use of noninvasive functional and molecular imaging modalities, which is capable of yielding a large amount of high-quality experimental data per protocol by increasing the number of quantitative data collections and by guiding tissue sampling and allowing a rapid and effective combination of analyses to be conducted [17].

Several imaging modalities have been developed, to date, to allow direct or indirect measurement of tumor oxygenation, with a few of these remaining less mature for clinical application. Of these, EPR spectroscopy, which involves the use of unpaired electron species to obtain images and spectra, is currently being explored in animals as a means to provide a quantitative measure of tissue oxygenation [18]. Although this modality has considerable potential to be developed as a tumor oximeter, i.e., in monitoring changes after tumor oxygenation [19], a suitable paramagnetic marker with low toxicity for human remains yet to become available. The need for appropriate EPR instrumentation in the clinical setting also prevents this promising modality from becoming widespread [20]. Photoacoustic tomography (PAT) is also available for imaging blood oxygenation using the differential optical contrast between O_2Hb and dHb. PAT has been implemented for imaging cerebral blood oxygenation of rats *in vivo*, demonstrating that PAT is capable of capturing the changes from hyperoxia to hypoxia [21], while no study reported on its clinical application.

4.1. Magnetic resonance imaging

BOLD-MRI is shown to have potential as a diagnostic modality for tumor hypoxia [22]. Hemoglobin occurs as deoxyhemoglobin in oxygen-deficient states, where not oxyhemoglobin but paramagnetic deoxyhemoglobin can increase the transverse relaxation of the surrounding protons [23]. BOLD-MRI employs deoxyhemoglobin-derived endogenous signals as image contrast to depict changes in oxygenation in blood. Decreased oxygenation in blood results in decreased signal intensity in T2-weighted images, and this correlation between the BOLD-MRI signal and vascular oxygenation allows pO_2 to be directly estimated. This has indeed led to numerous studies being conducted to investigate carbogen breathing in mice, oxygenation in tumor models [24], and kidney function in patients [22, 25, 26] using the modality as a noninvasive technique with high spatial and temporal resolution [22]. As with phosphorescence and near-infrared fluorescence imaging, the major disadvantage of BOLD-MRI is that it reflects change in oxygen tension in vasculature but not those in tissues. Again, not being a quantitative method, it may easily be affected by multiple factors such as flow effects, hematocrit, pH, and temperature [27].

^{19}F MRI involves the use of two types of markers, i.e., perfluorocarbons (PFCs) and fluorinated nitroimidazoles as contrast agents, which are not used in conventional T1-weighted MRI. While being highly hydrophobic, PFCs are highly oxygen soluble [28]. Due to the linear relationship between the ^{19}F spin lattice relaxation rate of PFCs and the dissolved oxygen concentration, the ^{19}F-based oximetry allows vascular oxygenation to be measured *in vivo* [29]. PFCs investigated to date include hexafluorobenzene (HFB) [30] and perfluoro-15-crown-5-ether (PF15C5) [31, 32], which are injectable intravenously or intratumorally. ^{19}F MRI is increasingly employed to detect changes in tumor oxygenation that occur in response to treatments that are radio-sensitizing and oxygen-augmenting [33]. The disadvantages of ^{19}F MRI are that flow artifacts affect the measurements and that, with some contrast agents, oxygen sensitivity is easily influenced by such conditions as temperature, dilution, pH, common proteins, and blood [34]. Following intravenous injection, most PFC contrast agent is extensively ingested by the reticuloendothelial system (RES) and their slow clearance may cause adverse reactions. Their intratumoral injection may also raise concern over its associated risk, e.g., embolism associated with accidental injection of PFC emulsion into the tumoral vein [35]. One major drawback of the nitroimidazole derivatives is their central nervous system (CNS) toxicity profile, with misonidazole shown to be associated with neuropathy and acute toxicity on the CNS [33].

"Vessel architectural imaging" (VAI) has recently been proposed as a new paradigm in MRI providing a basis for vessel caliber estimation [36] by incorporating an overlooked temporal shift in the MR signal, thus generating, unlike any other noninvasive imaging modality, new information on vessel type and function. Indeed, this new modality allowed an oral pan-vascular endothelial growth factor (pan-VEGF) receptor kinase inhibitor to be evaluated for its therapeutic efficacy in glioblastoma patients [37], demonstrating using VAI that anti-VEGF therapy not only normalizes tumor vasculature and alleviates edema but also prolongs survival in these patients.

4.2. Positron emission tomography

Efforts have recently been directed toward developing contrast agents for noninvasive hypoxia imaging with positron emission tomography (PET) and single-photon emission computed tomography (SPECT). Organic molecular markers labeled with positron-emitting radioisotopes are employed in PET imaging to allow the extent of tumor hypoxia to be measured. Commonly used radioisotopes include ^{18}F, ^{124}I, and $^{60/64}$Cu and the molecular markers to be labeled with these isotopes include 2-nitroimidazoles, e.g., fluoromisonidazole (FMISO), EF5, and fluoroetanidazole (FETA), nucleoside conjugates, e.g., iodoazomycin arabinoside (IAZA), and Cu(II)-diacetyl-bis (N4-methylthiosemicarbazone) (Cu-ATSM) [38–40]. These markers are shown not only to bind maximally to severely hypoxic cells to form such stable adducts as are detectable with a PET scanner but to provide a clear demarcation of hypoxic cells *in vivo* through their rapid reoxidization and removal from normal cells.

Of the first-generation nitroimidazoles, ^{18}F-labeled misonidazole (^{18}F-FMISO) is the most commonly used as being sensitive only to the presence of hypoxia in viable cells [41]. It is reported that a hypoxic state defined as <10 mmHg is required to induce significant ^{18}FMISO uptake [42]. ^{18}F-FMISO uptake is shown to vary widely depending on the type of patients and tumors, whereas ^{18}F-FMISO is shown to allow hypoxia to be detected in various tumors such as glioma, head and neck cancer, renal tumor, and non-small cell lung cancer [42–44]. A clinical trial of glioblastoma multiforme patients [45] demonstrated increased ^{18}F-FMISO uptake and retention on both post-treatment FMISO and FDG images, suggesting that reoxygenation did not take place. It is reported that the distribution of oxygen and hypoxia was increased and decreased, respectively, in non-small cell lung carcinomas following treatment, as assessed by sequential FMISO imaging [46]. Given that no correlation is shown between patient diagnosis and degree of decrease in FMISO uptake and retention, in selectively boosting the radiation dose to hypoxic subvolumes, there appears to be a larger role for serial imaging during treatment than for baseline volume measurement. Again, pretreatment FMISO uptake/retention and survival has been shown to be correlated and allow treatment failure to be predicted [45, 47]. However, ^{18}F-FMISO may not be readily available for use in other cancers [42, 48].

The second-generation nitroimidazoles include 18F-fluorerythronitroimidazole (FETNIM) [49, 50], FETA [51], and EF5 [52, 53], which are more water soluble and not readily suscepti-ble to degradation by most oxidizing mechanisms in place in humans. ^{18}F-EF5 was tested in clinical trials for its feasibility as an imaging agent for hypoxia [54] and was shown to be hypoxia-specific, with its increased uptake shown to be correlated with the extent of tumor and high risk of metastasis in cancer patients [52], suggesting its usefulness in identifying high-risk candidates for clinical trials evaluating the influence of early chemotherapy on the occurrence of metastasis [55]. ^{18}F-FAZA has great promise as an imaging agent for tumor hypoxia due to its faster diffusion into cells and faster clearance from normal tissues than ^{18}F-FMISO [56]. PET imaging using ^{18}F-FMISO demonstrated very high tracer uptake in all seven patients with high-grade gliomas evaluated, showing the potential of ^{18}F-FMISO as an imaging agent in assessing hypoxia in this tumor type [57].

4.3. Phosphorescence imaging

Phosphorescence imaging with injection of porphyrin complex (Oxyphor) into the vasculature also allows tumor vascular pO_2 to be measured [58, 59]. Recently, a general approach has been proposed through which to construct phosphorescent nanosensors with tunable spectral characteristics, varying degrees of quenching, and a high oxygen selectivity [60]. These probes are shown to exhibit excellent performance in measuring vascular pO_2 in the rat brain with *in vivo* microscopy [60]. NIRS are also available for analysis of tumor oxygenation *in vivo* based on recorded spectral changes by hemoglobin in the vasculature [61–63]. Kim and Liu [64] demonstrated in an animal study that NIRS is associated with comparable efficacy to that with electrode measurements in evaluating tumor hypoxia. They showed that either carbogen (95% CO_2 and 5% O_2) or 100% oxygen inhalation could improve the vascular oxygen level of rat breast tumors. However, both phosphorescence imaging and NIRS are not readily trans-latable into clinical applications due to their low spatial resolution, light scattering, limited path length, low sensitivity, and susceptibility to environmental influence.

4.4. Visible light spectroscopy

In the search for noninvasive, continuous modalities for monitoring ischemia, electrical bioimpedance cardiac output monitoring has been proposed but shown to be incompatible with the thermodilution methods [65, 66]. Again, while near-infrared spectroscopy (NIRS) [67] is shown to respond to both hypoxemia [68, 69] and ischemia [70–72], its clinical use has been limited to large organs, such as the brain [73, 74, 85–87] with its broad normal ranges reported to be between 48% and 88% [75, 76]. Similarly, wide normal ranges are reported for sublingual capnography [77–79]. Also available, albeit invasive are polarographic oximetry probes [80] and fiber-enabled pulmonary catheters.

Visible light spectroscopy (VLS) appears to be similar to NIRS on some counts [81] with its mean VLS StO2 shown to be not significantly different from NIRS StO2 reported in human studies [67–76]. Again, the fractional contribution of venous blood to the cerebral NIRS signal has been reported to be 0.84 ± 0.21 ranging from 0.60 to 1.00 [82–84]. Using central venous and pulse oximetry saturation as estimates for local venous and arterial saturation, it is shown to be not significantly different at 0.89 ± 0.04. It is suggested that the two modalities cover similar microvascular compartments.

At the same time, VLS is shown to be superior to NIRS in monitoring tissues that lend themselves to monitoring, thus suggesting a more versatile role for VLS in patient treatment [81]. The NIRS light sources and detectors require to be spaced 2–5 cm apart or more to illuminate and monitor a large, homogenous tissue volume (>30 ml), thus making NIRS with its long and bulky sensors unsuitable for monitoring tissue regions, e.g., thin tissues such as gastrointestinal mucosa or small tumors. In contrast, the visible light used in VLS is shown to be strongly absorbed by tissue and VLS measurement to be highly localized thus making VLS unsuitable for transcranial use or use over thick skin dominated by surface tissue properties. Using VLS, a rapid real-time drop in tumor oxygenation was detected during local ischemia following clamping or epinephrine administration [85], with the tissue oximetry performed during endoscopy demonstrating a significantly lower tissue oxygenation (StO_2) in tumors (46% ± 22%) than in normal mucosa (72% ± 4%) ($P < 0.0001$). Thus, VSL tissue oximetry may be able to distinguish neoplastic tissue with a high specificity to aid in the endoscopic detection of gastrointestinal tumors. Again, of note, chronic gastrointestinal ischemia was also detected using the same method [86] (**Figure 1**).

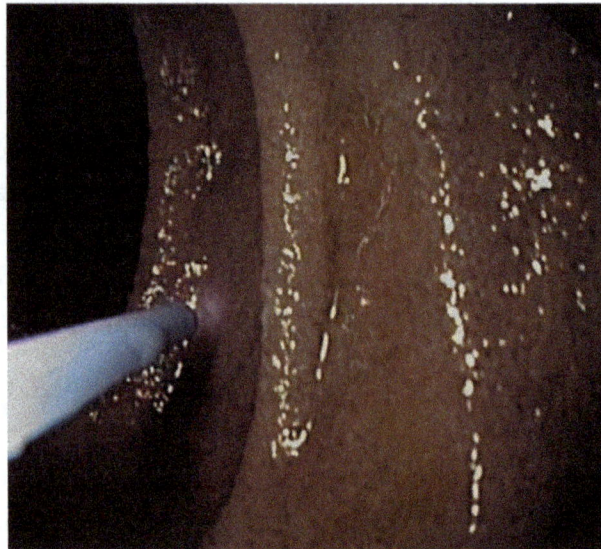

Figure 1. VLS measurements using a fiber-optic catheter-based VLS oximeter. The catheter is passed through the accessory channel of the endoscope and positioned about 1–5 mm above the mucosa.

5. Hypoxia imaging endoscopy with no phosphor

Kaneko et al. [87] reported hypoxia imaging endoscopy equipped with a laser light source. In this system, signals from the laser light passed through the processor were calculated as StO_2. The measurement range of StO_2 was from 0% to 100% in contactless of tumor or normal mucosa under endoscopic observation. Display imaging was performed with the use of laser light alone without phosphor, provided a display of overlay and pseudocolor images. The laser light used was not near-infrared but ranged within visible light wavelengths. In principle, this utilized the difference in absorption coefficient between oxyhemoglobin and deoxyhemoglobin. Two challenges were identified, however, in deriving the StO_2 of tissue in alimentary tracts from differences in absorption spectra between oxyhemoglobin and deoxyhemoglobin using small numbers of wavelengths. First, there is not only a small difference in optical absorption spectra in the visible light region but also a narrow bandwidth between isosbestic points. Second, the reflectance of a tissue depends on hematocrit (Hct) as well as StO_2, given that light absorption increases as hemoglobin density increases.

An imaging system equipped with laser diodes of 445 and 473 nm and a white fluorescent pigment body was therefore developed. Hypoxia imaging with this system rendered visible an alimentary tract tumor in real time and allowed the whole tumor to be visualized. With the tumor surface and normal mucosa rendered visible, no heterogeneity was seen with the use of this system. In the first-in-human clinical trial, early cancers of the esophagus, stomach, and colorectum were detected as hypoxic areas (**Figure 2**). Furthermore, colorectal adenomas with histologically low-grade atypia were also detected as hypoxic areas and no complications were reported in the patients with visualization of these tumors in real-time hypoxia imaging which involved only laser light without injection or oral administration of phosphor. As mentioned above, it will be expected that the hypoxia imaging endoscopy is shown to be superior to VLS or NIRS in measuring StO_2 of surface of tumor and normal mucosa.

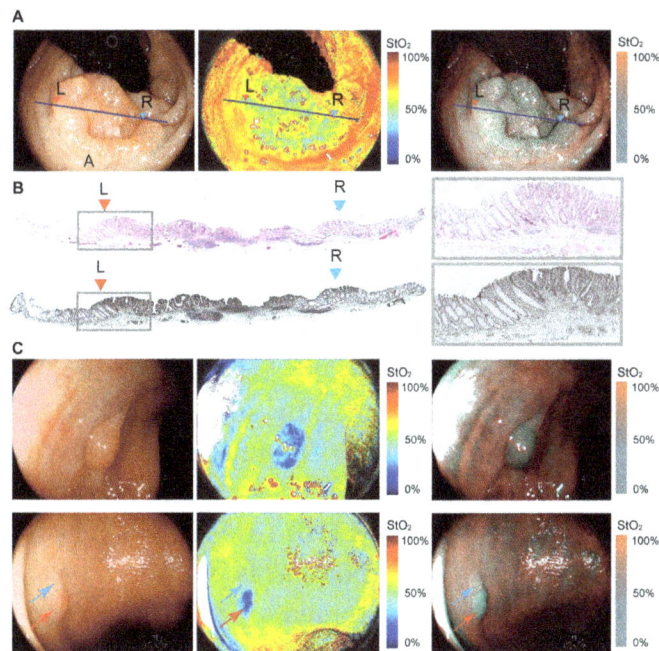

Figure 2. StO_2 maps obtained in human subject research. (A) White light image by endoscopic observation in rectal adenocarcinoma (left). Line (L-R) corresponds to cross section of pathological diagnosis. StO_2 map visualized by laser endoscope system (middle: pseudocolor StO_2 image; right: StO_2 overlay image). (B) Cross-sectional appearance stained with H&E (upper) and HIF1 alpha antibody (lower) corresponding to the hypoxic area visualized with StO_2 map. (C) Endoscopic images of a colorectal adenoma (upper) showing clear hypoxia: white light image (upper left), pseudocolor StO_2 map (upper middle) and overlayed image (upper right). Another case of a colonic lesion (lower) consisting of an adenoma (red arrow) and a hyperplasia (blue arrow): white light image (lower left), pseudocolor StO_2 map (lower middle) and overlayed image (lower right). Only the adenoma was detected as hypoxia.

6. Indirect hypoxia evaluation

Proteins and genes whose expression is associated with hypoxia have potential as endogenous molecular markers of hypoxia and have been explored over the years; meanwhile, hypoxia-specific agents have also been explored and shown to be useful in monitoring hypoxia [88]. Immunohistochemical (IHC) staining for hypoxia marker adducts in situ is also available to provide indirect quantitative information on the relative oxygenation of tissue at a cellular resolution. IHC approaches have a role to play particularly *in vitro* studies, including assays of human biopsy specimens. Given the complex biology of tumor hypoxia for which no single marker is expected to have a strong prognostic power in clinical practice, efforts have been directed toward combining various markers to create a prognostic profile of hypoxia [89].

6.1. Hypoxia-inducible factor 1

Optical imaging has had an important role to play in evaluating hypoxia, especially in biopsy specimens. With the introduction of transgenes with the hypoxia responsive element as promoter sequences coupled to reporter genes, e.g., luciferase reporter gene [90, 91] or green fluorescent protein (GFP) [92], a number of modalities have been developed to allow HIF-1 activity to be directly measured. Of these, a HIF-1-dependent promoter-regulated luciferase reporter gene, shown to produce a 100-fold increased luciferase response to hypoxia, has been used to evaluate anti-hypoxia therapy for its efficacy in animals [93]. Again, an imaging probe has been developed for HIF-1-active cells using a PTD-ODD fusion protein. given that, being involved in the same ODD control as HIF-1α, PTD-ODD fusion proteins are thought likely to be co-localized with HIF-1α [93–96]. First developed as a model probe, PTD-ODD-enhanced GFP-labeled with near-infrared fluorescent dye Cy5.5 was shown to permeate cell membrane with high efficiency, with its stability controlled in an oxygen concentration-dependent manner; to accumulate in hypoxic tumor cells with HIF-1 activity, thus allowing the hypoxic tumor cells with HIF-1 activity to be imaged in contrast to the surrounding cells under aerobic conditions [96]. Bioluminescence imaging has also been used to noninvasively depict HIF-1α as it is upregulated *in vivo* following chemotherapy, suggesting that this modality may prove useful in the evaluation of emerging anti-HIF-1 therapeutics [97]. While these imaging tools have a role to play in elucidating the biology of hypoxia and mechanisms of tumor response to therapy, heterogeneous gene responses to HIF-1 pose challenges to these HIF-1-targeted modalities. Furthermore, only weak correlation has been shown between HIF-1α expression and oxygen electrode or PET imaging measurements [98, 99], thus throwing in doubt the value of HIF-1α quantification as a measure of hypoxia.

6.2. Carbonic anhydrase IX

Downstream of HIF-1, carbonic anhydrase 9 (CA IX), a member of the CA family known to exist in cytosolic, membrane-associated, mitochondrial, and secreted carbonic anhydrases (CAs), may represent an alternative target [100]. A membrane-associated enzyme involved in the respiratory gas exchange and acid-base balance, CA IX is shown to be found less abundantly in normal tissue and only in gastric mucosa, small intestine, and muscle. Under hypoxic conditions, CA IX is shown to be overexpressed in different types of cancer [101], with the staining pattern shown to be more generalized in VHL-associated tumors and focal-perinecrotic in non-VHL-associated tumors [102].

CA IX has been imaged with fluorescent-labeled sulfonamides in a tumor xenograft model to allow hypoxic and (re)-oxygenated cells to be distinguished [103], which demonstrated that CA IX required exposure to hypoxia for its binding and retention—a finding confirmed by an *in vivo* imaging study [103]. In renal-cell carcinoma xenografts, a G250 monoclonal antibody against CA IX was shown to significantly inhibit tumor growth [104]. Again, phase II clinical trials employed G250-based radioimmunoimaging to detect primary and metastatic lesions as well as to guide radioimmunotherapy after labeling G250 with therapeutic radioisotopes, which included ^{177}Lu, ^{90}Y, or ^{186}Re [105]. High-affinity human monoclonal antibodies (A3 and CC7) specific to human CA IX were developed using phage display technology [106] and these reagents may have a role to play in a wide range of settings, including noninvasive imaging of hypoxia and drug delivery [106]. In this regard, combining CA IX and a proliferation marker may prove helpful in identifying proliferating cells under hypoxic conditions [107, 108], while no correlation is shown between the amount of CA IX and direct oxygen measurement with a needle electrode [109].

Furthermore, hypoxia markers have been identified and shown to be induced by hypoxia and expressed in human tumors, including VEGF and GLUTs, both of which are upregulated by increased activity of HIF-1 under hypoxic conditions [110]. Imaging strategies targeting these proteins have also been explored for their ability to assess tumor vasculature and proliferation, while the relationship between pO_2 values and protein expression levels remains unclear [111].

7. Heterogeneity of tumor

Tissue oxygenation is shown to be highly heterogeneous due to the presence of both highly oxygenated arterial vascular regions and poorly oxygenated tissues and cells. Spatial and temporal heterogeneity also contribute to the complexity of the issue. Heterogeneity is thus a major factor in hypoxia measurement that affects our ability to stratify patients and predict outcomes using the imaging technologies available, and its biological implications need to be further explored, and effective approaches to assessing heterogeneity remain to be established. Hypoxia imaging endoscopy allowed early cancers of the pharynx, esophagus, stomach, and colorectum to be captured in whole for the first time [87], with no heterogeneity found in nearly all early cancers or colorectal neoplasia detected. Given that tissue heterogeneity may vary between early, advanced, and metastatic tumors, however, it remains crucial to elucidate tissue heterogeneity as it is associated with tumor progression.

8. Future of hypoxia measuring methods

Given the wide variety of techniques available for assessing hypoxia, e.g., polarographic needle electrodes, IHC staining, PET, MRI, optical imaging with NIR fluorescence or bioluminescence, visible light spectroscopy, and hypoxia imaging endoscopy, it remains critically important to determine their relative advantages and disadvantages for clinical application. Improvements in hypoxia measuring techniques will hinge primarily on which techniques are chosen and how these techniques are applied in the clinic. Clearly, the best of these are expected to be sensitive to the biological sequel of hypoxia, and the ideal one expected to be clinically safe, readily available, minimally invasive, and free from radiation exposure, while at the same time providing high resolution and ease of use. In addition, NIR over 1000 nm wavelength, the so-called biological window, will be promising, because this wavelength area is good for tissue permeability due to reducing both light scattering and infrared absorption [112].

In the endoscopic fields of alimentary tracts, the existing diagnosis for neoplasia is based on the morphologic features of the tumor. However, imaging of a tumor focused on its function or metabolism yields a novel set of data. Hypoxia imaging endoscope system equipped with a laser source allows oxygen saturation to be shown with two types of overlay and pseudocolor images displayed one on top of the other [87]. Available for handling similarly to conventional endoscopy, this modality is easy to treat with and completely safe without being invasive. Of the large number of patients with cancers in the alimentary tract, such as oral cavity, esophagus, stomach, and colorectum in the world, a majority with advanced cancer patients receives chemotherapy, radiotherapy, and combination therapy. In this regard, this modality is expected to allow not only hypoxic states but also hyperoxic states of tumor to be detected in these patients, thus contributing to selection of therapy or drug as well as evaluation of their therapeutic efficacy. Furthermore, this modality will serve as a screening method facilitating detection of early cancer. Advances in research into hypoxia and intratumoral microvessels of tumor with this endoscopic modality are expected and lead to development of new drugs. Thus, the proposed laser source-equipped hypoxia endoscope system appears to have the potential to redraw the endoscopic landscape.

9. Conclusions and perspectives

Tumor hypoxia assessment allows cancer patients to be followed up early after treatment initiation and drug resistance and radioresistance to be predicted. Current insights into the molecular mechanisms of hypoxia have indeed led to novel probes being developed for noninvasive imaging of hypoxia. Again, real-time hypoxic imaging in digestive endoscopy was obtained using such laser light as remains within visible light wavelengths, with no use of any probes. For innovation of endoscopy, it was elucidated that most of all early cancers and precursor lesions have already been to hypoxic state. This is a cutting edge finding. This imaging technology highlights a novel aspect of cancer biology as a potential biomarker which may come to be widely used in cancer diagnosis and treatment effect prediction. These approaches appear to have great promise and further studies on the predictive value of hypoxia measurement in tumors may help identify independent predictive marker of hypoxia as well as optimal parameters for assessing hypoxia. It remains to be clarified whether these new agents may help reduce hypoxic disease or whether they are available for hypoxia imaging.

Author details

Kazuhiro Kaneko[1], Hiroshi Yamaguchi[2] and Tomonori Yano[1*]

*Address all correspondence to: toyano@east.ncc.go.jp

1 Division of Science and Technology for Endoscopy, National Cancer Center Hospital East, Chiba, Japan

2 Imaging Technology Center, FUJIFILM Corporation, Tokyo, Japan

References

[1] Vaupel P, Mayer A (2007) Hypoxia in cancer: significance and impact on clinical outcome. Cancer Metastasis Rev 26:225–239

[2] Fukumura D, Jain RK (2007) Tumor microvasculature and microenvironment: targets for anti-angiogenesis and normalization. Microvasc Res 74:72–84

[3] Vaupel P, Mayer A, Hockel M (2004) Tumor hypoxia and malignant progression. Methods Enzymol 381:335–354

[4] Gray LH, Conger AD, Ebert M, Hornsey S, Scott OCA (1953) The concentration of oxygen dissolved in tissues at the time of irradiation as a factor in radiotherapy. Br J Radiol 26:638–648

[5] Matthews NE, Adams MA, Maxwell LR, Gofton TE, Graham CH (2001) Nitric oxide-mediated regulation of chemosensitivity in cancer cells. J Natl Cancer Inst 93:1879–1885

[6] Nordsmark M, Bentzen SM, Rudat V et al (2005) Prognostic value of tumor oxygenation in 397 head and neck tumors after primary radiation therapy. An international multi-center study. Radiother Oncol 77:18–24

[7] Brizel DM, Sibley GS, Prosnitz LR, Scher RL, Dewhirst MW (1997) Tumor hypoxia adversely affects the prognosis of carcinoma of the head and neck. Int J Radiat Oncol Biol Phys 38:285–289

[8]   Hockel M, Vorndran B, Schlenger K, Baussmann E, Knapstein PG (1993) Tumor oxygenation: a new predictive parameter in locally advanced cancer of the uterine cervix. Gynecol Oncol 51:141–149

[9]   Nordsmark M, Loncaster J, Chou SC et al (2001) Invasive oxygen measurements and pimonidazole labeling in human cervix carcinoma. Int J Radiat Oncol Biol Phys 49:581–586

[10] Nordsmark M, Overgaard J (2000) A confirmatory prognostic study on oxygenation status and loco-regional control in advanced head and neck squamous cell carcinoma treated by radiation therapy. Radiother Oncol 57:39–43

[11] Evans SM, Judy KD, Dunphy I et al (2004) Hypoxia is important in the biology and aggression of human glial brain tumors. Clin Cancer Res 10:8177–8184

[12] Powell ME, Collingridge DR, Saunders MI et al (1999) Improvement in human tumour oxygenation with carbogen of varying carbon dioxide concentrations. Radiother Oncol 50:167–171

[13] Gatenby RA, Moldofsky PJ, Weiner LM (1988) Metastatic colon cancer: correlation of oxygen levels with I-131 F(ab')2 uptake. Radiology 166:757–759

[14] Brizel DM, Scully SP, Harrelson JM et al (1996) Radiation therapy and hyperthermia improve the oxygenation of human soft tissue sarcomas. Cancer Res 56:5347–5350

[15] Pauwels EK, Mariani G (2007) Assessment of tumor tissue oxygenation: agents, methods and clinical significance. Drug News Perspect 20:619–626

[16] Massoud TF, Gambhir SS (2007) Integrating noninvasive molecular imaging into molecular medicine: an evolving paradigm. Trends Mol Med 13:183–191

[17] Willmann JK, van Bruggen N, Dinkelborg LM, Gambhir SS (2008) Molecular imaging in drug development. Nat Rev Drug Discov 7:591–607

[18] Swartz HM, Clarkson RB (1998) The measurement of oxygen *in vivo* using EPR techniques. Phys Med Biol 43:1957–1975

[19] Matsumoto K, English S, Yoo J et al (2004) Pharmacokinetics of a triarylmethyl-type paramagnetic spin probe used in EPR oximetry. Magn Reson Med 52:885–892

[20] Krohn KA, Link JM, Mason RP (2008) Molecular imaging of hypoxia. J Nucl Med 49(Suppl 2):129S–148S

[21] Wang X, Xie X, Ku G, Wang LV, Stoica G (2006) Noninvasive imaging of hemoglobin concentration and oxygenation in the rat brain using high-resolution photoacoustic tomography. J Biomed Opt 11:024015

[22] Padhani A (2010) Science to practice: what does MR oxygenation imaging tell us about human breast cancer hypoxia? Radiology 254:1–3

[23] Howe FA, Robinson SP, McIntyre DJ, Stubbs M, Griffiths JR (2001) Issues in flow and oxygenation dependent contrast (FLOOD) imaging of tumours. NMR Biomed 14:497–506

[24] Stubbs M (1999) Application of magnetic resonance techniques for imaging tumour physiology. Acta Oncol 38:845–853

[25] Tumkur SM, Vu AT, Li LP, Pierchala L, Prasad PV (2006) Evaluation of intra-renal oxygenation during water diuresis: a time-resolved study using BOLD MRI. Kidney Int 70:139–143

[26] O'Connor JP, Naish JH, Parker GJ et al (2009) Preliminary study of oxygen-enhanced longitudinal relaxation in MRI: a potential novel biomarker of oxygenation changes in solid tumors. Int J Radiat Oncol Biol Phys 75:1209–1215

[27] Mason RP (2006) Non-invasive assessment of kidney oxygenation: a role for BOLD MRI. Kidney Int 70:10–11

[28] Thomas SR, Pratt RG, Millard RW et al (1996) *In vivo* PO_2 imaging in the porcine model with perfluorocarbon F-19 NMR at low field. Magn Reson Imaging 14:103–114

[29] Mason RP, Shukla H, Antich PP (1993) *In vivo* oxygen tension and temperature: simultaneous determination using 19F NMR spectroscopy of perfluorocarbon. Magn Reson Med 29:296–302

[30] Zhao D, Ran S, Constantinescu A, Hahn EW, Mason RP (2003) Tumor oxygen dynamics: correlation of *in vivo* MRI with histological findings. Neoplasia 5:308–318

[31] van der Sanden BP, Heerschap A, Simonetti AW et al Characterization and validation of noninvasive oxygen tension measurements in human glioma xenografts by 19F-MR relaxometry. Int J Radiat Oncol Biol Phys 44:649–658

[32] McNab JA, Yung AC, Kozlowski P (2004) Tissue oxygen tension measurements in the Shionogi model of prostate cancer using 19F MRS and MRI. Magma 17:288–295

[33] Davda S, Bezabeh T (2006) Advances in methods for assessing tumor hypoxia *in vivo*: implications for treatment planning. Cancer Metastasis Rev 25:469–480

[34] Yu JX, Kodibagkar VD, Cui W, Mason RP (2005) 19F: a versatile reporter for non-invasive physiology and pharmacology using magnetic resonance. Curr Med Chem 12:819–848

[35] Hunjan S, Zhao D, Constantinescu A et al (2001) Tumor oximetry: demonstration of an enhanced dynamic mapping procedure using fluorine-19 echo planar magnetic resonance imaging in the Dunning prostate R3327-AT1 rat tumor. Int J Radiat Oncol Biol Phys 49:1097–1108

[36] Emblem KE, Mouridsen K, Bjornerud A et al (2013) Vessel architectural imaging identifies cancer patient responders to anti-angiogenic therapy. Nat Med; doi:10.1038/nm.3289

[37]   Batchelor TT, Sorensen AG, di Tomaso E et al (2007) AZD2171, a pan-VEGF receptor tyrosine kinase inhibitor, normalizes tumor vasculature and alleviates edema in glioblastoma patients. Cancer Cell 11:83–95

[38]   Rasey JS, Koh WJ, Evans ML et al (1996) Quantifying regional hypoxia in human tumors with positron emission tomography of [18F] fluoromisonidazole: a pretherapy study of 37 patients. Int J Radiat Oncol Biol Phys 36:417–428

[39]   Lehtio K, Eskola O, Viljanen T et al (2004) Imaging perfusion and hypoxia with PET to predict radiotherapy response in head-and-neck cancer. Int J Radiat Oncol Biol Phys 59:971–982

[40]   Souvatzoglou M, Grosu AL, Roper B et al (2007) Tumour hypoxia imaging with [18F] FAZA PET in head and neck cancer patients: a pilot study. Eur J Nucl Med Mol Imaging 34:1566–1575

[41]   Koh WJ, Rasey JS, Evans ML et al (1992) Imaging of hypoxia in human tumors with [F-18] fluoromisonidazole. Int J Radiat Oncol Biol Phys 22:199–212

[42]   Lee ST, Scott AM (2007) Hypoxia positron emission tomography imaging with 18f-fluoromisonidazole. Semin Nucl Med 37:451–461

[43]   Gagel B, Reinartz P, Demirel C et al (2006) [18F] fluoromisonidazole and [18F] fluoro-deoxyglucose positron emission tomography in response evaluation after chemo-/radiotherapy of non-small-cell lung cancer: a feasibility study. BMC Cancer 6:51

[44]   Eschmann SM, Paulsen F, Reimold M et al (2005) Prognostic impact of hypoxia imaging with 18F-misonidazole PET in non-small cell lung cancer and head and neck cancer before radiotherapy. J Nucl Med 46:253–260

[45]   Rajendran JG, Mankoff DA, O'Sullivan F et al (2004) Hypoxia and glucose metabolism in malignant tumors: evaluation by [18F] fluoromisonidazole and [18F] fluorodeoxy-glucose positron emission tomography imaging. Clin Cancer Res 10:2245–2252

[46]   Koh WJ, Bergman KS, Rasey JS et al (1995) Evaluation of oxygenation status during fractionated radiotherapy in human nonsmall cell lung cancers using [F-18] fluoromi-sonidazole positron emission tomography. Int J Radiat Oncol Biol Phys 33:391–398

[47]   Rajendran JG, Wilson DC, Conrad EU et al (2003) [18F] FMISO and [18F] FDG PET imaging in soft tissue sarcomas: correlation of hypoxia, metabolism and VEGF expression. Eur J Nucl Med Mol Imaging 30:695–704

[48]   Bentzen L, Keiding S, Nordsmark M et al (2003) Tumour oxygenation assessed by 18F-fluoromisonidazole PET and polarographic needle electrodes in human soft tissue tumours. Radiother Oncol 67:339–344

[49]   Lehtio K, Oikonen V, Gronroos T et al (2001) Imaging of blood flow and hypoxia in head and neck cancer: initial evaluation with [15O] H_2O and [18F] fluoroerythronitroi-midazole PET. J Nucl Med 42:1643–1652

[50] Yang DJ, Wallace S, Cherif A et al (1995) Development of F-18-labeled fluoroerythro-nitroimidazole as a PET agent for imaging tumor hypoxia. Radiology 194:795–800

[51] Barthel H, Wilson H, Collingridge DR et al (2004) *In vivo* evaluation of [18F] fluoroeta-nidazole as a new marker for imaging tumour hypoxia with positron emission tomography. Br J Cancer 90:2232–2242

[52] Ziemer LS, Evans SM, Kachur AV et al (2003) Noninvasive imaging of tumor hypoxia in rats using the 2-nitroimidazole 18F-EF5. Eur J Nucl Med Mol Imaging 30:259–266

[53] Evans SM, Kachur AV, Shiue CY et al (2000) Noninvasive detection of tumor hypoxia using the 2-nitroimidazole [18F] EF1. J Nucl Med 41:327–336

[54] Komar G, Seppanen M, Eskola O et al (2008) 18F-EF5: a new PET tracer for imaging hypoxia in head and neck cancer. J Nucl Med 49:1944–1951

[55] Evans SM, Fraker D, Hahn SM et al (2006) EF5 binding and clinical outcome in human soft tissue sarcomas. Int J Radiat Oncol Biol Phys 64:922–927

[56] Kumar P, Emami S, Kresolek Z et al (2009) Synthesis and hypoxia selective radiosen-sitization potential of beta-2-FAZA and beta-3-FAZL: fluorinated azomycin beta-nucleosides. Med Chem 5:118–129

[57] Postema EJ, McEwan AJ, Riauka TA et al (2009) Initial results of hypoxia imaging using 1-alpha-D: -(5-deoxy-5-[18F]-fluoroarabinofuranosyl)-2-nitroimidazole (18F-FAZA). Eur J Nucl Med Mol Imaging 36:1565–1573

[58] Rumsey WL, Vanderkooi JM, Wilson DF (1988) Imaging of phosphorescence: a novel method for measuring oxygen distribution in perfused tissue. Science 241:1649–1651

[59] Vinogradov SA, Grosul P, Rozhkov V et al (2003) Oxygen distributions in tissue measured by phosphorescence quenching. Adv Exp Med Biol 510:181–185

[60] Lebedev AY, Cheprakov AV, Sakadzic S et al (2009) Dendritic phosphorescent probes for oxygen imaging in biological systems. ACS Appl Mater Interfaces 1:1292–1304

[61] Pennekamp CW, Bots ML, Kappelle LJ, Moll FL, de Borst GJ (2009) The value of near-infrared spectroscopy measured cerebral oximetry during carotid endarterectomy in perioperative stroke prevention. A review. Eur J Vasc Endovasc Surg 38:539–545

[62] Jobsis FF (1977) Non-invasive, infra-red monitoring of cerebral O_2 sufficiency, blood volume, HbO_2-Hb shifts and blood flow. Acta Neurol Scand Suppl 64:452–453

[63] Hull EL, Conover DL, Foster TH (1999) Carbogen-induced changes in rat mammary tumour oxygenation reported by near infrared spectroscopy. Br J Cancer 79:1709–1716

[64] Kim JG, Liu H (2008) Investigation of biphasic tumor oxygen dynamics induced by hyperoxic gas intervention: the dynamic phantom approach. Appl Opt 47:242–252

[65] Barry BN, Mallick A, Bodenham AR, Vucevic M (1997) Lack of agreement between bioimpedance and continuous thermodilution measurement of cardiac output in intensive care unit patients. Crit Care 1:71–74

[66] Imhoff M, Lehner JH, Lohlein D (2000) Noninvasive whole-body electrical bioimpedance cardiac output and invasive thermodilution cardiac output in high-risk surgical patients. Crit Care Med 28:2812–2818

[67] Kurth CD, Steven JM, Benaron D, Chance B (1993) Near-infrared monitoring of the cerebral circulation. J Clin Monit 9:163–170

[68] Watkin SL, Spencer SA, Dimmock PW, Wickramasinghe YA, Rolfe P (1999) A comparison of pulse oximetry and near infrared spectroscopy (NIRS) in the detection of hypoxaemia occurring with pauses in nasal airflow in neonates. J Clin Monit Comput 15:441–447

[69] El-Desoky AE, Jiao LR, Havlik R, Habib N, Davidson BR, Seifalian AM (2000) Measurement of hepatic tissue hypoxia using near infrared spectroscopy: comparison with hepatic vein oxygen partial pressure. Eur Surg Res 32:207–214

[70] Fortune PM, Wagstaff M, Petros AJ (2001) Cerebro-splanchnic oxygenation ratio (CSOR) using near infrared spectroscopy may be able to predict splanchnic ischaemia in neonates. Intensive Care Med 27:1401–1407

[71] Fukui D, Urayama H, Tanaka K, Kawasaki S (2002) Use of near-infrared spectroscopic measurement at the buttocks during abdominal aortic surgery. Circ J 66:1128–1131

[72] DeBlasi RA, Quaglia E, Gasparetto A, Ferrari M (1992) Muscle oxygenation by fast near infrared spectrophotometry (NIRS) in ischemic forearm. Adv Exp Med Biol 316:163–172

[73] Shin'oka T, Nollert G, Shum-Tim D, du Plessis A, Jonas RA (2000) Utility of near-infrared spectroscopic measurements during deep hypothermic circulatory arrest. Ann Thorac Surg 69:578–583

[74] Vernieri F, Rosato N, Pauri F, Tibuzzi F, Passarelli F, Rossini PM (1999) Near infrared spectroscopy and transcranial Doppler in monohemispheric stroke. Eur Neurol 41:159–162

[75] Kurth CD, Steven JL, Montenegro LM, Watzman HM, Gaynor JW, Spray TL, Nicolson SC (2001) Cerebral oxygen saturation before congenital heart surgery. Ann Thorac Surg 72:187–192

[76] Misra M, Stark J, Dujovny M, Widman R, Ausman JI (1998) Transcranial cerebral oximetry in random normal subjects. Neurol Res 20:137–141

[77] Marik PE (2001) Sublingual capnography: A clinical validation study. Chest 120:923–27

[78] Povoas HP, Weil MH, Tang W, Sun S, Kamohara T, Bisera J (2001) Decreases in mesenteric blood flow associated with increases in sublingual pCO_2 during hemorrhagic shock. Shock 15:398–402

[79] Know, now. Sublingual CO_2. CapnoProbe Sublingual (SL) System brochure. Pleasanton, California, Nellcor Puritan Bennett, 2002, p 4

[80] Movsas B, Chapman JD, Hanlon AL, Horwitz EM, Pinover WH, Greenberg RE, Stobbe C, Hanks GE (2001) Hypoxia in human prostate carcinoma: An Eppendorf PO_2 study. Am J Clin Oncol 24:458–461

[81] Benaron DA, Parachikov IH, Friedland S et al (2004) Continuous, noninvasive, and localized microvascular tissue oximetry using visible light spectroscopy. Anesthesiology 100(6)

[82] Brun NC, Moen A, Borch K, Saugstad OD, Greisen G (1997) Near-infrared monitoring of cerebral tissue oxygen saturation and blood volume in newborn piglets. Am J Physiol 273(part 2):H682–H686

[83] Watzman HM, Kurth CD, Montenegro LM, Rome J, Steven JM, Nicolson SC (2000) Arterial and venous contributions to near-infrared cerebral oximetry. Anesthesiology 93:947–953

[84] Fantini S (2002) A haemodynamic model for the physiological interpretation of *in vivo* measurements of the concentration and oxygen saturation of haemoglobin. Phys Med Biol 47:N249–N257

[85] Maxim PG, Carson JJ, Benaron DA et al (2005) Optical detection of tumors *in vivo* by light tissue oximetry. Technol Cancer Res Treat 4:227–234.

[86] Noord DV, Sana A, Benaron DA et al (2011) Endoscopic visible light spectroscopy: a new, minimally invasive technique to diagnose chronic GI ischemia. Gastrointest Endosc 73:291–298

[87] Kaneko K, Yamaguchi H, Saito T et al (2014) Hypoxia imaging endoscopy equipped with laser light source from preclinical live animal study to first-in-human subject research. PLoS One 9(6):e99055. doi:10.1371/journal.pone.0099055

[88] Bussink J, Kaanders JH, van der Kogel AJ (2003) Tumor hypoxia at the micro-regional level: clinical relevance and predictive value of exogenous and endogenous hypoxic cell markers. Radiother Oncol 67:3–15

[89] Koukourakis MI, Bentzen SM, Giatromanolaki A et al (2006) Endogenous markers of two separate hypoxia response pathways (hypoxia inducible factor 2 alpha and carbonic anhydrase 9) are associated with radiotherapy failure in head and neck cancer patients recruited in the CHART randomized trial. J Clin Oncol 24:727–735

[90] Shibata T, Giaccia AJ, Brown JM (2000) Development of a hypoxia-responsive vector for tumor-specific gene therapy. Gene Ther 7:493–498

[91]   Payen E, Bettan M, Henri A et al (2001) Oxygen tension and a pharmacological switch in the regulation of transgene expression for gene therapy. J Gene Med 3:498–504

[92]   Vordermark D, Shibata T, Brown JM (2001) Green fluorescent protein is a suitable reporter of tumor hypoxia despite an oxygen requirement for chromophore formation. Neoplasia 3:527–534

[93]   Harada H, Kizaka-Kondoh S, Hiraoka M (2005) Optical imaging of tumor hypoxia and evaluation of efficacy of a hypoxia-targeting drug in living animals. Mol Imaging 4:182–193

[94]   Harada H, Hiraoka M, Kizaka-Kondoh S (2002) Antitumor effect of TAT-oxygen-dependent degradation-caspase-3 fusion protein specifically stabilized and activated in hypoxic tumor cells. Cancer Res 62:2013–2018

[95]   Harada H, Kizaka-Kondoh S, Hiraoka M (2006) Mechanism of hypoxia-specific cytotoxicity of procaspase-3 fused with a VHL-mediated protein destruction motif of HIF-1alpha containing Pro564. FEBS Lett 580:5718–5722

[96]   Harada H, Kizaka-Kondoh S, Li G et al (2007) Significance of HIF-1-active cells in angiogenesis and radioresistance. Oncogene 26:7508–7516

[97]   Viola RJ, Provenzale JM, Li F et al (2008) *In vivo* bioluminescence imaging monitoring of hypoxia-inducible factor 1alpha, a promoter that protects cells, in response to chemotherapy. AJR Am J Roentgenol 191:1779–1784

[98]   Mayer A, Wree A, Hockel M et al (2004) Lack of correlation between expression of HIF-1alpha protein and oxygenation status in identical tissue areas of squamous cell carcinomas of the uterine cervix. Cancer Res 64:5876–5881

[99]   Lehmann S, Stiehl DP, Honer M et al (2009) Longitudinal and multimodal *in vivo* imaging of tumor hypoxia and its downstream molecular events. Proc Natl Acad Sci USA 106:14004–14009

[100] Potter CP, Harris AL (2003) Diagnostic, prognostic and therapeutic implications of carbonic anhydrases in cancer. Br J Cancer 89:2–7

[101] Ivanov S, Liao SY, Ivanova A et al (2001) Expression of hypoxia-inducible cell-surface transmembrane carbonic anhydrases in human cancer. Am J Pathol 158:905–919

[102] Wykoff CC, Beasley NJ, Watson PH et al Hypoxia-inducible expression of tumor-associated carbonic anhydrases. Cancer Res 60:7075–7083

[103] Dubois L, Lieuwes NG, Maresca A et al (2009) Imaging of CA IX with fluorescent labelled sulfonamides distinguishes hypoxic and (re)-oxygenated cells in a xenograft tumour model. Radiother Oncol 92:423–428

[104] van Dijk J, Uemura H, Beniers AJ et al Therapeutic effects of monoclonal antibody G250, interferons and tumor necrosis factor, in mice with renal-cell carcinoma xenografts. Int J Cancer 56:262–268

[105] Stillebroer AB, Oosterwijk E, Oyen WJ, Mulders PF, Boerman OC (2007) Radiolabeled antibodies in renal cell carcinoma. Cancer Imaging 7:179–188

[106] Ahlskog JK, Schliemann C, Marlind J et al (2009) Human monoclonal antibodies targeting carbonic anhydrase IX for the molecular imaging of hypoxic regions in solid tumours. Br J Cancer 101:645–657

[107] Hoogsteen IJ, Marres HA, Wijffels KI et al (2005) Colocalization of carbonic anhydrase 9 expression and cell proliferation in human head and neck squamous cell carcinoma. Clin Cancer Res 11:97–106

[108] Kim SJ, Shin HJ, Jung KY et al (2007) Prognostic value of carbonic anhydrase IX and Ki-67 expression in squamous cell carcinoma of the tongue. Jpn J Clin Oncol 37:812–819

[109] Mayer A, Hockel M, Vaupel P (2005) Carbonic anhydrase IX expression and tumor oxygenation status do not correlate at the microregional level in locally advanced cancers of the uterine cervix. Clin Cancer Res 11:7220–7225

[110] Macheda ML, Rogers S, Best JD (2005) Molecular and cellular regulation of glucose transporter (GLUT) proteins in cancer. J Cell Physiol 202:654–662

[111] Jonathan RA, Wijffels KI, Peeters W et al (2006) The prognostic value of endogenous hypoxia-related markers for head and neck squamous cell carcinomas treated with ARCON. Radiother Oncol 79:288–297

[112] Anderson RR, Parrish JA (1981) The optics of human skin. J Invest Dermat 77:13–19

5

Arterial Oxygen Saturation During Ascent to 5010 m: Heart Rate and AMS Scores

Christopher B. Wolff, Annabel H. Nickol and

David J. Collier

Abstract

The hypothesis here is that tissues exposed to the hypoxia of altitude have increased blood flow so that the rate of arrival of oxygen is as rapid as normal. If the ascent is too rapid, the system starts to fail. The study involves an ascent to high altitude (5010 m) during which 59 subjects recorded their resting arterial oxygen saturation (SaO_2), heart rate (HR) and Lake Louise acute mountain sickness (AMS) scores, twice daily. During the major ascent SaO_2 fell progressively. In 42 subjects, HR increased in a highly significant, negative, relationship to SaO_2. In 10 subjects heart rate (HR) remained unchanged. Three subjects showed extreme HR variability. Data were incomplete in four subjects. For nine of the subjects, showing the progressive HR versus SaO_2 correlation during ascent, the sequence terminated with a lower HR than would be expected from the correlation so far. Individual AMS scores showed no correlation with SaO_2 but averaged values from 19 of the subjects from each 'one night' stopover; showed a strong, negative, correlation. Average stopover HR values correlated negatively with the average SaO_2 values. Cardiac output (CO) is likely to have increased during ascent as HR increased, since there is a progressive relationship between HR and cardiac output (CO). Hence, despite the progressive fall in SaO_2, tissue oxygen delivery (DO_2) would have remained close to normal in the 42 subjects who showed the significant HR: SaO_2 relationship.

Keywords: high altitude, SaO_2, heart rate, acute mountain sickness, oxygen delivery

1. Introduction

During ascent to high altitude, the fractional concentration of oxygen in the atmospheric gas is unchanged but overall barometric pressure falls. This means that there are less oxygen molecules per unit volume, so the activity, or oxygen partial pressure, falls. Breathing will only compensate for this, with a closer approach to normal concentration of oxygen in the blood (known as 'content,' CaO_2), if it is increased. Initially, lowered oxygen in the lung and hence in the blood causes blood flow to the brain to increase, washing out carbon dioxide (CO_2) from the brain environment. The increase in blood flow allows the rate of arrival of oxygen at the brain to normalize, the higher flow compensating for the lower CaO_2. So the rate of arrival of oxygen (oxygen delivery, DO_2) is sustained at or near the normal rate—three times the rate of cerebral oxygen consumption cerebral metabolic rate for oxygen, $CMRO_2$ [1]. However, the lower CO_2 in the brain, and resulting alkalinity, inhibits breathing via the central chemoreceptor, counteracting the stimulating effect of low oxygen at the peripheral arterial chemoreceptor. There is therefore an initial pause in ventilatory stimulation. Over 2–5 days, for a subject remaining at the same altitude, brain inhibition is removed as acidity is corrected. This restores the central chemoreceptor level of respiratory stimulus (removal of inhibition). So now the ventilatory stimulus from the peripheral arterial chemoreceptor activity stimulates ventilation, with improvement in the arterial oxygen level [1]. Since these effects are operating at the same time as subjects ascend, with environmental oxygen falling progressively, arterial oxygen content (CaO_2) and oxygen saturation (SaO_2) usually fall progressively during ascent.

Since individual breathing responses (known as ventilatory responses) vary between individuals the progressive drop in CaO_2 also varies between individuals. Most of the oxygen in the blood is carried on hemoglobin in the red cells and low CaO_2 is paralleled by lower arterial oxygen saturation of the hemoglobin (SaO_2). With little change in hemoglobin concentration (Hb) during ascent, SaO_2 therefore provides a guide to CaO_2 change. If there was no change in cardiac output (CO) the rate of oxygen delivery to the tissues ($DO_2 = CO \times CaO_2$) would fall in proportion to the fall in SaO_2. Here we are interested in the possibility that there may be compensatory increases in CO helping to sustain a more normal DO_2. During ascent, the use of a pulse oximeter provides SaO_2 and also gives the heart rate (HR). Cardiac output is equal to stroke volume (SV) times HR, that is, $CO = HR \times SV$. With only modest changes in SV during ascent HR changes can therefore act as a surrogate for CO changes. Increases in HR as SaO_2 falls during ascent would suggest that CO increases too. Increases in CO as SaO_2/CaO_2 fall will mean that there is compensatory response helping to maintain DO_2. It is therefore important to see whether there is a significant HR increase in relation to falling SaO_2 and to see whether this occurs in all or some subjects. Increases in heart rate can therefore be used as an indirect indicator of any cardiac output increase mitigating DO_2 reduction.

In a recent high-altitude study [2], undertaken in South America, eight normal subjects acclimatized to moderately high altitude during an initial 5-day sojourn at Cusco (3324 m). This was followed by two brief ascents to around 5000 m over a 4-week period. The preliminary acclimatization and brief ascents meant the subjects were likely to be less stressed by their hypoxic exposure than occurs with progressive ascents from sea level. Total time at high altitude was 28 days, the largest proportion at Cusco. SaO_2 and HR were recorded twice daily. For seven of the subjects, there was a highly significant relationship between HR and SaO_2, with the highest HR accompanying the lowest SaO_2 value. The remaining subject sustained near normal SaO_2 and HR. HR × SaO_2 (assumed to give a value changing in relation to DO_2) remained near constant throughout the trek in all subjects. Since HR × SaO_2 will have a similar trend to CO × CaO_2, DO_2 will have been well sustained despite the varying degrees of hypoxia. Despite apparently relatively good DO_2 maintenance, for these subjects, individual mean acute mountain sickness (AMS) scores correlated significantly with mean SaO_2 values both at rest and with mild exercise (30 cm step up over 2 min).

In a second high-altitude study, undertaken by 14 schoolboys and their teacher, an ascent was made to Annapurna base camp (4130 m) [3]. There was no preliminary acclimatization and, due to shortage of stopover sites, the final two ascent stages were large. The subjects each recorded SaO_2 and HR soon after arrival at each new altitude both at rest and with mild exercise. Not all subjects showed individually significant HR versus SaO_2 changes, but the overview across subjects (mean values at each altitude) was highly significant both for rest and exercise. Of interest was the fact that, for exercise, HR × SaO_2, otherwise constant, showed a large fall for the last ascent stage and base camp. Anecdotally, most subjects suffered considerable AMS symptoms during the 1 day stop at base camp. A plot of the mean values of HR versus SaO_2 for exercise shows a highly significant trend (**Figure 1**), but the HR value for base camp gives a point lower than expected from the rest of the values trend for HR versus SaO_2. This may well represent a failure of DO_2 compensation.

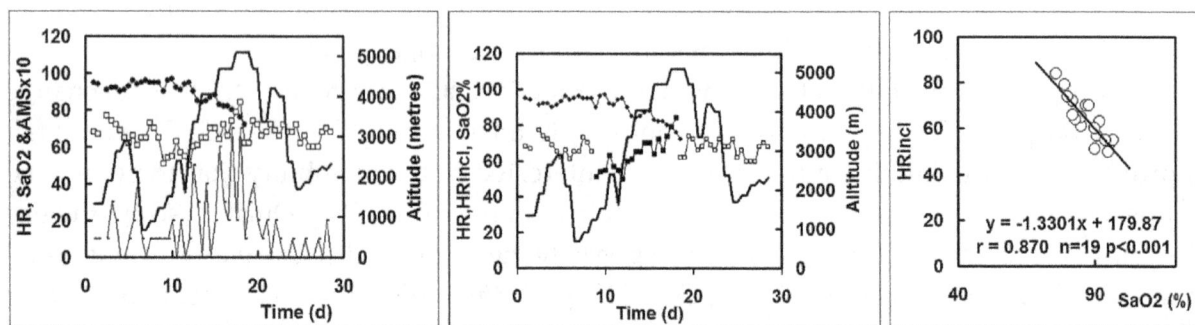

Figure 1. Data from this subject (15) illustrates rising HR during ascent. On the left HR (open squares), SaO_2 (filled circles) and AMS × 10 scores (mini flags) are shown (left hand axis) with altitude (right hand axis, continuous line). The middle plot shows the ascending values of HR as filled squares and omits the AMS scores. The plot on the right shows the ascending HR values plotted against SaO_2—slope significant at the $p < 0.001$ level.

1.1. Reasons why DO_2 control is important

Surprisingly, oxygen combines extreme toxicity with capability to provide energy more efficiently than other biochemical means utilized by other species. The ready conversion of oxygen to dangerous free radicals is largely prevented in our cells by the specific energy-generating biochemical sequences, especially featuring the Krebs cycle. There is an optimum rate at which oxygen flows to a particular tissue and this bears a constant relationship to the rate at which oxygen is utilized (VO_2). Hence, we have values for DO_2/VO_2 which are normally sustained at values specific to the tissue: for the brain 3:1, for heart 1.6:1 and at exercise rates below competitive levels skeletal muscle sustains a ratio 1.5:1 [4]. Maintaining these DO_2 values not only provides sufficient oxygen but also avoids an excess, which would endanger toxicity. Inadequacy of oxygen supply can endanger life following surgery partly from a tendency for an oxygen debt to develop during an operation. This results from reduced arterial pressure since some of the arterial volume escapes into veins relaxed by the anesthesia. The reduced pressure lowers cardiac output so that DO_2 falls, hence development of an oxygen debt [5].

Cerebral arterial blood flow and metabolic rate obtained by Severinghaus et al. [6] were further examined and showed that cerebral oxygen delivery was sustained after ascent to 3100 m, over the next 5 days. There was an initial fall in SaO_2 and compensatory rise in cerebral blood flow. The acclimatization process allowed the initially lowest SaO_2 to improve over the 5 days at altitude [7, 8].

2. Methods

Fifty-nine normal subjects undertook the trek to Kanchenjunga base camp (altitude 5010 m) from Kathmandu (1345 m). The first leg by plane took them to Tumlingtar (470 m) and then they made an initial partial ascent to 2900 m. There was then a descent to 675 m by the 7th day. From there, the rest of the trek (the main ascent) took around 14 days (a conservative ascent profile of just over 300 m per day). Parties of 7–11 subjects set off from Kathmandu separated by a few days. Each group was accompanied by porters and cooks who went ahead each day to prepare the next stopover site. Porters and yaks carried most of the research equipment for other studies and much of the individual luggage, largely housed in individual 60 L barrels. This meant that each subject carried a low-weight 'day pack.' Each subject measured their arterial saturation (SaO_2) and heart rate (HR) using a (Nonin, model 9500, Nonin Medical Inc. MIN, USA) oximeter. The evening measurement was made after at least 5 min rest, seated in the mess tent prior to supper. Readings were made after around 1 min to allow stability. A second measurement of SaO_2 and HR was made in the morning at each stopover site. Again, each measurement was made after at least 5 min rest in the mess tent prior to breakfast. At both morning and evening sessions, each subject filled in individual 'altitude sickness scores' for each of five symptom complexes (head, guts, tired, dizzy, sleep). Each category belongs to the mode of acute mountain sickness (AMS) assessment known as the Lake Louise consensus AMS scoring system [9]. The numerical system requires scores of 0–3 for each category. The AMS score is the total of the values entered in each category. For each category, zero represents no effect and for three, the symptom in the category is severe. Hence, the total possible range, theoretically, for a given score is from 0 to 15. A subject is deemed to be sick, however, with AMS with scores above 3.

3. Results

AMS scores showed no obvious trends during the major ascent for any individual, whereas SaO_2 fell during ascent in all cases (where the data had been recorded—a few subjects omitted variable amounts of data). The heart rate, however, showed an obvious progressively increasing trend in 42 individuals. For 10 subjects, there was no HR change during ascent.

Figure 1 shows a particularly clear example of increasing HR and decreasing SaO_2 for one individual during the major ascent. The AMS score is included in the left-hand panel and omitted in the middle panel, where the square HR symbol during ascent is filled in, to emphasis the progressively increasing HR. In the right-hand panel, HR from the ascent is plotted against SaO_2, showing the highly significant trend in this subject. For the 42 subjects showing increasing HR during ascent and falling SaO_2, individual least squares regression plots (HR versus SaO_2) give significance levels (p values). The degree of the HR versus SaO_2 relationship significance is shown for each subject in **Table 1**, according to the subject's identification number. Nineteen subjects (32%) showed significance at the 0.001 level; 17 (29%) at the 0.01 level and for 6 subjects (10%) significance level was only 0.05. The status for each of the remaining subjects is also shown: four subjects with poor data (very few recorded points or none at all), three subjects with apparently random data (labeled 'variability') and the ten subjects in whom HR was effectively unchanged. **Figure 2** shows HR, SaO_2, AMS score and altitude against time for three of the subjects in whom there was an unchanging HR. The first stopped recording prior to reaching base camp, the second stopped recording at base camp and the third continued, at least HR recording, even during descent.

Significance	Subject No.	Total	Percent
<0.001	1,3,6,8,20,25,26,27,30,32,34,36,40,48, 51,54,55,56,57	19	32
<0.01	4,16,17,21,22,23,24,31,33,35,39,43,45,46,47,50,52	17	29
<0.05	14,28,49,53,58,59	6	10
Ns			29
Poor data	2,5,13,29	4	
Variability	12,18,11	3	
Constant HR	7,9,10,15,19,37,38,41,42,44	10	

Table 1. Listing of all subjects according to (a) whether they showed a significant relationship between HR and SaO_2 during ascent in the upper part of the table ($p < 0.001$, $p < 0.01$ and $p < 0.05$) and (b) those without a significant relationship (poor data, variability or a constant HR).

In the face of any clear individual indication of progress of AMS scores during ascent, it was important to see whether the expected general tendency held good. Mean values for AMS scores and for HR and SaO_2 were calculated for 19 subjects (numbers 1–19) at each altitude. Mean AMS increased progressively with increasing altitude and was significantly related to SaO_2 (**Figure 3**, middle panel). This simply confirms the trend expected with ascent to altitude.

Mean arterial oxygen saturation at each one-night stopover fell progressively during ascent (**Figure 3**, left panel, $SaO_2\% = -0.0043 \times$ altitude (m) + 102.24; $R^2 = 0.972$) though there was considerable variation for the mean values at each stopover site. The error bars show the maximum and minimum individual values.

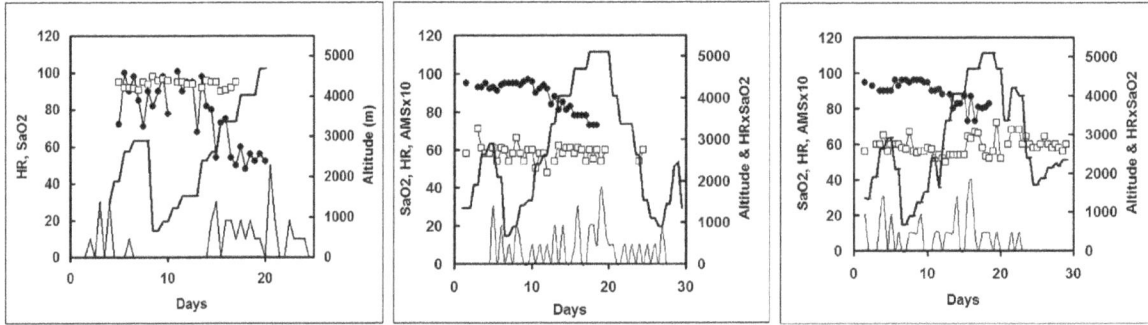

Figure 2. Plots against time of HR (open squares), SaO_2 (filled circles), AMS score (mini-flag) and altitude (continuous line) against time. Each is an example of data from a subject in whom HR remained near constant (subjects, 15, 44 and 38).

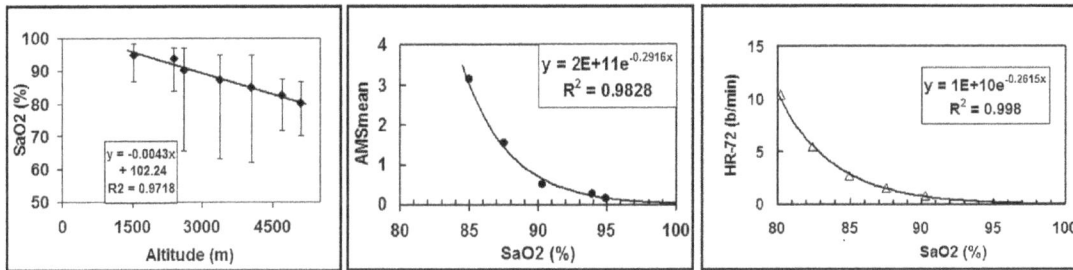

Figure 3. Mean values at each altitude of, $SaO_2\%$, AMS score and HR. The left panel shows SaO_2 against altitude with maximum and minimum values as 'error bars.' The middle panel shows mean AMS score against SaO_2 for one-night stopovers during the major ascent. The right-hand panel shows mean (HR - 72) plotted against $SaO_2\%$ above the first two stopovers of the major ascent. The points are from the lowest altitudes were probably from subjects who were not fully rested).

For mean HR (minus 72 as an assumed normal at sea level), values at each stopover site show a smooth relationship to SaO_2 for altitudes above 2400 m (**Figure 3**, right-hand panel). The higher mean HR at lower SaO_2 is consistent with the tendency for an increasing heart rate during ascent, found for most individuals.

Most subjects in the present study ($n = 42$, 71%) showed the significant HR: SaO_2 relationship. The trend relative to SaO_2 was sustained in 33 subjects; however, for nine subjects (numbered: 20, 25, 48, 50, 52, 53, 55, 56 and 57), the trend ended at the lowest SaO_2 with a lower HR than predicted by the trend to date. **Figure 4** shows an example (subject 25). HR (open rectangles) changes in the figure during base camp to larger open circles, where the points are obviously lower than expected from the trend during ascent. Although anecdotal, it may be no coincidence that the AMS scores are at their maximum at the same time.

Most subjects in the present study ($n = 42$, 71%) showed the significant HR: SaO_2 relationship. The trend relative to SaO_2 was sustained in 33 subjects; however, for nine subjects (numbered: 20, 25, 48, 50, 52, 53, 55, 56 and 57), the trend ended at the lowest SaO_2 with a lower HR than predicted by the trend to date. **Figure 4** shows an example (subject 25). HR (open rectangles) change in the figure during base camp to larger open circles, where the points are obviously lower than expected from the trend during ascent. Although anecdotal, it may be no coincidence that the AMS scores are at their maximum at the same time.

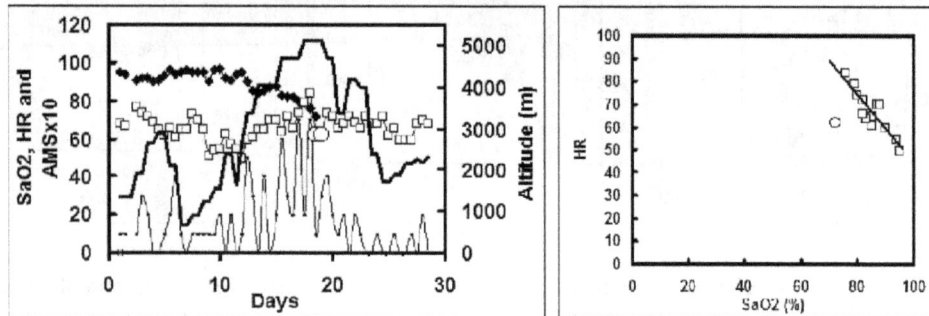

Figure 4. Example of late fall in HR. For subject 25, there was a steady rise in HR (left figure, open squares) during ascent (the period 9–18 days—from 1235 m to base camp at 5100 m). The next two values of HR after reaching base camp (large open circles) were significantly reduced. SaO_2 (filled diamonds) had fallen as usual during ascent. On the left, altitude is shown as a continuous line and AMS score (×10) shows as a thin jagged line. The plot on the right shows HR during the ascent plotted against SaO_2. The open circle represents the one of the two lower HR values for which SaO_2 was recorded. The lowered HR is thought to reflect impaired compensation for hypoxia.

4. Discussion

This HR, SaO_2 and AMS data, collected during a high-altitude trek to Kanchenjunga base camp in 1998, has shown important variations in individual responses. These differences raise questions concerning physiological mechanisms, such as the reason why a significant proportion of subjects (10 out of a total of 59 or 52 if we exclude 3 with inadequate data and variability —see **Table 1**) maintained a constant resting HR, despite falling SaO_2 during ascent. In contrast, in most subjects (42), HR increased in relation to falling SaO_2. Despite inspection of the individual time-based plots of AMS scores, there seemed no help there with its prediction, though there was, of course, the overall upward trend in the average AMS scores during ascent, accompanying lowered SaO_2 (**Figure 3**, middle panel).

A highly significant difference in vulnerability to acute mountain sickness (AMS) has been shown to be related to differences in the type of ACE gene (angiotensin-converting enzyme) carried by the subject. It is part of the renin-angiotensin system, which regulates blood pressure and the balance of fluids and salts in the body. Those with so-called 'double insertion' of the ACE gene experience far less trouble with high-altitude ascent than do those with 'double deletion.' Subjects with the mixed 'insertion/deletion' properties are intermediate [10]. It seems likely that good compensation with maintained DO_2 will be the background reason for the altitude advantage of those with double insertion ACE gene but this, of course, would need detailed examination in a major study. It is also possible that the subjects who sustained a constant heart rate with progressive lowering of SaO_2 belong to the double deletion group. Specific measurement would be required in the study to answer this question. There seems no known difference in responses to hypoxic exposure between men and women.

The significant inverse correlation between HR and SaO_2 in 42 subjects is consistent with the DO_2 priority of body tissues, illustrated for skeletal muscle [11], the brain [7, 8] and heart [4] and demonstrated for the whole body [12] in subjects breathing 12% oxygen—resting DO_2 for each individual was the same on 12% oxygen as on air, despite variations in SaO_2 in each individual on 12% oxygen.

It has been pointed out that HR usually increases as CO increases, but there may not have been complete DO_2 compensation in those who increased their HR during ascent. It is possible that the CO increase falls short of sustaining normal DO_2. Again, it would be useful to know whether the compensation indicated by the HR increase with falling SaO_2 is actually complete.

The depression of HR below that expected from the trend, usually found when it occurs, close to or actually at base camp was most likely to reflect inadequate DO_2. If this did represent a significant fall in DO_2 such subjects could be more vulnerable to AMS. For the subject, illustrated AMS scores were already increasing. It would be helpful in confirmation or refutation of assertions about HR if CO (in preference to HR) could be measured during ascent. Suitable portable equipment is awaited though none is at present on the horizon.

4.1. The value of the study

It is hoped that the illustration here of a variety of different features of the responses of individuals to the hypoxic environment of altitude will help guide future investigation and throw light on mechanisms responsible for AMS.

The study reported here is consistent with the ability of the body to sustain normal and adequate rates of oxygen delivery to the tissues. This has been shown to be limited by the severity of the hypoxic exposure with variation between subjects as to whether the limit is reached, the level of SaO_2 at which it happens, and the fact that a significant proportion of subjects do not make the compensatory adjustments seen in the majority.

The novelty of this study is the new insight that the heart rate increase is a reflection of increased cardiac output sustaining a compensatory rate of oxygen delivery to the tissues. When the heart rate fails to increase as expected from results to date it may be a clue that compensation is failing.

Acknowledgements

Thanks are due to Medical Expeditions (Altitude Education and Research Charity). This work was facilitated by the NIHRB Biomedical Research Unit in Cardiovascular Disease at Barts.

Author details

Christopher B. Wolff[1*], Annabel H. Nickol[2] and David J. Collier[1]

*Address all correspondence to: chriswolff@doctors.org.uk

1 William Harvey Heart Centre, Barts and the London School of Medicine and Dentistry, Queen Mary University of London, London, UK

2 Oxford Centre, for Respiratory Medicine, Churchill Hospital, Oxford, UK

References

[1] Wolff CB. Physiological processes during respiratory acclimatization to low inspired oxygen. In: Mountains: Geology, Topography and Environmental Concern. Goncalves AJB and Vieria AAB, Nova publishers, Hauppauge, New York 2014, Ch. 11.

[2] Brierley G, Parks T, Wolff CB. The relationship of acute mountain sickness to arterial oxygen saturation at altitudes of 3324 to 5176 m. Adv Exp Med Biol. 2012;737:207–212.

[3] Holdsworth L and Wolff CB. Oxygen delivery deficit in exercise with rapid ascent to high altitude. Adv Exp Med Biol. 2013;765:95–99.

[4] Wolff CB Normal cardiac output, oxygen delivery and oxygen extraction. Adv Exp Med Biol. 2007;599:169–182.

[5] Shoemaker WC, Appel PL, Kram HB. Role of oxygen debt in the development of organ failure, sepsis and death in high-risk surgical patients, Chest. 1992;102:208–215.

[6] Severinghaus JW, Chiodi H, Eger EI, Brandstater B, Hornbein TF. Cerebral blood flow in man at high altitude. Circ Res. 1966;19:274–282.

[7] Wolff CB. Cerebral blood flow and oxygen delivery at high altitude. High Altd Med Biol. 2000;1(1):33–38.

[8] Wolff CB, Barry P, Collier DJ. Cardiovascular and respiratory adjustments at altitude sustain cerebral oxygen delivery – Severinghaus revisited. Comp Bioch and Physiol Part A. 2002;132:221–229.

[9] Hackett PH and Oeltz O. The Lake Louis Consensus on the definition and quantification of altitude illness. In: Hypoxia and Mountain Medicine, edited by Sutton JR, Coates G and Houston CS. Burlington: Queen City Printers, 1992, pp 327–330.

[10] Montgomery HE, Marshall RM, Hemingway H Myerson S, Clarkson P, Dollery C et al. Human gene for physical performance. Nature (London). 1998;393:221–222

[11] Wolff CB. Cardiac output, oxygen consumption and muscle oxygen delivery in submaximal exercise: normal and low O_2 states. Adv Exp Med Biol. 2003;510:279–284.

[12] Bell M, Thake CD, Wolff CB. Effect of Inspiration of 12% O_2 (balance N_2) on cardiac output, respiration, oxygen saturation and oxygen delivery. Adv Exp Med Biol. 2011;915:327–332.

6

Hypoxia and Pulmonary Hypertension

Nicoletta Charolidi and Veronica A. Carroll

Abstract

Vasoconstriction in response to low oxygen tension (hypoxia) in pulmonary arteries is an important physiological adaptation to reroute blood flow to areas of higher oxygenation for effective gaseous exchange. However, chronic hypoxia is a common feature of lung disease, such as chronic obstructive pulmonary disease (COPD). Hypoxic stress triggers cellular phenotypic alterations including increased proliferation and migration of vascular smooth muscle cells (VSMCs), as well as synthesis of extracellular matrix (ECM) proteins that remodel lung vasculature. Remodelling of vessels increases the risk of pulmonary hypertension (PH)—elevated pulmonary arterial pressure—and eventually right heart failure. This chapter will summarise the major pathways and mechanisms involved in hypoxia-driven pulmonary hypertension (PH).

Keywords: hypoxia, pulmonary hypertension, HIF-1α, HIF-2α, mTOR, VHL

1. Introduction

The main function of the cardiovascular system is to circulate and deliver oxygen to metabolically active tissues of the body. At physiologically normal oxygen levels, the pulmonary vasculature of healthy individuals is highly distensible, allowing the cardiac output to adjust to levels of activity. In varying degrees of oxygen availability, as in different altitudes, adaptive cardiovascular responses are employed. In acute hypoxia (short, transient reduction in oxygen tension), the pulmonary vascular bed constricts rapidly [1]. When oxygen levels are restored, it dilates again in a swift and reversible manner. With a sustained hypoxic exposure (hours to days), the response is different. There is a loss of pulmonary distensibility, increased arterial pressure, tachycardia and increased workload for the right cardiac ventricle. In return to normoxic conditions, there is, at least in the short term, a limited reversibility of these effects. The Operation Everest II study [2] demonstrated this phenomenon by monitoring the pulmonary vascular pressure of healthy individuals who were exposed to progressive partially pressured oxygen over a period of a few weeks. However, for high-altitude populations, such as the Tibetans, this is not the case. Due to natural selection and adaptation over many thousands of years living under low oxygen conditions, Tibetans have altered oxygen-sensing mechanisms and pulmonary vascular resistance to sustained hypoxia (discussed later in this chapter) [3].

Healthy, native sea-level dwellers, who move to high altitude, develop high pulmonary arterial pressure, but with time, in the majority of cases, it stabilises and becomes well tolerated [4]. By contrast, people with pre-existing lung pathologies, such as chronic obstructive pulmonary disease (COPD), cystic fibrosis, idiopathic pulmonary fibrosis, bronchiectasis or restrictive chest wall abnormalities, are at risk of developing pulmonary hypertension (PH). Chronic PH lowers quality of life and decreases life expectancy for the affected individuals [5–8].

The pathophysiology of hypoxia-associated PH is characterised by extensive vascular remodelling that leads to arterial narrowing rather than reversible vessel vasoconstriction (**Figure 1**). Processes that take place include endothelial cell dysfunction, muscularisation of normally non-muscular arteries, phenotypic switching and proliferation of vascular smooth muscle cells (VSMCs), increased extracellular matrix deposition and erythrocytosis [7, 9, 10]. In this chapter, recent developments in mechanistic aspects underlying hypoxia-induced pathophysiological changes in PH will be briefly summarised.

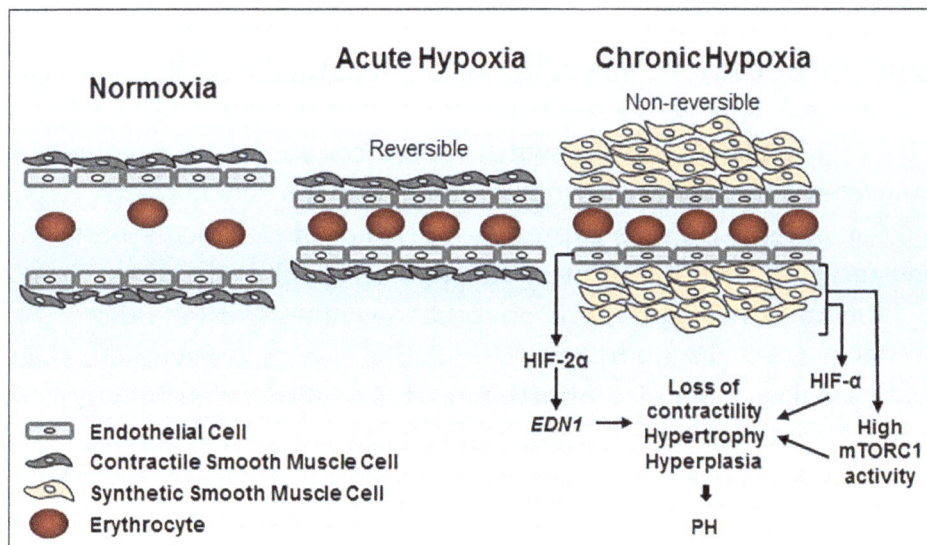

Figure 1. Schematic representation of pulmonary arterial responses to normoxia, acute hypoxia and chronic hypoxia. With acute and chronic hypoxia, the pulmonary artery undergoes vasoconstriction. In the case of acute hypoxia, the artery can reversibly dilate. But in chronic hypoxia, the artery undergoes nonreversible vascular remodelling characterised by intimal thickening due to VSMC dedifferentiation (loss of contractility, hypertrophy and hyperplasia). Additionally, there is distal muscularisation of non-muscular vessels, a settled-in endothelial cell dysfunction and erythrocytosis. Activation of HIF-1α and HIF-2α as well as over-activation of mTORC1 contributes to VSMC dedifferentiation and the establishment of hypoxic PH. Abbreviations: HIF-1α, hypoxia-inducible factor 1α; HIF-2α, hypoxia-inducible factor 2α; mTORC1, mechanistic target of rapamycin complex 1; PH, pulmonary hypertension.

2. Role of endothelial cell dysfunction

Endothelial cells in pulmonary vessels first sense hypoxic stress. Having a role in maintaining homeostasis, endothelial cells contribute to reducing the vascular tone in order for vasoconstriction to take place and regulate vessel adaptation to increased blood flow [11]. In healthy individuals, the endothelium is responsible for the balanced expression of vasoactive mediators that have either vasodilator ability, such as nitric oxide (NO) and prostacyclin (PGI_2), or vasoconstrictive properties, such as endothelin-1 (ET-1) [11–14]. ET-1 is released abluminally and triggers vasoconstriction through binding to its VSMC receptors ET_A and ET_B [15]. However, when ET-1 binds to its endothelial ET_B receptor, it can induce vasodilation through NO and PGI_2 recruitment [15], while this route also serves for ET-1 clearance from the lung [16].

In pathological PH, as in COPD, endothelial cell dysfunction is one of the major contributing factors for the progression of the condition. It has been found that endothelial NO synthase (eNOS), the enzyme responsible for NO production, as well as prostacyclin synthase, the enzyme responsible for PGI_2 production, is markedly diminished in patients with COPD [12, 17]. Furthermore, ET-1 has been reported to have an increased expression in the lungs of patients with PH and is a therapeutic target [14]. ET-1, as well as being a potent vasoconstrictor, is also a VSMC mitogen, acting through smooth muscle ET_A and ET_B receptors [15]. So in effect, during hypoxic endothelial dysregulation, the pathogenic excess of ET-1 maintains vessel constriction and VSMC proliferation.

3. Phenotypic switching of vascular smooth muscle cells

In hypoxia, the highly plastic VSMCs switch from a contractile to a synthetic phenotype, which is characterised by increased proliferation and extracellular matrix deposition [18]. Differentiated smooth muscle cells express a repertoire of contractile proteins, signalling molecules and receptors for their primary function of vessel contraction. These contractile VSMCs have little capacity for proliferation, protein synthesis or migration [18]. However, pulmonary VSMCs, under chronic hypoxic stimulation, switch to a synthetic state exhibiting hypertrophy, hyperplasia, loss of contractility and migration, contributing to the enlargement of the arterial intimal layer (**Figure 1**) and in the muscularisation of non-muscular pulmonary vessels [9]. Additionally, there is a deposition of collagen and elastic fibres. In extreme cases, the excessive VSMC proliferation can progress from vascular lesions to calcification. These phenomena seem to correlate with the degree of PH extent and COPD severity [19–21].

The endothelial dysfunction that takes place in PH may also contribute to the dedifferentiation and proliferation of VSMCs [22]. Specifically, dysregulated endothelial cells can cause alterations in AKT signalling in VSMCs, which in turn triggers their phenotypic switch [23]. This pathway is also affected by aberrant regulation of the mechanistic target of rapamycin (mTOR) pathway (discussed later in this chapter).

4. Hypoxia and pulmonary hypertension

The major cellular oxygen-sensing mechanism implicated in hypoxia-induced pulmonary hypertension is the hypoxia-inducible factor (HIF) pathway. HIFs are transcription factors that induce the activation of some several hundred genes in response to hypoxia [24]. Initially identified as regulators of erythropoietin (EPO), the hormone responsible for increased red blood cells in response to low oxygen levels, HIFs have since been found to regulate expression of genes that are important for angiogenesis, cellular metabolism, cardiovascular development and cardiovascular control [24–26].

In low oxygen conditions, HIFs bind DNA as heterodimeric complexes of alpha (HIF-α) and beta (HIF-β) subunits, with HIF-α being the subunit regulated by oxygen tension [27]. Higher animals have a series of isoforms for each of the HIF subunits as a result of gene evolutionary duplications [24]. In humans, there are three paralogs of HIF-α—HIF-1α, HIF-2α and HIF-3α—with the first two members being the best characterised [24, 25]. The expression of HIF-1α and HIF-2α is differentially regulated, while their balance is believed to be important for tissue-specific differences in oxygen sensing [25]. They both bind to the same DNA consensus (RCGTG) in hypoxia-response elements of the genome, but they only induce partially overlapping sets of genes [27, 28].

In normoxic conditions, the HIF-α subunit is hydroxylated by Fe(II) prolyl hydroxylase domain (PHD) enzymes (PHD1, PHD2 and PHD3 or otherwise known as Egln2, Egln1 and Egln3) that use 2-oxoglutarate and Fe^{2+} as substrates [29]. After hydroxylation by PHDs, HIF-α is recognised and bound by the von Hippel-Lindau (VHL) protein, a ubiquitin E3 ligase, which marks HIF-α for proteasomal degradation. In hypoxia, PHD enzymes are inactive allowing HIF-α subunits to translocate to the nucleus and activate HIF target genes. HIFs are further regulated by factor-inhibiting HIF (FIH)-mediated asparaginyl hydroxylation, which impairs their recruitment to transcriptional complexes [30].

Mouse models of HIF-1α and HIF-2α have illustrated that the HIF pathway is critically important for the pulmonary hypoxic response and the development of PH. Heterozygous deficiency of either HIF-1α or HIF-2α allele in mice does not affect their life span, and these animals are largely normal in unstressed, normal oxygen conditions. In response to chronic hypoxia (10% for 3 weeks), HIF-$1\alpha^{+/-}$ mice exhibit an attenuated PH with a low rise in right ventricular pressure and right ventricular hypertrophy [31]. Interestingly, heterozygous HIF-$2\alpha^{+/-}$ mice, exposed to 10% oxygen for 10 weeks, showed a complete lack of any PH manifestation [32]. Of note, animals with hetero- or homozygous mutations in stabilising HIF-2α spontaneously developed progressive PH [33]. These studies all indicate a pathological role of both HIF-α subunits in PH development.

Cell-type-specific inactivation of HIF-α with the use of a variety of promoters has also been studied but with some variable results, which may be due to the method of HIF-α manipulations and/or the use of different mouse strains [34–36]. Nevertheless, there seems to be a clear link between HIFs and PH, since studies from human genetics, including several populations that have adapted to different altitudes, have demonstrated the importance of HIF-2α in pulmonary response to hypoxia and PH pathophysiology [37].

The Tibetans, who have lived for at least 25,000 years in 4000 m elevation and continuously inspired partially pressured oxygen (~80 mmHg), have been identified to have a number of single-nucleotide polymorphisms in close-to-one-another loci near the gene *EPAS1*, which encodes HIF-2α [38]. HIF-2α is the subunit responsible for EPO regulation and in turn erythropoiesis. Tibetans manifest blunted PH and reduced erythropoiesis at high altitude. At sea level, they manifest a lower pulmonary arterial pressure in response to hypoxia when compared with other populations [39, 40]. Recently, a missense mutation in PHD2 (*EGLN1*) was identified which allows for increased PHD2 activity under hypoxic conditions, thereby decreasing HIF-α stabilisation and reducing erythropoiesis at altitude [41].

Further evidence for a role for HIF-2α in PH comes from another human genetic study, which showed that an activating HIF-2α mutation (G$\rightarrow$A substitution in position 2097) caused erythrocytosis with elevated total red cell volume and PH in an affected family [42].

5. VHL and pulmonary hypertension

The VHL protein is a tumour suppressor and an essential component for the clearance of HIF-α through the ubiquitin-proteasomal degradation pathway [24, 43]. A number of VHL mutations have been described that result in aberrant induction of HIF target genes, due to the loss of function of VHL and in turn to the loss of HIF-α regulation. VHL mutations are associated with VHL syndrome, which is a hereditary condition, characterised by highly vascularised tumours within specific tissues, including the renal, retinal and central nervous system [44]. However, a small number of VHL mutations (R200W, D126N, S183L, D126N) are associated with development of Chuvash polycythemia (CP) [45–47]. CP is a rare autosomal recessive condition that is endemic to the population in Chuvashia, Russia and in the island of Ischia, Italy [46, 48]. Chuvash patients manifest increased haemoglobin and haematocrit with elevated levels of EPO, as well as increased expression of vascular endothelial growth factor (VEGF) and ET-1, which are HIF-α target genes [45–49]. In addition, these patients are highly susceptible to both arterial and venous thrombosis and can develop mild to severe PH [45–49].

The importance of HIF-2α isoform in the regulation of pulmonary vascular control has also been demonstrated by the use of a mouse model of CP [50]. This model carries a hypomorphic VHL allele (with an R200W substitution) and recapitulates all symptoms of the human CP phenotype. Interestingly, when these mice are crossed with HIF-2$\alpha^{+/-}$ or HIF-1$\alpha^{+/-}$ strains for heterozygous deficiency in either of the two HIF-α, they manifest an ameliorated PH phenotype for suppressed HIF-2α, but not for HIF-1α.

Comparison of CP and HIF-2α gain-of-function mutation human phenotypes has additionally shown that the latter condition somehow manifests more moderate symptoms than the first. The explanation for this may be that, in CP, both HIF-α subunits are upregulated, and therefore, there may be an additive effect [51]. Furthermore, VHL has a number of HIF-α-independent functions that may also play a role in the CP phenotype.

6. New advances: hypoxic induction of zinc transporters

Zinc, an essential dietary element, plays an important cytoprotective role for the lung by sheltering the pulmonary epithelium from extrinsic activation of apoptotic pathways following acute lung injury [52]. Zinc transporters are responsible for zinc cellular uptake and homeostasis [53]. A recent linkage analysis study that compared a PH-resistant rat strain, Fisher 344 (F344), with the Wistar Kyoto (WKY) strain identified the gene *Slc39a12*, which encodes the ZIP12 zinc transporter, as a major regulator of hypoxia-induced pulmonary vascular remodelling [53]. In the F344 strain, this gene lacks a crucial thymidine, which leads to a frameshift mutation in exon 11 and renders translation of the protein redundant. ZIP12 is normally expressed in endothelial, interstitial and VSMCs, but its expression increases in remodelled pulmonary vessels following hypoxia-induced PH [53]. ZIP12 is likely a HIF target gene since both HIF-1α and HIF-2α were detected bound to ZIP12 hypoxia-response element. The investigators of this study further generated a ZIP12$^{-/-}$ rat model for comparison with the original F344 and WKY strains and found that genetic disruption of ZIP12 recapitulates the phenotype of the PH-resistant F344 strain under conditions of hypoxia.

Zinc-binding motifs have been considered as potential PH drug-therapeutic targets with phosphodiesterase type 5 (PDE5) and histone deacetylases as examples [54, 55]. Zinc is a structural component of a number of intracellular enzymes, transcription factors, other proteins and cofactors and is a putative drug target for PH.

7. Role of hypoxia-inducible microRNAs in pulmonary hypertension

MicroRNAs (miRNAs) are small non-coding RNA molecules (about 21 nucleotides long) that regulate gene expression post-transcriptionally. Hypoxic stimulation of a variety of human cell types has shown induction of more than 90 miRNAs [56], with altered expression of some of these miRNAs involved in VSMC remodelling and endothelial cell dysfunction in PH [57].

MiRNAs that have been causally implicated in PH include miR-204, miR-138, miR-21 and miR-130/miR-301, among others (**Table 1**). MiR-204 has been shown to be downregulated in VSMCs of patients suffering from PH, as well as in mouse models of the disease [58, 59]. The degree of miR-204 suppression has been found to be inversely proportional to the degree of pulmonary artery resistance and pressure, while compensating for the loss of miR-204 through nebulisation in PH patients has been shown to reverse the VSMC proliferative and anti-apoptotic phenotype [59]. MiR-204 is involved in the activation of the nuclear factor of activated T cell (NFAT) pathway, the Rho pathway, VSMC proliferation and resistance to apoptosis, as well as downregulation of transcripts such as bone morphogenetic protein receptor type II (BMPR2) and interleukin-6 (IL-6) [60–62]. Also, miR-204 regulates the expression of the Runt-related transcription factor 2 (RUNX2), which has been shown to stabilise HIF-1α in chondrocytes by competing with VHL [20, 63]. In the context of hypoxia, RUNX2 is upregulated, since miR-204 is downregulated, and therefore sustains HIF-1α activation,

MicroRNA	Change in PH	Target transcripts	Cellular function, process or pathway affected	Ref.
miR-204	↓	BMPR2, IL-6, RUNX2 among others	Activation of NFAT pathway, VSMC proliferation, resistance to apoptosis, Rho pathway, HIF-1α pathway	[20, 58–63]
miR-138	↑	HIF-1α, S100A1	HIF-1α pathway, endothelial regulation of vasomotor tone	[64]
miR-21	↑	PDCD4, SPRY2, PPARα	VSMC proliferation, resistance to apoptosis	[61, 65–67]
miR-130/301	↑	PPARγ which leads to subordinate gene targets and other miRNAs	Master regulator of cell proliferation and apoptosis in PH ↓ miR-204	[68]

Table 1. MicroRNAs that are causally implicated in PH.

which in turn contributes to aberrant VSMC proliferation, resistance to apoptosis and their transdifferentiation to osteoblast-like cells [20].

MiR-138 is upregulated by hypoxia and suppresses HIF-1α [64]. However, its upregulation also contributes to endothelial cell dysfunction in PH by downregulating the small EF-hand Ca^{2+}-binding protein S100A1 that relays Ca^{2+} oscillations, controlling vascular tone responses [64].

MiR-21 expression has been found to be upregulated in both pulmonary VSMC and endothelial cells during hypoxic conditions [61, 65]. This upregulation, in turn, leads to downregulation of programmed cell death protein 4 (PDCD4), sprouty homolog 2 (SPRY2) and peroxisome proliferator-activated receptor-α (PPARα), which when dysregulated play a role in the increased proliferation and resistance to apoptosis [65–67]. Treatment of mice with anti-miR-21 during hypoxia showed an improvement in distal pulmonary artery muscularisation [69]. However, miR-21 has also been shown to have a protective effect during PH [61]. Using VHL-null mice, IL-6 transgenic mice, pulmonary vessels from patients with PH as well as deficient (miR-21$^{-/-}$) or miR-21 overexpression (miR-21$^{+/+}$) mouse models, it has been demonstrated that miR-21 loss of function causes onset of PH [61]. Specifically, miR-21 deletion showed exaggerated pulmonary vascular remodelling, whereas in mice overexpressing miR-21, these disease-associated phenotypes were abolished [61].

The family of miR-130/301 is also upregulated in pulmonary VSMCs and the endothelium in hypoxia, as well as in the lungs of mice with PH due to chronic hypoxic exposure [68]. This upregulation is mediated by HIF-2α and Oct-4. MiR-130/301 is a master regulator miRNA subordinating other miRNA pathways, and, for instance, it suppresses miR-204 [68].

miR-223, miR-17, miR-130, miR-145, miR-424 and miR503 are also involved in the pathophysiology of PH (reviewed in Ref. [70]). So far, PH animal models have helped greatly in these studies, but the exact role and balance for each of these miRNAs in human PH have not been fully elucidated.

8. mTOR signalling in hypoxia-induced pulmonary hypertension

Mechanistic target of rapamycin (mTOR) is a cellular hub that controls growth factor signalling and nutrient sensing to regulate cell growth, proliferation, metabolism and survival [71]. mTOR is a protein kinase that is the catalytic component of two functionally distinct complexes, mTOR complex 1 (mTORC1) and mTOR complex 2 (mTORC2) [72, 73]. mTORC1 is composed of mTOR, Raptor, LST8/GβL, PRAS40 and DEP domain containing mTOR-interacting protein (DEPTOR), and its activity is stimulated by growth factor signals to regulate protein synthesis through 4E-BP1/BP2 and the S6 kinases, S6K1 and S6K2 [74, 75]. By contrast, mTORC2, which comprises mTOR, Rictor, LST8/GβL, DEPTOR, SIN1 and PRR5, regulates cytoskeletal organisation [76, 77] and has a role in phosphorylation of protein kinase C (PKC), protein kinase B (PKB) and serum- and glucocorticoid-induced protein kinase (SGK) to promote cell survival and cell cycle progression [78–80].

Aberrant mTOR activity has a well-characterised role in promoting proliferative diseases including cancer and smooth muscle cell pathologies [71]. mTORC1 signalling is activated following vascular injury promoting Vinhibitor, rapamycin, promotes smooth muscle cell (SMC) remodelling. Accordingly, mTOR inhibitors are widely used in drug-eluting stents to prevent restenosis. In addition, mTOR also regulates the differentiation state of VSMCs since the mTOR inhibitor, rapamycin, promotes SMC differentiation and expression of contractile proteins [81]. mTORC1 activity is low in differentiated contractile VSMCs but becomes activated by growth factors and is thought to contribute to the change towards a synthetic phenotype that is characterised by increased SMC proliferation and migration. As such, rapamycin analogues may have therapeutic potential for treating PH.

The relationship between hypoxic conditions and mTOR is complex and depends, in part, on cellular context. Many cell types respond to prolonged periods of hypoxia by inactivating energy-intensive processes such as protein synthesis and proliferation, and accordingly mTOR is downregulated [82]. By contrast, the vasculature responds to long-term hypoxia by promoting new blood vessel growth—angiogenesis, which in turn, restores O$_2$ to deprived tissues. Hypoxic stress is a key driving force in the vascular remodelling observed in pulmonary hypertension, and HIFs activate pulmonary artery endothelial and smooth muscle cell proliferation, which is mediated by both mTORC1 and mTORC2 [83–85]. Currently, the mechanisms by which hypoxia/HIFs signal to activate mTOR in ECs and VSMCs are poorly understood [86–90].

9. Conclusion

Severe PH associated with hypoxic lung disease is a life-threatening condition with poor survival rates. Despite significant advances in targeted therapeutics for PH, randomised clinical trial data for this particular group of patients are scarce, and it is not clear whether endothelin receptor antagonists will benefit patients with hypoxia-associated PH. Importantly, recent genetic studies identifying mutations in the oxygen-sensing machinery have provided new mechanistic insights into the aetiology of PH. Further studies are required to determine whether specific targeting of HIF-2α will provide additional therapeutic benefit for this complex disease.

Author details

Nicoletta Charolidi and Veronica A. Carroll*

*Address all correspondence to: vcarroll@sgul.ac.uk

Vascular Biology Research Centre, Molecular and Clinical Sciences Research Institute, St George's, University of London, London, UK

References

[1] Euler U, Liljestrand G. Observations on the pulmonary arterial blood pressure in the cat. Acta Physiol Scand. 1946;12:301–20.

[2] Groves BM, Reeves JT, Sutton JR, Wagner PD, Cymerman A, Malconian MK, et al. Operation Everest II: elevated high-altitude pulmonary resistance unresponsive to oxygen. J Appl Physiol (1985). 1987 Aug;63(2):521–30.

[3] Aldenderfer M. Peopling the Tibetan plateau: insights from archaeology. High Alt Med Biol. 2011;12(2):141–7.

[4] West JB, American College of Physicians, American Physiological Society. The physiologic basis of high-altitude diseases. Ann Intern Med. 2004 Nov 16;141(10):789–800.

[5] Seeger W, Adir Y, Barberà JA, Champion H, Coghlan JG, Cottin V, et al. Pulmonary hypertension in chronic lung diseases. J Am Coll Cardiol. 2013 Dec 24;62 (25 Suppl):D109–16.

[6] Wells JM, Washko GR, Han MK, Abbas N, Nath H, Mamary AJ, et al. Pulmonary arterial enlargement and acute exacerbations of COPD. N Engl J Med. 2012 Sep 6;367(10):913–21.

[7] Blanco I, Piccari L, Barberà JA. Pulmonary vasculature in COPD: the silent component. Respirology. 2016 Aug;21(6):984–94.

[8] Wells JM, Farris RF, Gosdin TA, Dransfield MT, Wood ME, Bell SC, et al. Pulmonary artery enlargement and cystic fibrosis pulmonary exacerbations: a cohort study. Lancet Respir Med. 2016 Aug;4(8):636–45.

[9] Stenmark KR, Fagan KA, Frid MG. Hypoxia-induced pulmonary vascular remodeling: cellular and molecular mechanisms. Circ Res. 2006 Sep 29;99(7):675–91.

[10] Kylhammar D, Rådegran G. The principal pathways involved in the in vivo modulation of hypoxic pulmonary vasoconstriction, pulmonary arterial remodelling and pulmonary hypertension. Acta Physiol (Oxf). 2016 Jul 6;Epub ahead of print.

[11] Stamler JS, Loh E, Roddy MA, Currie KE, Creager MA. Nitric oxide regulates basal systemic and pulmonary vascular resistance in healthy humans. Circulation. 1994 May;89(5):2035–40.

[12] Tuder RM, Cool CD, Geraci MW, Wang J, Abman SH, Wright L, et al. Prostacyclin synthase expression is decreased in lungs from patients with severe pulmonary hypertension. Am J Respir Crit Care Med. 1999 Jun;159(6):1925–32.

[13] Barberà JA, Roger N, Roca J, Rovira I, Higenbottam TW, Rodriguez-Roisin R. Worsening of pulmonary gas exchange with nitric oxide inhalation in chronic obstructive pulmonary disease. Lancet (London, England). 1996 Feb 17;347(8999):436–40.

[14] Giaid A, Yanagisawa M, Langleben D, Michel RP, Levy R, Shennib H, et al. Expression of endothelin-1 in the lungs of patients with pulmonary hypertension. N Engl J Med. 1993 Jun 17;328(24):1732–9.

[15] Bialecki RA, Fisher CS, Murdoch WW, Barthlow HG, Bertelsen DL. Functional comparison of endothelin receptors in human and rat pulmonary artery smooth muscle. Am J Physiol. 1997 Feb;272(2 Pt 1):L211–8.

[16] Fukuroda T, Fujikawa T, Ozaki S, Ishikawa K, Yano M, Nishikibe M. Clearance of circulating endothelin-1 by ETB receptors in rats. Biochem Biophys Res Commun. 1994 Mar 30;199(3):1461–5.

[17] Yang Q, Shigemura N, Underwood MJ, Hsin M, Xue H-M, Huang Y, et al. NO and EDHF pathways in pulmonary arteries and veins are impaired in COPD patients. Vascul Pharmacol. 2012;57(2–4):113–8.

[18] Owens GK, Kumar MS, Wamhoff BR. Molecular regulation of vascular smooth muscle cell differentiation in development and disease. Physiol Rev. 2004 Jul;84(3):767–801.

[19] Carlsen J, Hasseriis Andersen K, Boesgaard S, Iversen M, Steinbrüchel D, Bøgelund Andersen C. Pulmonary arterial lesions in explanted lungs after transplantation correlate with severity of pulmonary hypertension in chronic obstructive pulmonary disease. J Heart Lung Transplant. 2013 Mar;32(3):347–54.

[20] Ruffenach G, Chabot S, Tanguay VF, Courboulin A, Boucherat O, Potus F, et al. Role for Runt-related transcription factor 2 in proliferative and calcified vascular lesions in pulmonary arterial hypertension. Am J Respir Crit Care Med. 2016 Nov 15;194(10)1273–85.

[21] Santos S, Peinado VI, Ramírez J, Melgosa T, Roca J, Rodriguez-Roisin R, et al. Characterization of pulmonary vascular remodelling in and patients with mild COPD. Eur Respir J. 2002 Apr;19(4):632–8.

[22] Powell RJ, Cronenwett JL, Fillinger MF, Wagner RJ, Sampson LN. Endothelial cell modulation of smooth muscle cell morphology and organizational growth pattern. Ann Vasc Surg. 1996 Jan;10(1):4–10.

[23] Brown DJ, Rzucidlo EM, Merenick BL, Wagner RJ, Martin KA, Powell RJ. Endothelial cell activation of the smooth muscle cell phosphoinositide 3-kinase/Akt pathway promotes differentiation. J Vasc Surg. 2005 Mar;41(3):509–16.

[24] Bishop T, Ratcliffe PJ. HIF hydroxylase pathways in cardiovascular physiology and medicine. Circ Res. 2015 Jun 19;117(1):65–79.

[25] Semenza GL. Oxygen sensing, homeostasis, and disease. N Engl J Med. 2011 Aug 11;365(6):537–47.

[26] Maxwell PH, Pugh CW, Ratcliffe PJ. Inducible operation of the erythropoietin 3′ enhancer in multiple cell lines: evidence for a widespread oxygen-sensing mechanism. Proc Natl Acad Sci U S A. 1993 Mar 15;90(6):2423–7.

[27] Hu CJ, Wang LY, Chodosh LA, Keith B, Simon MC. Differential roles of hypoxia-inducible factor 1alpha (HIF-1alpha) and HIF-2alpha in hypoxic gene regulation. Mol Cell Biol. 2003 Dec;23(24):9361–74.

[28] Schödel J, Oikonomopoulos S, Ragoussis J, Pugh CW, Ratcliffe PJ, Mole DR. High-resolution genome-wide mapping of HIF-binding sites by ChIP-seq. Blood. 2011 Jun 9;117(23):e207–17.

[29] Bruick RK, McKnight SL. A conserved family of prolyl-4-hydroxylases that modify HIF. Science. 2001 Nov 9;294(5545):1337–40.

[30] Mahon PC, Hirota K, Semenza GL. FIH-1: a novel protein that interacts with HIF-1alpha and VHL to mediate repression of HIF-1 transcriptional activity. Genes Dev. 2001 Oct 15;15(20):2675–86.

[31] Yu AY, Shimoda LA, Iyer NV, Huso DL, Sun X, McWilliams R, et al. Impaired physiological responses to chronic hypoxia in mice partially deficient for hypoxia-inducible factor 1alpha. J Clin Invest. 1999 Mar;103(5):691–6.

[32] Brusselmans K, Compernolle V, Tjwa M, Wiesener MS, Maxwell PH, Collen D, et al. Heterozygous deficiency of hypoxia-inducible factor-2alpha protects mice against pulmonary hypertension and right ventricular dysfunction during prolonged hypoxia. J Clin Invest. 2003 May;111(10):1519–27.

[33] Tan Q, Kerestes H, Percy MJ, Pietrofesa R, Chen L, Khurana TS, et al. Erythrocytosis and pulmonary hypertension in a mouse model of human HIF2A gain of function mutation. J Biol Chem. 2013 Jun 14;288(24):17134–44.

[34] Ball MK, Waypa GB, Mungai PT, Nielsen JM, Czech L, Dudley VJ, et al. Regulation of hypoxia-induced pulmonary hypertension by vascular smooth muscle hypoxia-inducible factor-1α. Am J Respir Crit Care Med. 2014 Feb 1;189(3):314–24.

[35] Kim Y-M, Barnes EA, Alvira CM, Ying L, Reddy S, Cornfield DN. Hypoxia-inducible factor-1α in pulmonary artery smooth muscle cells lowers vascular tone by decreasing myosin light chain phosphorylation. Circ Res. 2013 Apr 26;112(9):1230–3.

[36] Skuli N, Liu L, Runge A, Wang T, Yuan L, Patel S, et al. Endothelial deletion of hypoxia-inducible factor-2alpha (HIF-2alpha) alters vascular function and tumor angiogenesis. Blood. 2009 Jul 9;114(2):469–77.

[37] Semenza GL. Hypoxia-inducible factors in physiology and medicine. Cell. 2012 Feb 3;148(3):399–408.

[38] Beall CM, Cavalleri GL, Deng L, Elston RC, Gao Y, Knight J, et al. Natural selection on EPAS1 (HIF2alpha) associated with low hemoglobin concentration in Tibetan highlanders. Proc Natl Acad Sci U S A. 2010 Jun 22;107 25 :11459–64.

[39] Petousi N, Croft QP, Cavalleri GL, Cheng HY, Formenti F, Ishida K, et al. Tibetans living at sea level have a hyporesponsive hypoxia-inducible factor system and blunted physiological responses to hypoxia. J Appl Physiol. 2014 Apr 1;116(7):893–904.

[40] Simonson TS, Yang Y, Huff CD, Yun H, Qin G, Witherspoon DJ, et al. Genetic evidence for high-altitude adaptation in Tibet. Science. 2010 Jul 2;329(5987):72–5.

[41] Lorenzo FR, Huff C, Myllymäki M, Olenchock B, Swierczek S, Tashi T, et al. A genetic mechanism for Tibetan high-altitude adaptation. Nat Genet. 2014;46(9):951–6.

[42] Gale DP, Harten SK, Reid CDL, Tuddenham EG, Maxwell PH. Autosomal dominant erythrocytosis and pulmonary arterial hypertension associated with an activating HIF2 alpha mutation. Blood. 2008 Aug 1;112(3):919–21.

[43] Maxwell PH, Wiesener MS, Chang GW, Clifford SC, Vaux EC, Cockman ME, et al. The tumour suppressor protein VHL targets hypoxia-inducible factors for oxygen-dependent proteolysis. Nature. 1999 May 20;399(6733):271–5.

[44] Chittiboina P, Lonser RR. Von Hippel-Lindau disease. Handb Clin Neurol. 2015;132:139–56.

[45] Sarangi S, Lanikova L, Kapralova K, Acharya S, Swierczek S, Lipton JM, et al. The homozygous VHL(D126N) missense mutation is associated with dramatically elevated erythropoietin levels, consequent polycythemia, and early onset severe pulmonary hypertension. Pediatr Blood Cancer. 2014 Nov;61(11):2104–6.

[46] Ang SO, Chen H, Hirota K, Gordeuk VR, Jelinek J, Guan Y, et al. Disruption of oxygen homeostasis underlies congenital Chuvash polycythemia. Nat Genet. 2002 Dec;32(4):614–21.

[47] Bond J, Gale DP, Connor T, Adams S, de Boer J, Gascoyne DM, et al. Dysregulation of the HIF pathway due to VHL mutation causing severe erythrocytosis and pulmonary arterial hypertension. Blood. 2011 Mar 31;117(13):3699–701.

[48] Perrotta S, Nobili B, Ferraro M, Migliaccio C, Borriello A, Cucciolla V, et al. Von Hippel-Lindau-dependent polycythemia is endemic on the island of Ischia: identification of a novel cluster. Blood. 2006 Jan 15;107(2):514–9.

[49] Smith TG, Brooks JT, Balanos GM, Lappin TR, Layton DM, Leedham DL, et al. Mutation of von Hippel-Lindau tumour suppressor and human cardiopulmonary physiology. PLoS Med. 2006 Jul;3(7):e290.

[50] Hickey MM, Richardson T, Wang T, Mosqueira M, Arguiri E, Yu H, et al. The von Hippel-Lindau Chuvash mutation promotes pulmonary hypertension and fibrosis in mice. J Clin Invest. 2010 Mar;120(3):827–39.

[51] Formenti F, Beer PA, Croft QP, Dorrington KL, Gale DP, Lappin TRJ, et al. Cardiopulmonary function in two human disorders of the hypoxia-inducible factor (HIF) pathway: von Hippel-Lindau disease and HIF-2alpha gain-of-function mutation. FASEB J. 2011 Jun;25`6`:2001–11.

[52] Zalewski PD, Forbes IJ, Betts WH. Correlation of apoptosis with change in intracellular labile Zn(II) using zinquin [(2-methyl-8-p-toluenesulphonamido-6-quinolyloxy)acetic acid], a new specific fluorescent probe for Zn(II). Biochem J. 1993 Dec 1;296(Pt 2):403-8.

[53] Zhao L, Oliver E, Maratou K, Atanur SS, Dubois OD, Cotroneo E, et al. The zinc transporter ZIP12 regulates the pulmonary vascular response to chronic hypoxia. Nature. 2015 Aug 20;524(7565):356–60.

[54] Zhao L, Mason NA, Morrell NW, Kojonazarov B, Sadykov A, Maripov A, et al. Sildenafil inhibits hypoxia-induced pulmonary hypertension. Circulation. 2001 Jul 24;104(4):424–8.

[55] Zhao L, Chen CN, Hajji N, Oliver E, Cotroneo E, Wharton J, et al. Histone deacetylation inhibition in pulmonary hypertension: therapeutic potential of valproic acid and suberoylanilide hydroxamic acid. Circulation. 2012 Jul 24;126(4):455–67.

[56] Kozomara A, Griffiths-Jones S. miRBase: annotating high confidence microRNAs using deep sequencing data. Nucleic Acids Res. 2014 Jan;42(Database issue):D68–73.

[57] White K, Loscalzo J, Chan SY. Holding our breath: the emerging and anticipated roles of microRNA in pulmonary hypertension. Pulm Circ. 2012 Jul;2(3):278–90.

[58] Caruso P, MacLean MR, Khanin R, McClure J, Soon E, Southgate M, et al. Dynamic changes in lung microRNA profiles during the development of pulmonary hypertension due to chronic hypoxia and monocrotaline. Arterioscler Thromb Vasc Biol. 2010 Apr;30(4):716–23.

[59] Courboulin A, Paulin R, Giguère NJ, Saksouk N, Perreault T, Meloche J, et al. Role for miR-204 in human pulmonary arterial hypertension. J Exp Med. 2011 Mar 14;208(3):535–48.

[60] Bonnet S, Rochefort G, Sutendra G, Archer SL, Haromy A, Webster L, et al. The nuclear factor of activated T cells in pulmonary arterial hypertension can be therapeutically targeted. Proc Natl Acad Sci U S A. 2007 Jul 3;104(27):11418–23.

[61] Parikh VN, Jin RC, Rabello S, Gulbahce N, White K, Hale A, et al. MicroRNA-21 integrates pathogenic signaling to control pulmonary hypertension: results of a network bioinformatics approach. Circulation. 2012 Mar 27;125(12):1520–32.

[62] Tuder RM, Marecki JC, Richter A, Fijalkowska I, Flores S. Pathology of pulmonary hypertension. Clin Chest Med. 2007 Mar;28(1):23–42, vii.

[63] Lee SH, Che X, Jeong JH, Choi JY, Lee YJ, Lee YH, et al. Runx2 protein stabilizes hypoxia-inducible factor-1α through competition with von Hippel-Lindau protein (pVHL) and stimulates angiogenesis in growth plate hypertrophic chondrocytes. J Biol Chem. 2012 Apr 27;287(18):14760–71.

[64] Sen A, Ren S, Lerchenmüller C, Sun J, Weiss N, Most P, et al. MicroRNA-138 regulates hypoxia-induced endothelial cell dysfunction by targeting S100A1. PLoS One. 2013 Nov 11;8(11):e78684.

[65] Sarkar J, Gou D, Turaka P, Viktorova E, Ramchandran R, Raj JU. MicroRNA-21 plays a role in hypoxia-mediated pulmonary artery smooth muscle cell proliferation and migration. Am J Physiol Lung Cell Mol Physiol. 2010 Dec;299(6):L861–71.

[66] Cheng Y, Zhu P, Yang J, Liu X, Dong S, Wang X, et al. Ischaemic preconditioning-regulated miR-21 protects heart against ischaemia/reperfusion injury via anti-apoptosis through its target PDCD4. Cardiovasc Res. 2010 Aug 1;87(3):431–9.

[67] Davis BN, Hilyard AC, Lagna G, Hata A. SMAD proteins control DROSHA-mediated microRNA maturation. Nature. 2008 Jul 3;454(7200):56–61.

[68] Bertero T, Lu Y, Annis S, Hale A, Bhat B, Saggar R, et al. Systems-level regulation of microRNA networks by miR-130/301 promotes pulmonary hypertension. J Clin Invest. 2014 Aug;124(8):3514–28.

[69] Yang S, Banerjee S, Freitas Ad, Cui H, Xie N, Abraham E, et al. miR-21 regulates chronic hypoxia-induced pulmonary vascular remodeling. Am J Physiol Lung Cell Mol Physiol. 2012 Mar 15;302(6):L521–9.

[70] Mohsenin V. The emerging role of microRNAs in hypoxia-induced pulmonary hypertension. Sleep Breath. 2016 Sep;20(3):1059–67.

[71] Laplante M, Sabatini DM. mTOR signaling in growth control and disease. Cell. 2012 Apr 13;149(2):274–93.

[72] Sciarretta S, Volpe M, Sadoshima J. Mammalian target of rapamycin signaling in cardiac physiology and disease. Circ Res. 2014 Jan 31;114(3):549–64.

[73] Ratcliffe PJ. Oxygen sensing and hypoxia signalling pathways in animals: the implications of physiology for cancer. J Physiol. 2013 Apr 15;591(8):2027–42.

[74] Corradetti MN, Guan KL. Upstream of the mammalian target of rapamycin: do all roads pass through mTOR?. Oncogene. 2006 Oct 16;25(48):6347–60.

[75] Sengupta S, Peterson TR, Sabatini DM. Regulation of the mTOR complex 1 pathway by nutrients, growth factors, and stress. Mol Cell. 2010 Oct 22;40(2):310–22.

[76] Sarbassov DD, Ali SM, Kim DH, Guertin DA, Latek RR, Erdjument-Bromage H, et al. Rictor, a novel binding partner of mTOR, defines a rapamycin-insensitive and raptor-independent pathway that regulates the cytoskeleton. Curr Biol. 2004 Jul 27;14(14):1296–302.

[77] Liu L, Das S, Losert W, Parent CA. mTORC2 regulates neutrophil chemotaxis in a cAMP- and RhoA-dependent fashion. Dev Cell. 2010 Dec 14;19(6):845–57.

[78] Sarbassov DD, Guertin DA, Ali SM, Sabatini DM. Phosphorylation and regulation of Akt/PKB by the rictor-mTOR complex. Science. 2005 Feb 18;307(5712):1098–101.

[79] García-Martínez JM, Alessi DR. mTOR complex 2 (mTORC2) controls hydrophobic motif phosphorylation and activation of serum- and glucocorticoid-induced protein kinase 1 (SGK1). Biochem J. 2008 Dec 15;416(3):375–85.

[80] Alessi DR, Andjelkovic M, Caudwell B, Cron P, Morrice N, Cohen P, et al. Mechanism of activation of protein kinase B by insulin and IGF-1. EMBO J. 1996 Dec 2;15(23):6541–51.

[81] Martin KA, Rzucidlo EM, Merenick BL, Fingar DC, Brown DJ, Wagner RJ, et al. The mTOR/p70 S6K1 pathway regulates vascular smooth muscle cell differentiation. Am J Physiol Cell Physiol. 2004 Mar;286(3):C507–17.

[82] Brugarolas J, Lei K, Hurley RL, Manning BD, Reiling JH, Hafen E, et al. Regulation of mTOR function in response to hypoxia by REDD1 and the TSC1/TSC2 tumor suppressor complex. Genes Dev. 2004 Dec 1;18(23):2893–904.

[83] Humar R, Kiefer FN, Berns H, Resink TJ, Battegay EJ. Hypoxia enhances vascular cell proliferation and angiogenesis in vitro via rapamycin (mTOR)-dependent signaling. FASEB J. 2002 Jun;16(8):771–80.

[84] Goncharov DA, Kudryashova TV, Ziai H, Ihida-Stansbury K, DeLisser H, Krymskaya VP, et al. Mammalian target of rapamycin complex 2 (mTORC2) coordinates pulmonary artery smooth muscle cell metabolism, proliferation, and survival in pulmonary arterial hypertension. Circulation. 2014 Feb 25;129(8):864–74.

[85] Krymskaya VP, Snow J, Cesarone G, Khavin I, Goncharov DA, Lim PN, et al. mTOR is required for pulmonary arterial vascular smooth muscle cell proliferation under chronic hypoxia. FASEB J. 2011 Jun;25(6):1922–33.

[86] Goncharova EA. mTOR and vascular remodeling in lung diseases: current challenges and therapeutic prospects. FASEB J. 2013 May;27(5):1796–807.

[87] Dai Z, Li M, Wharton J, Zhu MM, Zhao Y-Y. Prolyl-4 hydroxylase 2 (PHD2) deficiency in endothelial cells and hematopoietic cells induces obliterative vascular remodeling and severe pulmonary arterial hypertension in mice and humans through hypoxia-inducible factor-2α. Circulation. 2016 Jun 14;133(24):2447–58.

[88] Houssaini A, Abid S, Derumeaux G, Wan F, Parpaleix A, Rideau D, et al. Selective tuberous sclerosis complex 1 gene deletion in smooth muscle activates mammalian target of rapamycin signaling and induces pulmonary hypertension. Am J Respir Cell Mol Biol. 2016 Sep;55(3):352–67.

[89] Wessler JD, Steingart RM, Schwartz GK, Harvey BG, Schaffer W. Dramatic improvement in pulmonary hypertension with rapamycin. Chest. 2010 Oct;138(4):991–3.

[90] Seyfarth H-J, Hammerschmidt S, Halank M, Neuhaus P, Wirtz HR. Everolimus in patients with severe pulmonary hypertension: a safety and efficacy pilot trial. Pulm Circ. 2013 Sep;3(3):632–8.

7

Hypoxia in Mesenchymal Stem Cell

Wahyu Widowati, Dwi Davidson Rihibiha,

Khie Khiong, M. Aris Widodo,

Sutiman B. Sumitro and Indra Bachtiar

Abstract

Mesenchymal stem cells (MSCs) are non-hematopoietic multipotent stem cells with self-renewal properties and ability to differentiate into a variety of mesenchymal tissues. This chapter overviews effects of hypoxia on MSCs, makes it promising therapy to various diseases. Cultivation of MSCs under hypoxic condition results in variety of outcome that is important to be noted in clinical use. In most studies, hypoxic condition appears to increase proliferation, differentiation, and immune regulatory performance of MSCs without affecting its characteristic. Those benefits are therefore utilized in clinical application. However, there are also studies that report on negative effects of hypoxia in MSCs such as chromosomal instability. Molecular mechanism of MSCs in hypoxic condition is provided for better understanding, which is crucial for further development with better outcome.

Keywords: mesenchymal stem cells, hypoxia

1. Introduction

In these days, stem cell therapy is becoming more believable in treating degenerative diseases compared to conventional medicine. Various diseases such as diabetes, myocardial infarction, spinal cord injury, stroke, and Parkinson's and Alzheimer's diseases have become more prevalent with increasing life expectancy. It has been estimated that in the United States alone, ~128 million individuals would benefit from regenerative stem cell therapy during their lifetime. Mesenchymal stem cells (MSCs) have been highly utilized to treat degenerative diseases among other stem cells. These cells are found in tissues such as bone marrow, adipose tissue, umbilical cord, and dental pulp. Self-renewal and multipotency are the key features of MSCs that make it promising tool. These properties have raised interest on researchers for finding appropriate method to optimize the genetic and environmental factors, which later enhance the biological activities of MSCs.

Many researches have been conducted in the last two decades to study the complex processes in stem cell maintenance. The role of hypoxic conditions (usually 2–9% O_2 concentration) on stem cell biology is very interesting subject due to its beneficial effects. Thus, cultivation of MSCs under hypoxia is currently studied to obtain better understanding, as well as further development to generate better outcome.

2. Mesenchymal stem cell

About 130 years ago, German pathologist Conheim proposed the presence of non-hematopoietic stem cells in the bone marrow that contributes to wound healing in numerous peripheral tissues. Later in the early 1970s, Friedenstein and colleagues demonstrated that the rodent bone marrow had fibroblastoid cells with clonogenic potential *in vitro* [1, 2]. In the study, after the non-adherent cells were removed a few hours later, spindle-like cells, which were morphologically heterogeneous, appeared to attach to the plastic, capable of forming colonies. These cells could also make bone and reconstitute a hematopoietic microenvironment in subcutaneous transplants. Moreover, they could regenerate heterotopic bone tissue in serial transplants, thus indicated their self-renewal potential. Over the years, many studies have investigated these findings and found that these cells were also present in the human bone marrow and could be sub-passaged and differentiated *in vitro* into a variety of the mesenchymal lineages such as osteoblasts, chondrocytes, adipocytes, and myoblasts [3–7]. It has been further renamed as "mesenchymal stem cell" or MSC [4].

MSCs or MSC-like cells are also found in fat, umbilical cord blood, amniotic fluid, placenta, dental pulp, tendons, synovial membrane, and skeletal muscle, yet the complete equivalency of such populations remains unclear [8–16]. Characteristic of MSCs according to The International Society for Cell Therapy [17] consists of (1) adherence to plastic in standard culture conditions; (2) expression of the surface molecules CD73, CD90, and CD105 in the absence of CD34, CD45, HLA-DR, CD14 or CD11b, CD79a, or CD19 surface molecules; and (3) a capacity for differentiation to osteoblasts, adipocytes, and chondroblasts *in vitro*. These criteria were established to standardize human MSC isolation but may not apply uniformly to other species. For instance, marker expression and behavior in murine MSCs were different compared to human MSCs [18]. Certain *in vivo* surface markers may no longer be expressed after Transplantation, although new markers are obtained during expansion. In study done by Jones et al., MSC uniformly expressed HLA-DR (a marker that should not be expressed on MSCs by the above definition) while also expressing CD90 and CD105, adhering to plastic in culture, and differentiating into osteoblasts, adipocytes, and chondroblasts [19]. Indeed, clear definition of MSC-specific characteristics is difficult to apply in both human and animal models.

3. Hypoxia in mesenchymal stem cell

Numerous *in vitro* studies have been conducted in the last two decades to observe the complex processes in stem cell maintenance. However, the role of physiologically hypoxic conditions (usually 2–9% O_2 concentration) on stem cell biology received very little attention. O_2 concentration is an environmental factor that plays a vital role on stem cell fate and function [20]. Stem cells are typically cultured under the ambient O_2 concentration without paying attention to the metabolic milieu of the niche in which they normally grow [21]. The effects of different O_2 levels in MSC culture were first studied in 1958, when Cooper et al. and Zwartouw and Westwood observed that some cells proliferated more rapidly under low O_2 tension levels compared to normal atmospheric levels [22, 23]. MSCs are present in perivascular niches in close association with blood vessels in virtually all tissues [11, 16, 24] and have been compared to pericytes [25]. Even though MSCs are located close to vascular structures, the different tissues where these stem cells are found exhibit low oxygen tensions [26–29]. Therefore, it is possible that maintaining MSCs in an undifferentiated state may require a hypoxic environment, in addition to other factors.

The higher O_2 concentration might cause environmental stress to the *in vitro* cultured MSCs. Recent studies have presented significant evidences regarding the negative outcome under ambient O_2 concentration on MSCs, including early senescence, longer population doubling (PD) time, DNA damage [30, 31], and poor engraftment following transplantation [32, 33]. These have shown the influential effect of O_2 concentration on MSCs biology and raised serious concern over its therapeutic efficiency and biosafety. Thus, the effect of different O_2 concentration on MSCs biology is further discussed based on recent research outcomes.

4. Characteristic of MSCs in hypoxic condition

As described above, MSC immunophenotype is characterized by the expression of CD73, CD90, CD105, CD106, CD146, and MHC class I molecules, and the absence of markers such as CD45 and CD34 or MHC class II molecules [17]. Many studies suggest that hypoxia has no effect on MSCs characteristic, indicated by surface markers. According to one study by Holzwarth et al., there were no significant differences in the expression of cell surface markers after 14 days of culture at 1% when compared to 20% of O_2 [34]. Referring to study carried out by Nekanti et al., WJ-MSCs cultured under both hypoxia and normoxia for 10 passages were positive for CD44, CD73, CD90, CD105, and CD166 and negative for CD34, CD45, and HLA-DR, and there was no significant difference between the two populations [35]. These results are also supported by study carried out by Widowati et al. The surface marker of WJ-MSCs of P4 and P8 both normoxic and hypoxic 5% O_2 were not significantly different. WJ-MSCs were positive for CD105, CD73, and CD90 and negative for CD34, CD45, CD14, CD19, and HLA-II [36].

Morphology changes are also documented in MSCs under hypoxia. Referring to Nekanti et al., WJ-MSC cultured under hypoxia showed a higher amount of large, flattened cells both at early and late passages, compared to normoxic cultures. The enlargement in cell size under hypoxia might be due to a natural response to low oxygen, in which increased surface area would allow for an increase in oxygen diffusion rate [35].

5. MSCs proliferation in hypoxic condition

Capability for self-renewal is a key feature of stem cells. An increased proliferation rate is necessary for more efficient use of stem cells in regenerative therapies. Fehrer et al. demonstrated that bone marrow-derived MSCs (BM-MSCs) cultured in 3% O_2 concentration showed significant increased *in vitro* proliferative lifespan, with ~10 additional population doublings (PDs) (28.5 ± 3.8 PD in 20% O_2 and 37.5 ± 3.4 PD in 3% O_2) before reaching senescence compared to cells cultured in the ambient O_2 environment [31]. In addition, early passaged MSCs cultured in hypoxic conditions also exhibit increased proliferative lifespan along with significant difference in population doubling [30]. Furthermore, it is possible to harvest more than 1×10^9 MSCs from the first five passages cultured in 3% O_2, whereas in ambient condition only 2×10^7 cells can be obtained [30]. Higher *in vitro* expansion rate in hypoxic conditions has also been reported by other researchers [37–39]. Such *in vitro* culture environment also allows to maintain a higher proportion of rapidly self-renewing MSCs for a longer period of time [40]. Other study showed that the increased hypoxic (O_2 2.5%) condition was the best microenvironment for stem cell proliferation compared to normoxic and hypoxic (O_2 5%) for cells at a high passage (P7, P8) [41].

However, various responses of stem cells under hypoxia have been reported [42]. Those differences in cellular responses on hypoxia might be associated with degrees and durations of hypoxia, as well as other cell conditions. Oxygen tension in the stem cell niche for MSCs is suggested to be various from 1 to 7% [43]. A study by Holzwarth et al. showed that rates of MSCs proliferation were reduced after 7 days of culture under hypoxia at 21, 5, 3, and 1% O_2. In their study, only 1.37% of the cells entered the G2/M phase in hypoxic cultures (1% O_2) after 7 days, compared to 2.50% at hyperoxic culture (21% O_2). Reduced O_2 concentrations were therefore confirmed to inhibit cell proliferation as indicated by reduced number of cells in the G2/M phase [34].

6. Chromosomal stability of MSCs in hypoxic condition

Some recent studies have found that human mesenchymal stem cells (hMSCs) retained chromosomal stability following long-term culture *in vitro* [44–46]. Hypoxic environments have shown to increase mutation frequencies in cancer cell lines and trigger genomic rearrangements [47, 48]. It is suggested that oxygen concentration has a major impact on karyotypic aberration. Referring to study of Ueyama et al., chromosomal instability is associated with repeated cell division. A high frequency of chromosomal abnormality breakpoints in common fragile sites (CFSs) was detected by karyotypic analysis (e.g., 2q33, 7q11, 7q36, 8q22.1, 8q24.1,

11p15.1, 19q13) [49]. Generally, chromosomes have fragile sites that are prone to exhibiting gaps and breaks during metaphase [50], in which chromosome rearrangement occurs in cultured cells. Fragile sites are categorized into two main classes, common and rare, according to their frequency in the population [51]. In Ueyama study, several genes involved in regulation of the cell cycle, transcription and cell adhesion, are located in that region with a frequency of 6, 5, and 2%, respectively. In particular, the 11p15.5 domain known as an important tumor suppressor gene region such as tetraspanin 32 (TSPAN32) and tumor-suppressing subtransferable candidate 4 (TSSC4) is present in this region. Alterations in this region have been associated with some neoplasia. It is suggested that the deletion of contiguous genes may induce a multisystem developmental disorder and that these alterations might influence normal functioning and cell survival.

Sex chromosome aneuploidy was also one of the most observed aberrational karyotypes. Frequency of sex chromosome in cultured lymphocytes was significantly higher in females than in males, and that loss of Y chromosomes correlated with age in human bone marrow cells [52, 53]. There are several factors influencing karyotypic stability such as hypoxic culture conditions, donor age, and multiple passages. Karyotypic aberrations increased with passage number and hMSCs undergo spontaneous transformation with tumorigenic potential, especially in later passages under hypoxic culture conditions in hMSCs of elderly donors [49]. Shortly, monitoring of chromosomal stability in culture expanded hMSCs is required prior to exposure to human beings, in order to detect mutations and potentially immortalized clones and to prevent transplant-associated tumor formation.

7. MSCs plasticity in hypoxic condition

The multilineage potential of MSCs is one of the reasons underlying their use in regenerative medicine [54]. Results of MSC differentiation into other lineages diverse according to several studies [34, 55, 56]. Some *in vitro* studies have shown that cultures with low O_2 concentrations stimulated cells to differentiate into adipogenic, osteogenic, or chondrogenic cells. Previous study showed that Rat mesenchymal stem cells (rMSCs) cultured in 5% oxygen produced more bone than cells cultured in 20% O_2 throughout their cultivation time, as indicated by increased markers of osteogenesis, including alkaline phosphatase activity, calcium content, and von Kossa staining. These markers were usually elevated above basal levels when cells were switched from control to low oxygen at first passage and decreased for cells switched from low to control oxygen [57]. Hypoxia appears to exert a potent lipogenic effect independent of PPAR-γ2 maturation pathway [58]. The level of differentiated antigen H-2Dd and the number of G2/S/M phase cells increased evidently under 8% O_2 condition. Also, the proportion of wide, flattened, and epithelial-like cells increased significantly in MSCs. When cultured in adipogenic medium, there was a fivefold to sixfold increase in the number of lipid droplets under hypoxic conditions compared with that in normoxic culture. Oct4 was downregulated under 8% O_2 condition but still expressed after adipocyte differentiation in normoxic culture and treated with hypoxia-mimicking agents, cobalt chloride ($CoCl_2$) and deferoxamine mesylate

(DFX). These findings indicate that hypoxia enhances MSC differentiation and hypoxia and hypoxia-mimicking agents generate different effects on MSC differentiation [59].

Conversely, some others have reported suppressive effects of low O_2 tension levels on the plasticity of MSCs. Differentiation capacity into adipogenic progeny was diminished, and no osteogenic differentiation was detected at 3% oxygen. In turn, MSC that had previously been cultured at 3% oxygen could subsequently be stimulated to successfully differentiate at 20% oxygen [31]. Temporary exposure of MSCs to hypoxia resulted in (i) persistent (up to 14 days postexposure) downregulation of cbfa-1/Runx2, osteocalcin, and type I collagen and (ii) permanent (up to 28 days postexposure) upregulation of osteopontin mRNA expressions [60]. Another study by Widowati et al. showed both nor-WJ-MSCs and hypo-WJ-MSCs differenti-ated to osteocytes, chondrocytes, and adipocytes, although there was no significant difference among treatments [36]. Study conducted by Georgi et al. showed that molecular fingerprints of human MSCs, primary chondrocytes, and MSC/primary chondrocytes coculture differ when cultured in either normoxic (21% O_2) or hypoxic (2.5% O_2) conditions [61]. In the study, cartilage formation increased in cocultures of MSCs and primary chondrocytes was lost when the cells were cultured under hypoxia which was associated with a decrease in the mRNA expression of the chondrogenic marker SOX9 and FGF-1. This coincided with a significant decrease in lipids. Lipid profiles of normoxic and hypoxic cultures are different. The improved cartilage formation in cocultures of MSCs and chondrocytes may employ soluble factors, including small molecules, lipids, or proteins [62]. Lipids such as phospholipids, cholesterol, and diacylglycerols play significant roles in cellular signaling, membrane integrity, and metabolism [63]. Recent study described that short-term changes in sphingolipid metabolism resulted in long-term effects on the chondrogenic phenotype, and the stimulation of chondro-cytes with acylceramidase improves cartilage repair and MSC differentiation [64].

8. Immunomodulatory effects of MSCs in hypoxic condition

One of the key factors of MSC in therapeutics development is their known anti-inflammatory/ immunomodulatory properties. Clinical studies showed efficacy of MSC at inhibiting lethal, immune-based condition of graft versus host disease [65–70]. It has been reported that MSCs derived from adipose, bone marrow, and placenta have the capability to recover ischemic injury by increasing vascularization and reducing inflammation in ischemia-injured hindlimb, lung, heart, and brain [71–73]. Thus, these cells have been used in clinical trials to treat ischemic disease [74]. MSCs produce a broad variety of cytokines, chemokines, and growth factors that may potentially be involved in tissue repair. Hypoxia increases the production of several of these factors, although different responses are also noted in few studies. Referring to Chang et al., hypoxic preconditioning enhances the capacity of the secretome obtained from cultured human MSCs to release several of these factors and the therapeutic potential of the cultured MSC secretome in experimental TBI [75].

One of the most studied mechanisms of inflammation-induced MSC activity is treatment with interferon gamma (IFN-γ). This cytokine is usually secreted during inflammatory Th1 immune responses that are associated with autoimmunity mediated by cellular means, such as CD8 T cells and NK cells, which commonly occur in multiple sclerosis, diabetes type 1, and rheumatoid arthritis [76]. Treatment of IFN-γ in MSC has been reported to enhance the immunosuppressive activity through stimulation of the enzyme IDO [77–80]. MSC expression of the tryptophan-catabolizing enzyme indolamine 2,3 deoxygenase (IDO) was markedly upregulated under hypoxia [81]. IDO is critical in immune regulation by MSC through induction of T cell anergy [82] and stimulation of T regulatory cells (T-regs) [83, 84].

Moreover, IFN-γ induced secretion of other inhibitors of inflammation by MSCs, including the complement inhibitor factor H [85], as well as the immunomodulatory molecules TGF-β and HGF [86]. At a functional level, Noone et al. demonstrated that IFN-γ pretreatment of MSC resulted in protection of MSCs from NK-mediated killing via upregulation of prostaglandin E (PGE)-2 synthesis [87]. IFN-γ, along with necrosis factor-alpha (TNF-α), IL-1α, and IL-1β, induces Gal-9 in MSC [88].

Another inflammatory mediator known to induce regenerative activities in MSC is the macrophage-derived cytokine TNF-α. Pretreatment of TNF-α in MSCs provided superior angiogenic activity *in vitro*, as indicated by expression of VEGF, as well as *in vivo* in an animal model of critical limb ischemia, as compared to untreated MSCs [89]. In other study, TNF-α preconditioning increased proliferation, mobilization, and osteogenic differentiation of MSCs and upregulated bone morphogenetic protein-2 (BMP-2) protein level. Osteogenic differentiation of MSC induced by TNF-α was partially inhibited after BMP-2 knockdown by siRNA [90]. Lipopolysaccharide and toll-like receptor (TLR) agonists, as activators of innate immunity, are also responsible for regenerative activity of MSCs by inducing paracrine factors secretion such as VEGF [91]. IFN-γ and TLR also upregulate the glucocorticoids production, which decreases T cells stimulated by radiotherapy in colonic mucosa [92].

Akiyama et al. reported that MSCs induced T cell apoptosis via the Fas/FasL pathway [93]. Telomerase improved immunomodulatory properties of MSCs by upregulating FasL expression [94]. Dental follicle cells and cementoblasts have been reported to trigger apoptosis of ameloblast-lineage cells, as well as Hertwig's epithelial root sheath (HERS)/epithelial rests of Malassez (ERM) cells, via the Fas/FasL pathway during tooth development [95]. FasL regulated the immunomodulatory properties of Human gingiva-derived mesenchymal stem cells (hGMSCs), which is promoted by hypoxia. However, the underlying pathways of such event remain unclear. Further studies regarding the pathways involved in hGMSC-mediated immunomodulation are encouraged.

9. Molecular mechanism of MSCs in hypoxic condition

O_2 concentration in the stem cell niche (usually 2–9% O_2) is considered a driver of cell function [20]. Hypoxia plays a vital role in maintaining homeostasis within the body from the early stage of embryonic development. It facilitates proper embryonic development, maintains stem cell pluripotency, induces differentiation, and regulates the signaling of multiple cascades, including angiogenesis [96]. In hypoxic conditions, these functions are regulated by several transcription factors such as hypoxia-inducible factors (HIFs), prolyl hydroxylases (PHDs), factor-inhibiting HIF-1 (FIH-1), activator protein 1 (AP-1), nuclear factor (NF)-κB, p53, and c-Myc [97]. Although interaction among all of the transcription factors is required for cellular response, HIFs (especially HIF-1) are the key regulators of cellular response to hypoxia [98]. The discovery of HIF-1a by Greg Semenza provided profound insight into the cellular mechanisms that control hypoxic adaptation [99–101].

Generally, under hypoxic conditions, low O_2 level suppresses the prolyl hydroxylation that leads to HIF-1α accumulation and nuclear translocation [102]. After nuclear translocation, it binds with HIF-1β to form the heterodimer. Then, the HIF-1 heterodimer binds to a hypoxia-response element (HRE) in the target genes, associated with coactivators such as CBP/p300, and regulates the transcription (**Figure 1**) of as many as 70 genes involved in metabolism, angiogenesis, invasion/metastasis, and cell fate [103].

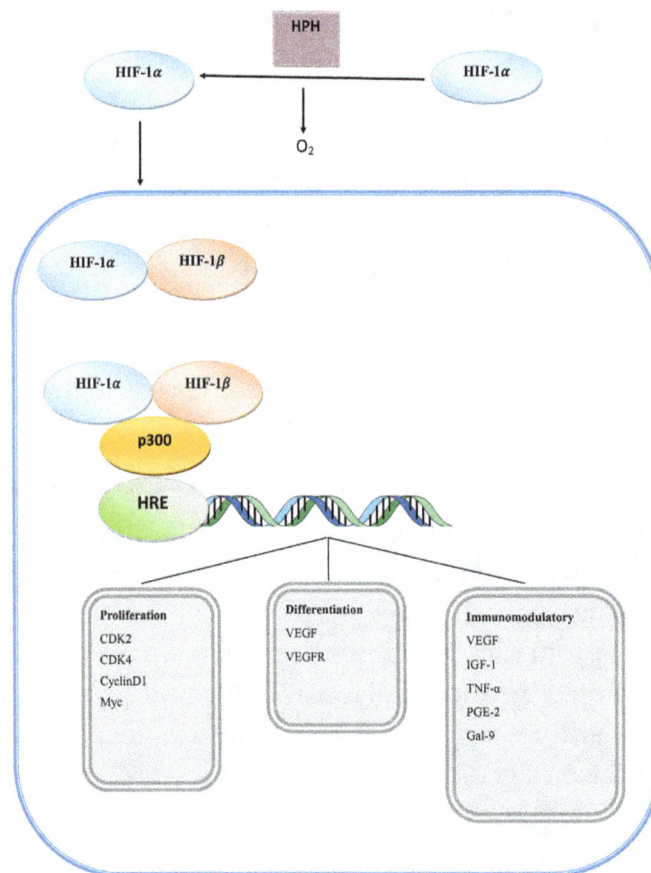

Figure 1. Regulation of hypoxia in MSCs. HIF, hypoxia-inducible factor; HPH, HIF-prolyl hydroxylases; HPE, HIF-prolyl hydroxylases; HRE, hypoxia-response element; CDK, cyclin-dependent kinase; VEGF, vascular endothelial growth factor; VEGFR, vascular endothelial growth factor receptor; IGF, insulin-like growth factor; TNF, tumor necrosis factor; PGE-2, prostaglandin E-2; Gal9, galectin-9. The prolyl hydroxylation process is suppressed due to lack of O_2 that leads HIF-1α accumulation and nuclear translocation after nuclear translocation, and it binds HIF-1β to form the heterodimer. Then, the HIF-1 heterodimer binds HRE in the genes target, associated with coactivators such as CBP/p300, and regulates the transcription of as many as 70 genes involved in proliferation, differentiation, and immunomodulatory.

In 2007, iPSCs were discovered by Shinya Yamanaka and colleagues, and the subsequent identification of the necessary transcriptional programs was required to maintain stem cells in a pluripotent state [104, 105]. The measurement of low partial pressures of oxygen in various stem cell niches raises question whether HIF-1a and iPSCs pathways were converged. It was described initially in Embryonic stem cells (ESCs) [106], hematopoietic stem cells (HSCs) [107], neural stem cells (NSCs) [108], and cancer stem cells (CSCs) [109], which now further expanded to include iPSCs [110]. Remarkably, Yamanaka first reprogrammed fibroblasts to iPSCs using only four transcription factors (Oct4, Sox2, c-Myc, and Klf4) [105] in the same year that Oct4 was shown to be a specific target gene of HIF-2a [111]. The correlation between HIF-2a and Oct4 has been proposed as underlying mechanism of stem cells response to hypoxic conditions in their niche and direct modification of stem cell function by low O_2. HIF-2a expression has recently been investigated in several stem cell lineages, and Oct4 expression is tightly regulated throughout embryogenesis. Loss or even decrease in Oct4 expression leads to differentiation [112]. Oct4 works in concert with Nanog and Sox2 to maintain stem cell identity and repress genes that promote differentiation [113]. The recent identification of HIF-2a upregulation by Oct4 in CSCs and ESCs underscores the importance of this axis in maintaining stemness in both development and disease.

It is known that phosphorylation of protein kinase B (Akt), a downstream gene of phosphatidylinositol 3-kinase (PI3K) signaling pathway, is an important step in signaling pathways that mediate cell proliferation [114, 115]. In PI3K/Akt pathway, a large number of substrates are phosphorylated, including HIF-1 [116]. Referring to study done by Rosová et al., the preculture of MSCs in hypoxia prior to injection activated the PI3K/Akt signaling pathway while maintaining their viability and cell cycle rates [117].

Hypoxia-mediated MSC differentiation by reducing apoptosis via activating the PI3K/Akt/FoxO pathway. Referring to Wang et al., MSCs underwent apoptosis upon induction for chondrogenic differentiation [118]. Apoptosis has been demonstrated as a general phenomenon that occurs during endochondral differentiation of chondrocytes [119]. One study demonstrated that chondrocytes progression to endochondral ossification employed higher FAS receptor and caspase protein as indicators of apoptosis [120]. Other studies showed that both the Wnt/beta-catenin and Indian hedgehog (Ihh) signaling pathways play important roles in endochondral ossification. Beta-catenin is needed at upstream of Ihh signaling for chondrocyte survival and inhibition of apoptosis [121]. The expression of Sox9, col2a1 and aggrecan in prechondrogenic cells 30 and chondrocytes 14 is regulated by PI3K/Akt pathway. It has also been demonstrated that PI3K/Akt regulated col2a1 and aggrecan by modulating Sox9 expression and transcriptional activity in nucleus pulposus cells 31.

Lee et al. [122] showed novel pathway for hypoxia-induced proliferation and migration in human mesenchymal stem cells that employ HIF-1α, FASN, and mTORC1O. Hypoxia treatment stimulates UCB-hMSC proliferation, along with the expression of two lipogenic enzymes: fatty acid synthase (FASN) and stearoyl-CoA desaturase-1 (SCD1). FASN is a key enzyme in UCB-hMSC proliferation and migration. Hypoxia-induced FASN expression was regulated by the HIF-1α/SCAP/SREBP1 pathway. Mammalian target of rapamycin (mTOR) was phosphorylated by hypoxia, whereas inhibition of FASN by cerulenin suppressed hypoxia-induced mTOR phosphorylation, as well as UCB-hMSC proliferation and migration. Hypoxia-induced proliferation and migration are significantly inhibited by raptor small interfering RNA. Hypoxia-induced mTOR also regulates CDK2, CDK4, cyclin D1, cyclin E, and F-actin expression as well as c-myc, p-cofilin, profilin, and Rho GTPase. Moreover, hypoxia-induced FASN stimulates FFA production as well as proliferation and migration. Several studies reported that FAS and FA derivatives inhibited and uncoupled oxidative phosphorylation of various cells [123–125]. Palmitic acid treatment rescues inhibition of mTOR phosphorylation as well as restriction of UCB-hMSC proliferation and migration. Change in cellular metabolite ratios may be another pathway, in addition to the HIF1a/SCAP/SREBP1 pathway, involved in the regulation of lipid metabolism in UCB-hMSCs. Some studies reported that alteration of cellular metabolite ratios, such as NADP/NADPH, by hypoxia has also an important role in the regulation of various stem cell functions such as cell cycle and self-renewal activities [126, 127].

10. Hypoxic MSCs in clinical application

MSCs possess anti-inflammatory/immunomodulatory properties, which are utilized in therapeutics development. Clinical studies on efficacy of MSCs have been shown to inhibit lethal, immune-based condition of graft versus host disease [65–70]. Moreover, MSCs derived from adipose, bone marrow, and placenta have the capability to recover ischemic injury by increasing vascularization and reducing inflammation in ischemia-injured hindlimb, lung, heart, and brain [71–73, 128]. These cells have been used in clinical trials to treat ischemic disease [74], and the safety of MSCs has been evaluated [129, 130]. There are several modified approaches, which have been proposed to improve the effect of MSCs on ischemia-related disease, such as over expression of angiogenesis-related genes such as bFGF on MSCs [131], combination with other cells such as endothelial cells [84], antioxidants such as melatonin [132], serum deprivation [72], and cell spheroids [133].

From isolation to engraftment, the MSCs usually pass through two different phases, consisting of *in vitro* culture condition (from isolation to transplantation) and *in vivo* or physiological condition (before isolation and after transplantation). At present, most of the expansion procedures of MSCs are performed under ambient O_2 concentration, where cells are exposed to 20% O_2, which is ~4–10 times more than the concentration of O_2 in their natural niches [134, 135]. Maintaining genetic stability has been a challenge during *in vitro* expansion of MSCs. Increased rates of aneuploidy, double-stranded DNA breakdown, and faster telomere shortening have been reported for MSCs cultured in ambient condition [30]. According to recent review, major causes behind aneuploidy were defective spindle assembly checkpoint, centrosome amplification, and merotelic attachments [136], which are caused by ROS [137]. ROS also acts in acceleration of telomere shortening and DNA breakdown [138, 139]. Correlation between telomere shortening and aneuploidy in embryonic and hepatocellular carcinoma cells has also been reported in recent studies [140, 141]. The higher ROS production due to the increased mitochondrial respiration during expansion of MSCs in ambient O_2 concentration might be the cause behind genetic instability in them. However, cells undergo anaerobic respiration during hypoxia, which lowers the ROS concentration within the cells. This might reduce the DNA damage, telomere shortening, and aneuploidy which in return may increase the biosafety of stem cell-based therapy.

The ability of stem or progenitor cells to home and engraft into target tissues after transplantation is the key to succeed in clinical application. The degree of homing and engraftment of MSCs in adult recipients is very low [142–144]. Hypoxic culture conditions may also provide a solution for more efficient engraftment. Recently, early passaged mouse BM-MSCs showed better engraftment than late passaged mouse BM-MSCs in *in vivo* model [145]. In other study, hypoxic preconditioned murine MSCs also enhanced skeletal muscle regeneration and improved blood flow and vascular formation compared to normoxic condition [146]. Furthermore, hypoxic conditions cause MSCs to grow faster [30] while maintaining a higher number of rapidly self-renewing cells [40]. Hypoxic environment also upregulated chemokine receptors CXCR4, CXCR7 and CX3CR1 [147, 148], and they may facilitate tissue-specific trafficking of MSCs. Thus, sufficient numbers of MSCs with a higher fraction of rapidly self-renewing cells are suggested, and highly expressed chemokine receptors on their surface can be obtained from the early passages of hypoxic cultures, which could increase the efficiency of damaged tissue-specific migration and engraftment following transplantation.

MSCs cultured under hypoxic conditions also increased in vascular endothelial growth factor receptor 1 (VEGFR1) expression and VEGF- or placental growth factor (PLGF)-dependent migration (Okuyama et al., 2006). Preconditioning with oxygen and combined glucose depletion also increased the survival of stem cell antigen (Sca)-1þ cells via PI3K/Akt-dependent caspase-3 downregulation and thereby increased the engraftment rate [149]. In addition to the increase in migration and survival, MSCs with hypoxic preconditioning have also been shown to enhance revascularization after transplantation for hindlimb ischemia [117]. Therefore, culturing MSCs in hypoxic conditions can also be considered as a solution for tissue-specific engraftment.

Hypoxia-stimulated immune regulation of MSCs has been observed in the situation of allogeneic use of BM-MSCs for stimulation of therapeutic angiogenesis. Recent study showed hypoxia-conditioned BM-MSCs from B6 mice repair limb of Balb/c mice compared to normoxic MSCs. Engraftment in allogeneic recipients increased by decreasing NK cells cytotoxicity and the accumulation of host-derived NK cells when transplanted *in vivo*. These allogeneic hypoxia-treated BM-MSCs increased CD31+ endothelial cells and αSMA+ and desmin + muscle cells, thereby enhancing angiogenesis and restoring muscle structure. Moreover, anti-NK antibodies along with normoxic MSCs enhanced angiogenesis and prevented limb amputation in allogeneic recipients with limb ischemia [150].

Some studies have shown that MSC transplantation contributes to tumor formation *in vivo* [24, 151, 152], whereas Furlani et al. reported that cultured MSCs with spontaneous transformations had no functional effects after intracardiac transplantation [153]. Further studies regarding tumorigenicity and safety of the stem cell-based products are encouraged. However, complexity of cell therapy requires more standards for advanced medicinal products [154]. Thus, especially in the field of regenerative medicine, concrete and specific standards and governmental support systems are necessary to promote their production [154].

11. Perspective of hypoxic MSCs

Hypoxic condition has been confirmed to enhance MSCs proliferation, differentiation, and immune regulatory performance. However, some studies have also reported opposite and negative effects. Different outcomes in each study raise interest in availability of more appropriate methods for cell cultures, which require further study in standardizing the culture of MSCs for use in cell therapy. Optimal conditions for the culture of MSCs have not yet been clearly defined, and it is very crucial to precisely determine the effects of hypoxia on MSCs differentiation, proliferation, and morphology, among other aspects. Moreover, hypoxic MSC-based therapies require a complete understanding of stem cell molecular mechanism. The clarity in stem cell regulation is important for further development such as periodic monitoring of chromosomal stability in culture prior to exposure to human to detect mutations and to prevent transplant-associated tumor formation, and also genetic engineering of physiology of MSCs to acquire better outcome.

12. Conclusion

The growing interest in the potential application of MSCs in regenerative medicine was followed by the several studies measuring the effects of low O_2 levels on the behavior and function of MSCs. Hypoxic condition appears to enhance MSCs proliferation, differentiation, and immune regulatory performance in damaged tissues without affecting its characteristic. However, there are also studies that report on negative effects of hypoxia in MSCs.

Author details

Wahyu Widowati[1*], Dwi Davidson Rihibiha[2], Khie Khiong[2], M. Aris Widodo[3],
Sutiman B. Sumitro[4] and Indra Bachtiar[5]

*Address all correspondence to: wahyu_w60@yahoo.com

1 Faculty of Medicine, Maranatha Christian University, Bandung, Indonesia

2 Biomolecular and Biomedical Research Center, Aretha Medika Utama, Bandung, Indonesia

3 Laboratory of Pharmacology, Faculty of Medicine, Brawijaya University, Malang, Indonesia

4 Department of Biology, Faculty of Mathematics and Natural Sciences, Brawijaya University, Malang, Indonesia

5 Stem Cell and Cancer Institute, Jakarta, Indonesia

References

[1] Friedenstein AJ. The development of fibroblast colonies in monolayer cultures of guinea-pig bone marrow and spleen cells. Cell Tissue Kinet. 1970;3:393–403. doi: 10.1111/j.1365-2184.1970.tb00347.x.

[2] Friedenstein AJ. Stromal mechanisms of bone marrow: cloning *in vitro* and retransplantation *in vivo*. Haematol Blood Transfus. 1980;25:19–29. doi:10.1007/978-3-642-67319-1_3.

[3] Bianco P, Robey PG, Simmons PJ. Mesenchymal stem cells: revisiting history, concepts, and assays. Cell Stem Cell. 2008;2:313–319. doi:10.1016/j.stem.2008.03.002.

[4] Caplan AI. Adult mesenchymal stem cells for tissue engineering versus regenerative medicine. J Cell Physiol. 2007;213:341–347. doi:10.1002/jcp.21200.

[5] Kolf CM, Cho E, Tuan RS. Biology of adult mesenchymal stem cells: regulation of niche, self-renewal and differentiation. Arthritis Res Ther. 2007;9:204. doi:10.1186/ar2116.

[6] Pittenger MF, Mackay AM, Beck SC, Jaiswal RK, Douglas R, Mosca JD, et al. Multilineage potential of adult human mesenchymal stem cells. Science. 1999;284:143–147. doi:10.1126/science.284.5411.143.

[7] Prockop DJ. "Stemness" does not explain the repair of many tissues by mesenchymal stem/multipotent stromal cells (MSCs). Clin Pharmacol Ther. 2007;82:241–243. doi: 10.1038/sj.clpt.6100313.

[8] Rogers I, Casper RF. Umbilical cord blood stem cells. Best Pract Res Clin Obstet Gynaecol. 2004;18:893–908. doi:10.1016/j.bpobgyn.2004.06.004.

[9] Bieback K, Kluter H. Mesenchymal stromal cells from umbilical cord blood. Curr Stem Cell Res Ther. 2007;2:310–323.

[10] Xu Y, Malladi P, Wagner DR, Longaker MT. Adipose-derived mesenchymal cells as a potential cell source for skeletal regeneration. Curr Opin Mol Ther. 2005;7:300–305. PMID:16121695.

[11] Shi S, Gronthos S. Perivascular niche of postnatal mesenchymal stem cells in human bone marrow and dental pulp. J Bone Miner Res. 2003;18:696–704. doi:10.1359/jbmr.2003.18.4.696.

[12] Tsai MS, Lee JL, Chang YJ, Hwang SM. Isolation of human multipotent mesenchymal stem cells from second-trimester amniotic fluid using a novel two-stage culture protocol. Hum Reprod. 2004;19:1450–1456. doi:10.1093/humrep/deh279.

[13] Bi Y, Ehirchiou D, Kilts TM, Inkson CA, Embree MC, Sonoyama W, et al. Identification of tendon stem/progenitor cells and the role of the extracellular matrix in their niche. Nat Med. 2007;13:1219–1227. doi:10.1038/nm1630.

[14] Igura K, Zhang X, Takahashi K, Mitsuru A, Yamaguchi S, Takashi TA. Isolation and characterization of mesenchymal progenitor cells from chorionic villi of human placenta. Cytotherapy. 2004;6:543–553. doi:10.1080/14653240410005366-1.

[15] De Bari C, Dell'accio F, Tylzanowski P, Luyten FP. Multipotent mesenchymal stem cells from adult human synovial membrane. Arthritis Rheum. 2001;44:1928–1942. doi: 10.1002/1529-0131(200108)44:8<1928::AID-ART331>3.0.CO;2-P.

[16] Crisan M, Deasy B, Gavina M, Zheng B, Huard J, Lazzari L, et al. Purification and long-term culture of multipotent progenitor cells affiliated with the walls of human blood vessels: myoendothelial cells and pericytes. Methods Cell Biol. 2008;86:295–309. doi: 10.1016/S0091-679X(08)00013-7.

[17] Dominici M, Le Blanc K, Mueller I, Slaper-Cortenbach I, Marini F, Krause D, et al. Minimal criteria for defining multipotent mesenchymal stromal cells: the international society for cellular therapy position statement. Cytotherapy. 2006;8:315–317. doi: 10.1080/14653240600855905.

[18] Peister A, Mellad JA, Larson BL, Hall BM, Gibson LF, Prockop DJ. Adult stem cells from bone marrow (MSCs) isolated from different strains of inbred mice vary in surface epitopes, rates of proliferation, and differentiation potential. Blood. 2004;103:1662–1668. doi:10.1182/blood-2003-09-3070.

[19] Jones EA, Kinsey SE, English A, Jones RA, Straszynski L, Meredith DM, et al. Isolation and characterization of bone marrow multipotential mesenchymal progenitor cells. Arthritis Rheum. 2002;46:3349–3360. doi:10.1002/art.10696.

[20] Simon MC, Keith B. The role of oxygen availability in embryonic development and stem cell function. Nat Rev Mol Cell Biol. 2008;9:285–296. doi:10.1038/nrm2354.

[21] Scadden DT. The stem-cell niche as an entity of action. Nature. 2006;441:1075–1079. doi: 10.1038/nature04957.

[22] Cooper PD, Burt AM, Wilson JN. Critical effect of oxygen tension on rate of growth of animal cells in continuous suspended culture. Nature. 1958;182:1508–1509. doi: 10.1038/1821508b0.

[23] Zwartouw HT, Westwood JC. Factors affecting growth and glycolysis in tissue culture. Br J Exp Pathol. 1958;39:529–539.

[24] Miura M, Miura Y, Padilla-Nash HM, Molinolo AA, Fu B, Patel V, et al. Accumulated chromosomal instability in murine bone marrow mesenchymal stem cells leads to malignant transformation. Stem Cells. 2006;24:1095–1093. doi:10.1634/stemcells.2005-0403.

[25] Kuhn NZ, Tuan RS. Regulation of stemness and stem cell niche of mesenchymal stem cells: implications in tumorigenesis and metastasis. J Cell Physiol. 2010;222:268–277. doi:10.1002/jcp.21940.

[26] Harrison JS, Rameshwar P, Chang V, Bandari P. Oxygen saturation in the bone marrow of healthy volunteers. Oxygen saturation in the bone marrow of healthy volunteers. Blood. 2002;99:394. PMID:11783438.

[27] Kofoed H, Sjontoft E, Siemssen SO, Olesen HP. Bone marrow circulation after osteotomy. Blood flow, pO2, pCO2, and pressure studied in dogs. Acta Orthop Scand. 1985;56:400–403.

[28] Matsumoto A, Matsumoto S, Sowers AL, Koscielniak JW, Trigg NJ, Kuppusamy P, et al. Absolute oxygen tension (pO(2)) in murine fatty and muscle tissue as determined by EPR. Magn Reson Med. 2005;54:1530–1535. doi:10.1002/mrm.20714.

[29] Pasarica M, Sereda OR, Redman LM, Albarado DC, Hymel DT, Roan LE, et al. Reduced adipose tissue oxygenation in human obesity: evidence for rarefaction, macrophage chemotaxis, and inflammation without an angiogenic response. Diabetes. 2009;58:718–725. doi:10.2337/db08-1098.

[30] Estrada JC, Albo C, Benguría A, Dopazo A, Lopez-Romero P, Carrera-Quintanar L, et al. Culture of human mesenchymal stem cells at low oxygen tension improves growth and genetic stability by activating glycolysis. Cell Death Differ. 2012;19:743–755. doi: 10.1038/cdd.2011.172.

[31] Fehrer C, Brunauer R, Laschober G, Unterluggauer H, Reitinger S, Kloss F, et al. Reduced oxygen tension attenuates differentiation capacity of human mesenchymal stem cells and prolongs their lifespan. Aging Cell. 2007;6:745–757. doi:10.1111/j. 1474-9726.2007.00336.x.

[32] Mohamadnejad M, Pournasr B, Bagheri M, Aghdami N, Shahsavani M, Hosseini LA, et al. Transplantation of allogeneic bone marrow mesenchymal stromal cell-derived hepatocyte-like cells in homozygous familial hypercholesterolemia. Cytotherapy. 2010;12:566–568. doi:10.3109/14653240903511143.

[33] Schachinger V, Erbs S, Elsasser A, Haberbosch W, Hambrecht R, Holschermann H. Intracoronary bone marrow-derived progenitor cells in acute myocardial infarction. N Engl J Med. 2006;355:1210–1221.

[34] Holzwarth C, Vaegler M, Gieseke F, Pfister SM, Handgretinger R, Kerst G, et al. Low physiologic oxygen tensions reduce proliferation and differentia-tion of human multipotent mesenchymal stromal cells. BMC Cell Biol. 2010;11:1–11. doi:10.1186/1471-2121-11-11.

[35] Nekanti U, Dastidar S, Venugopal P, Totey S, Ta M. Increased proliferation and analysis of differential gene expression in human Wharton's jelly-derived mesenchymal stromal cells under hypoxia. Int J Biol Sci. 2010;6:499–512.

[36] Widowati W, Wijaya L, Murti H, Widyastuti H, Agustina D, Laksmitawati DR, et al. Conditioned medium from normoxia (WJMSCs-norCM) and hypoxia-treated WJMSCs (WJMSCs-hypoCM) in inhibiting cancer cell proliferation. BGM. 2015;7:8–17.

[37] Basciano L, Nemos C, Foliguet L, de Isla N, de Carvalho M, Tran N, et al. Long term culture of mesenchymal stem cells in hypoxia promotes a genetic program maintaining their undifferentiated and multipotent status. BMC Cell Biol. 2011;12:1–12. doi: 10.1186/1471-2121-12-12.

[38] Grayson WL, Zhao F, Bunnell B, Ma T. Hypoxia enhances proliferation and tissue formation of human mesenchymal stem cells. Biochem Biophys Res Commun. 2007;358:948–953. doi:10.1016/j.bbrc.2007.05.054.

[39] Weijers EM, Van Den Broek LJ, Waaijman T, Van Hinsbergh VWM, Gibbs S, Koolwijk P. The influence of hypoxia and fibrinogen variants on the expansion and differentiation of adipose tissue-derived mesenchymal stem cells. Tissue Eng Part A. 2011;17:2675–2685. doi:10.1089/ten.tea.2010.0661.

[40] Saller MM, Prall WC, Docheva D, Schönitzer V, Popov T, Anz D, et al. Increased stemness and migration of human mesenchymal stem cells in hypoxia is associated with altered integrin expression. Biochem Biophys Res Commun. 2012;423:379–385. doi:10.1016/j.bbrc.2012.05.134.

[41] Widowati W, Wijaya L, Bachtiar I, Gunanegara RF, Sugeng SU, Irawan YA, et al. Effect of oxygen tension on proliferation and characteristics of Wharton's jelly-derived mesenchymal stem cells. BGM. 2014;6:43–48. doi:10.1016/j.bgm.2014.02.001.

[42] Pattappa G, Thorpe SD, Jegard NC, Heywood HK, de Bruijn JD, Lee DA. Continuous and uninterrupted oxygen tension influences the colony formation and oxidative metabolism of human mesenchymal stem cells. Tissue Eng Part C Methods. 2013;19:68–79. doi:10.1089/ten.TEC.2011.0734.

[43] Yew TL, Chang MC, Hsu YT, He FY, Weng WH, Tsai CC, et al. Efficient expansion of mesenchymal stem cells from mouse bone marrow under hypoxic conditions. J Tissue Eng Regen Med. 2013;7:984–993. doi:10.1002/term.1491.

[44] Rubio D, Garcia-Castro J, Martin MC, de la Fuente R, Cigudosa JC, Lloyd AC, et al. Spontaneous human adult stem cell transformation. Cancer Res. 2005;65:3035–3039. doi:10.1158/0008-5472.CAN-04-4194.

[45] Bernardo ME, Zaffaroni N, Novara F, Cometa AM, Avanzini MA, Moretta A, et al. Human bone marrow derived mesenchymal stem cells do not undergo transformation after long-term *in vitro* culture and do not exhibit telomere maintenance mechanisms. Cancer Res. 2007;67:9142–9149. doi:10.1158/0008-5472.CAN-06-4690.

[46] Zhang ZX, Guan LX, Zhang K, Wang S, Cao PC, Wang YH, et al. Cytogenetic analysis of human bone marrow-derived mesenchymal stem cells passaged *in vitro*. Cell Biol Int. 2007;31:645–648. doi:10.1016/j.cellbi.2006.11.025.

[47] Fischer U, Radermacher J, Mayer J, Mehraein Y, Meese E, et al. Tumor hypoxia: impact on gene amplification in glioblastoma. Int J Oncol. 2008;33:509–515. doi:10.3892/ijo_00000034.

[48] Coquelle A, Toledo F, Stern S, Bieth A, Debatisse M. A new role for hypoxia in tumor progression: induction of fragile site triggering genomic rearrangements and formation of complex DMs and HSRs. Mol Cell. 1998;2:259–265. doi:10.1016/S1097-2765(00)80137-9.

[49] Ueyama H, Horibe T, Hinotsu S, Tanaka T, Inoue T, Urushihara H, et al. Chromosomal variability of human mesenchymal stem cells cultured under hypoxic conditions. J Cell Mol Med. 2012;16:72–82. doi:10.1111/j.1582-4934.2011.01303.x.

[50] Sutherland GR. Chromosomal fragile sites. Genet Anal Biomol Eng. 1991;8:161–166. doi:10.1016/1050-3862(91)90056-W.

[51] Lukusa T, Fryns JP. Human chromosome fragility. Biochim Biophys Acta. 2008;1779:3–16. doi:10.1016/j.bbagrm.2007.10.005.

[52] Nowinski GP, Van Dyke DL, Tilley BC, Jacobsen G, Babu VR, Worsham MJ, et al. The frequency of aneuploidy in cultured lymphocytes is correlated with age and gender but not with reproductive history. Am J Hum Genet. 1990;46:1101–1111. PMCID:PMC1683821.

[53] Pierre RV, Hoagland HC. Age-associated aneuploidy: loss of Y chromosome from human bone marrow cells with aging. Cancer. 1972;30:889–894. doi:10.1002/1097-0142(197210)30:4<889::AID-CNCR2820300405>3.0.CO;2-1.

[54] Baksh D, Song L, Tuan RS. Adult mesenchymal stem cells: characterization, differentiation, and application in cell and gene therapy. J Cell Mol Med. 2004;8:301–316. doi:10.1111/j.1582-4934.2004.tb00320.x.

[55] Hung SP, Ho JH, Shih YR, Lo T, Lee OK. Hypoxia promotes proliferation and osteogenic differentiation potentials of human mesenchymal stem cells. J Orthop Res. 2012;30:260–266.doi:10.1002/jor.21517.

[56] Huang J, Deng F, Wang L, Xiang XR, Zhou WW, Hu N, et al. Hypoxia induces osteogenesis related activities and expression of core binding factor alpha1 in mesenchymal stem cells. Tohoku J Exp Med. 2011;224:7–12. doi:10.1620/tjem.224.7.

[57] Lennon DP, Edmison JM, Caplan AI. Cultivation of rat marrow-derived mesenchymal stem cells in reduced oxygen tension: effects on *in vitro* and *in vivo* osteochondrogenesis. J Cell Physio. 2001;187:345–355. doi:10.1002/jcp.1081.

[58] Fink T, Abildtrup L, Fogd K, Abdallah BM, Kassem M, Ebbesen P, Zachar V. Induction of adipocyte like phenotype in human mesenchymal stem cells by hypoxia. Stem Cells. 2004;22:1346–1355. doi:10.1634/stemcells.2004-0038.

[59] Ren H, Cao Y, Zhao Q, Li J, Zhou C, Liao L, et al. Proliferation and differentiation of bone marrow stromal cells under hypoxic conditions. Biochem Biophys Res Commun. 2006;347:12–21. doi:10.1016/j.bbrc.2006.05.169.

[60] Potier E, Ferreira E, Andriamanalijaona R, Pujol JP, Oudina K, Logeart-Avramoglou D, et al. Hypoxia affects mesenchymal stromal cell osteogenic differentiation

and angiogenic factor expression. Bone. 2007;40:1078–1087. doi:10.1016/j.bone. 2006.11.024.

[61] Georgi N, Cillero-Pastor B, Eijkel GB, Periyasamy PC, Kiss A, van Blitterswijk C, et al. Differentiation of mesenchymal stem cells under hypoxia and normoxia: lipid profiles revealed by time-of-flight secondary ion mass spectrometry and multivariate analysis. Anal Chem. 2015;87:3981–3988. doi:10.1021/acs.analchem.5b00114.

[62] Maumus M, Manferdini C, Toupet K, Peyrafitte JA, Ferreira R, Facchini A, et al. Adipose mesenchymal stem cells protect chondrocytes from degeneration associated with osteoarthritis. Stem Cell Res. 2013;11:834–844. doi:10.1016/j.scr.2013.05.008.

[63] Brown AJ. Cholesterol, statins and cancer. Clin Exp Pharmacol Physiol. 2007;34:135–141. doi:10.1111/j.1440-1681.2007.04565.x.

[64] Simonaro CM, Sachot S, Ge Y, He X, Deangelis VA, Eliyahu E, et al. Acid ceramidase maintains the chondrogenic phenotype of expanded primary chondrocytes and improves the chondrogenic differentiation of bone marrow-derived mesenchymal stem cells. PLoS One 2013;8:1–14. doi:10.1371/journal.pone.0062715.

[65] Ringden O, Uzunel M, Rasmusson I, Remberger M, Sundberg B, Lönnies H, Le Blanc K. Mesenchymal stem cells for treatment of therapy resistant graft versus host disease. Transplant. 2006;81:1390–1397. doi:10.1097/01.tp.0000214462.63943.14.

[66] Le Blanc K, Rasmusson I, Sundberg B, Götherström C, Hassan M, Uzunel M, et al. Treatment of severe acute graft versus host disease with third party haploidentical mesenchymal stem cells. Lancet. 2004;363:1439–1441. doi:10.1016/S0140-6736(04)16104-7.

[67] Le Blanc K, Frassoni F, Ball L, Locatelli F, Roelofs H, Lewis I, et al. Mesenchymal stem cells for treatment of steroid-resistant, severe, acute graft versus host disease: a phase II study. Lancet. 2008;371:1579–1586. doi:10.1016/S0140-6736(08)60690-X.

[68] Ning H, Yang F, Jiang M, Hu L, Feng K, Zhang J, et al. The correlation between cotransplantation of mesenchymal stem cells and higher recurrence rate in hematologic malignancy patients: outcome of a pilot clinical study. Leukemia. 2008;22:593–599. doi: 10.1038/sj.leu.2405090.

[69] Ball L, Bredius R, Lankester A, Schweizer J, van den Heuvel-Eibrink M, Escher H, et al. Third party mesenchymal stromal cell infusions fail to induce tissue repair despite successful control of severe grade IV acute graft-versus-host disease in a child with juvenile myelo-monocytic leukemia. Leukemia. 2008;22:1256–1257. doi:10.1038/sj.leu. 2405013.

[70] Muller I, Kordowich S, Holzwarth C, Isensee G, Lang P, Neunhoeffer F, et al. Application of multipotent mesenchymal stromal cells in pediatric patients following allogeneic stem cell transplantation. Blood Cells Mol Dis. 2008;40:25–32. doi:10.1016/j.bcmd. 2007.06.021.

[71] Liu J, Hao H, Xia L, Ti D, Huang H, Dong L, et al. Hypoxia pretreatment of bone marrow mesenchymal stem cells facilitates angiogenesis by improving the function of endothelial cells in diabetic rats with lower ischemia. PLoS One. 2015;10:1–18. doi:10.1371/journal.pone.0126715.

[72] Sun CK, Leu S, Hsu SY, Zhen YY, Chang LT, Tsai CY, et al. Mixed serum-derived and normal adipose-derived mesenchymal stem cells against acute lung ischemia reperfusion injury in rats. Am J Transl Res. 2015;7:209–231.

[73] Zhang GW, Gu TX, Guan XY, Sun XJ, Jiang DQ, Tang R, Qi X, Li XY. Delayed enrichment for c-kit and inducing cardiac differentiation attenuated protective effects of BMSCs transplantation in pig model of acute myocardial ischemia. Cardiovasc Ther. 2015;33:184–192. doi:10.1111/1755-5922.12131.

[74] Bura A, Planat-Benard V, Bourin P, Silvestre JS, Gross F, Grolleau JL, et al. Phase I trial: the use of autologous cultured adipose-derived stroma/stem cells to treat patients with non-revascularizable critical limb ischemia. Cytotherapy. 2014;16:245–257. doi:10.1016/j.jcyt.2013.11.011.

[75] Chang CP, Chio CC, Cheong CU, Chao CM, Cheng BC, Lin MT. Hypoxic preconditioning enhances the therapeutic potential of the secretome from cultured human mesenchymal stem cells in experimental traumatic brain injury. Clin Sci. 2013;124:165–176. doi:10.1042/CS20120226.

[76] Skurkovich B, Skurkovich S. Anti-interferon-gamma antibodies in the treatment of autoimmune diseases. Curr Opin Mol Ther. 2003;5:52–57. PMID:12669471.

[77] Croitoru-Lamoury J, Lamoury FMJ, Caristo M, Suzuki K, Walker D, Takikawa O, et al. Interferon-γ regulates the proliferation and differentiation of mesenchymal stem cells via activation of indoleamine 2,3 dioxygenase (IDO). PLoS One. 2011;6:1–13. doi:10.1371/journal.pone.0014698.

[78] Rong LJ, Chi Y, Yang SG, Chen DD, Chen F, Xu SX, et al. Effects of interferon-γ on biological characteristics and immunomodulatory property of human umbilical cord-derived mesenchymal stem cells. J Exp hematol Chin Assoc Pathophysiol. 2012;20:421–426.

[79] Kang JW, Koo HC, Hwang SY, Kang SK, Ra JC, Lee MH, et al. Immunomodulatory effects of human amniotic membrane-derived mesenchymal stem cells. J Vet Sci. 2012;13:23–31. doi:10.4142/jvs.2012.13.1.23.

[80] Lin W, Oh SKW, Choo ABH, George AJT. Activated T cells modulate immunosuppression by embryonic- and bone marrow-derived mesenchymal stromal cells through a feedback mechanism. Cytotherapy. 2012;14:274–284. doi:10.3109/14653249.2011.635853.

[81] Roemeling-Van Rhijn M, Mensah FKF, Korevaar SS, Leijs MJC, Van Osch GJVM, IJzermans JNM, et al. Effects of hypoxia on the immunomodulatory properties of

adipose tissue-derived mesenchymal stem cells. Front Immunol. 2013;4:1–8. doi: 10.3389/fimmu.2013.00203.

[82] English K, Tonlorenzi R, Cossu G, Wood KJ. Mesoangioblasts suppress T cell proliferation through IDO and PGE-2-dependent pathways. Stem Cells Dev. 2013;22:512–523. doi:10.1089/scd.2012.0386.

[83] Engela AU, Baan CC, Peeters AM, Weimar W, Hoogduijn MJ. Interaction between adipose-tissue derived mesenchymal stem cells and regulatory T cells. Cell Transplant. 2013;22:41–54. doi:10.3727/096368912X636984.

[84] Huang CC, Chen DY, Wei HJ, Lin KJ, Wu CT, Lee TY, et al. Hypoxia-induced therapeutic neovascularization in a mouse model of an ischemic limb using cell aggregates composed of HUVECs and cbMSCs. Biomaterials. 2013;34:9441–9550. doi:10.1016/j.biomaterials.2013.09.010.

[85] Tu Z, Li Q, Bu H, Lin F. Mesenchymal stem cells inhibit complement activation by secreting factor H. Stem Cells Dev. 2010;19:1803–1809. doi:10.1089/scd.2009.0418.

[86] Ryan JM, Barry F, Murphy JM, Mahon BP. Interferon-gamma does not break, but promotes the immunosuppressive capacity of adult human mesenchymal stem cells. Clin Exp Immunol. 2007;149:353–363. doi:10.1111/j.1365-2249.2007.03422.x.

[87] Noone C, Kihm A, English K, O'Dea S, Mahon BP. IFN-gamma stimulated human umbilical-tissue derived cells potently suppress NK activation and resist NK mediated cytotoxicity *in vitro*. Stem Cells Dev. 2013;15:3003–3014. doi:10.1089/scd.2013.0028.

[88] Gieseke F, Kruchen A, Tzaribachev N, Bentzien F, Dominici M, Müller I. Proinflammatory stimuli induce galectin-9 in human mesenchymal stromal cells to suppress T-cell proliferation. Eur J Immunol. 2013;43:2741–2749. doi:10.1002/eji.201343335.

[89] Kwon YW, Heo SC, Jeong GO, Yoon JW, Mo WM, Lee MJ, et al. Tumor necrosis factor-α-activated mesenchymal stem cells promote endothelial progenitor cell homing and angiogenesis. Biochim Biophys Acta. 2013;1832:2136–2144. doi:10.1016/j.bbadis.2013.08.002.

[90] Lu Z, Wang G, Dunstan CR, Chen Y, Lu WYR, Davies B, et al. Activation and promotion of adipose stem cells by tumour necrosis factor-alpha preconditioning for bone regeneration. J Cell Physiol. 2013;228:1737–1744. doi:10.1002/jcp.24330.

[91] Grote K, Petri M, Liu C, Jehn P, Spalthoff S, Kokemüller H, et al. Toll-like receptor 2/6-dependent stimulation of mesenchymal stem cells promotes angiogenesis by paracrine factors. Eur Cells Mater. 2013;26:66–79. PMID:24027020.

[92] Bessout R, Sémont A, Demarquay C, Charcosset A, Benderitter M, Mathieu N. Mesenchymal stem cell therapy induces glucocorticoid synthesis in colonic mucosa and suppresses radiation-activated T cells: new insights into MSC immunomodulation. Mucosal Immunol. 2014;7:656–669. doi:10.1038/mi.2013.85.

[93] Akiyama K, Chen C, Wang D, Xu X, Qu C, Yamaza T, et al. Mesenchymal stem cell induced immunoregulation involves FAS-ligand-/FAS-mediated T cell apoptosis. Cell Stem Cell. 2012;10:544–555. doi:10.1016/j.stem.2012.03.007.

[94] Chen C, Akiyama K, Yamaza T, You Y-O, Xu X, Li B, et al. Telomerase governs immunomodulatory properties of mesenchymal stem cells by regulating FAS ligand expression. EMBO Mol Med. 2014;6:322–334. doi:10.1002/emmm.201303000.

[95] Ding, SW. RNA-based antiviral immunity. Nat Rev Immunol. 2010;10:632–644. doi:10.1038/nri2824.

[96] Lin Q, Kim Y, Alarcon RM, Yun Z. Oxygen and cell fate decisions. Gene Regul Syst Bio. 2008;2:43–51. PMCID:PMC2733087.

[97] Kenneth NS, Rocha S. Regulation of gene expression by hypoxia. Biochem J. 2008;414:19–29. doi:10.1042/BJ20081055.

[98] Stamati K, Mudera V, Cheema U. Evolution of oxygen utilization in multicellular organisms and implications for cell signalling in tissue engineering. J Tissue Eng. 2011;2:1–12. doi:10.1177/2041731411432365.

[99] Semenza GL, Wang GL. A nuclear factor induced by hypoxia via de novo protein synthesis binds to the human erythropoietin gene enhancer at a site required for transcriptional activation. Mol Cell Biol. 1992;12:5447–5454.

[100] Wang GL, Jiang BH, Rue EA, Semenza GL. Hypoxia inducible factor 1 is a basic helix loop helix PAS heterodimer regulated by cellular O2 tension. Proc Natl Acad Sci. 1995;92:5510–5514. PMCID:PMC46495.

[101] Wang GL, Semenza GL. General involvement of hypoxia-inducible factor 1 in transcriptional response to hypoxia. Proc Natl Acad Sci. 1993;90:4304–4308. PMCID: PMC46495.

[102] Weidemann A, Johnson RS. Biology of HIF-1α. Cell Death Differ. 2008;15:621–627. doi:10.1038/cdd.2008.12.

[103] Brahimi-Horn MC, Pouyssegur J. Oxygen, a source of life and stress. FEBS Lett. 2007;581:3582–3591. doi:10.1016/j.febslet.2007.06.018.

[104] Takahashi K, Tanabe K, Ohnuki M, Narita M, Ichisaka T, Tomoda K, et al. Induction of pluripotent stem cells from adult human fibroblasts by defined factors. Cell. 2007;131:861–872. doi:10.1016/j.cell.2007.11.019.

[105] Takahashi K, Yamanaka S. Induction of pluripotent stem cells from mouse embryonic and adult fibroblast cultures by defined factors. Cell. 2006;126:663–676. doi:10.1016/j.cell.2006.07.024.

[106] Adelman DM, Maltepe E, Simon MC. Multilineage embryonic hematopoiesis requires hypoxic ARNT activity. Genes Dev. 1999;13:2478–2483.

[107] Cipolleschi MG, Dello Sbarba P, Olivotto M. The role of hypoxia in the maintenance of hematopoietic stem cells. Blood. 1993;8:2031–2037. PMID:8104535.

[108] Panchision DM. The role of oxygen in regulating neural stem cells in development and disease. J Cell Physiol. 2009;220:562–568. doi:10.1002/jcp.21812.

[109] Li Z, Bao S, Wu Q, Wang H, Eyler C, Sathornsumetee S, et al. Hypoxia-inducible factors regulate tumorigenic capacity of glioma stem cells. Cancer Cell. 2009;15:501–513. doi: 10.1016/j.ccr.2009.03.018.

[110] Yoshida Y, Takahashi K, Okita K, Ichisaka T, Yamanaka S. Hypoxia enhances the generation of induced pluripotent stem cells. Cell Stem Cell. 2009;5:237–241. doi: 10.1016/j.stem.2009.08.001.

[111] Covello KL, Kehler J, Yu H, Gordan JD, Arsham AM, Hu CJ, et al. HIF-2alpha regulates Oct-4: effects of hypoxia on stem cell function, embryonic development, and tumor growth. Genes Dev. 2006;20:557–570. doi:10.1101/gad.1399906.

[112] Boiani M, Eckardt S, Scholer HR, McLaughlin KJ. Oct4 distribution and level in mouse clones: consequences for pluripotency. Genes. 2002;16:1209–1219. doi:10.1101/gad.966002.

[113] Boyer LA, Lee TI, Cole MF, Johnstone SE, Levine SS, Zucker JP, et al. Core transcriptional regulatory circuitry in human embryonic stem cells. Cell. 2005;122:947–956. doi: 10.1016/j.cell.2005.08.020.

[114] Borgatti P, Martelli AM, Bellacosa A, Casto R, Massari L, Capitani S, et al. Translocation of AKT/PKB to the nucleus of osteoblast-like MC3T3-E1 cells exposed to proliferative growth factors. FEBS Lett. 2000;477:27–32.

[115] Jung F, Haendeler J, Goebel C, Zeiher AM, Dimmeler S. Growth factor-induced phosphoinositide 3-OH kinase/Akt phosphorylation in smooth muscle cells: induction of cell proliferation and inhibition of cell death. Cardiovasc Res. 2000;48:148–157. doi: 10.1016/S0008-6363(00)00152-8.

[116] Semenza GL. Targeting HIF-1 for cancer therapy. Nat Rev Cancer. 2003;3:721–732. doi: 10.1038/nrc1187.

[117] Rosová I, Dao M, Capoccia B, Link D, Nolta JA. Hypoxic preconditioning results in increased motility and improved therapeutic potential of human mesenchymal stem cells. Stem Cells. 2008;26:2173–2182. doi:10.1634/stemcells.2007-1104.

[118] Wang CY, Chen LL, Kuo PY, Chang JL, Wang YJ, Hung SC. Apoptosis in chondrogenesis of human mesenchymal stem cells: effect of serum and medium supplements. Apoptosis. 2010;15:439–449. doi:10.1007/s10495-009-0431-x.

[119] Cheung JO, Grant ME, Jones CJ, Hoyland JA, Freemont AJ, Hillarby MC. Apoptosis of terminal hypertrophic chondrocytes in an *in vitro* model of endochondral ossification. J Pathol. 2003;201:496–503. doi:10.1002/path.1462.

[120] Aizawa T, Kon T, Einhorn TA, Gerstenfeld LC. Induction of apoptosis in chondrocytes by tumor necrosis factor-alpha. J Orthop Res. 2001;19:785–796. doi:10.1016/ S0736-0266(00)00078-4.

[121] Mak KK, Chen MH, Day TF, Chuang PT, Yang Y. Wnt/beta-catenin signaling interacts differentially with Ihh signaling in controlling endochondral bone and synovial joint formation. Development. 2006;133:3695–3707. doi:10.1242/dev.02546.

[122] Lee HJ, Ryu JM, Jung YH, Oh SY, Lee SJ, Han HJ. Novel pathway for hypoxia-induced proliferation and migration in human mesenchymal stem cells: involvement of HIF-1α, FASN, and mTORC1. Stem Cells. 2015;33:2182-2195. doi:10.1002/stem.2020.

[123] Ventura FV, Ruiter JP, Ijlst L, Almeida IT, Wanders RJ. Inhibition of oxidative phosphorylation by palmitoyl-CoA in digitonin permeabilized fibroblasts: implications for long-chain fatty acid beta oxidation disorders. Biochim Biophys Acta. 1995;1272:14–20.

[124] Samartsev VN, Belosludtsev KN, Chezganova SA, Zeldi IP. Effect of ethanol on the palmitate induced uncoupling of oxidative phosphorylation in liver mitochondria. Biochemistry. 2002;67:1240–1247. doi:10.1023/A:1021397220815.

[125] Brustovetskii NN, Dedukhova VN, Egorova MV, Mokhova EN, Skulachev VP. Uncoupling of oxidative phosphorylation by fatty acids and detergents suppressed by ATP/ADP antiporter inhibitors. Biokhimiia. 1991;56:1042–1048.

[126] Cipolleschi MG, Marzi I, Santini R, Fredducci D, Vinci MC, D'Amico M, et al. Hypoxia-resistant profile implies vulnerability of cancer stem cells to physiological agents, which suggests new therapeutic targets. Cell Cycle. 2014;13:268–278. doi:10.4161/cc.27031.

[127] Marzi I, Cipolleschi MG, D'Amico M, Stivarou T, Rovida E, Vinci MC, et al. The involvement of a Nanog, Klf4 and c-Myc transcriptional circuitry in the intertwining between neoplastic progression and reprogramming. Cell Cycle. 2013;12:353–364. doi: 10.4161/cc.23200.

[128] Li D, Zhang M, Zhang Q, Wang Y, Song X, Zhang Q. Functional recovery after acute intravenous administration of human umbilical cord mesenchymal stem cells in rats with cerebral ischemia-reperfusion injury. Intractable Rare Dis Res. 2015;4:98–104. doi: 10.5582/irdr.2015.01010.

[129] Karussis D, Karageorgiou C, Vaknin-Dembinsky A, Gowda-Kurkalli B, Gomori JM, Kassis I, et al. Safety and immunological effects of mesenchymal stem cell transplantation in patients with multiple sclerosis and amyotrophic lateral sclerosis. Arch Neurol. 2010;67:1187–1194. doi:10.1001/archneurol.2010.248.

[130] Lalu MM, McIntyre L, Pugliese C, Fergusson D, Winston BW, Marshall JC, et al. Safety of cell therapy with mesenchymal stromal cells (safe cell): a systematic review and meta-analysis of clinical trials. PLoS One. 2012;7:1–21. doi:10.1371/journal.pone. 0047559.

[131] Zhang JC, Zheng GF, Wu L, Ou Yang LY, Li WX. Bone marrow mesenchymal stem cells overexpressing human basic fibroblast growth factor increase vasculogenesis in ischemic rats. Braz J Med Biol Res. 2014;47:886–894. doi:10.1590/1414-431X20143765.

[132] Yip HK, Chang YC, Wallace CG, Chang LT, Tsai TH, Chen YL, et al. Melatonin treatment improves adipose-derived mesenchymal stem cell therapy for acute lung ischemia-reperfusion injury. J Pineal Res. 2013;54:207–221. doi:10.1111/jpi.12020.

[133] Park IS, Chung PS, Ahn JC. Enhanced angiogenic effect of adipose-derived stromal cell spheroid with low-level light therapy in hind limb ischemia mice. Biomaterials. 2014;35:9280–9289. doi:10.1016/j.biomaterials.2014.07.061.

[134] Antoniou ES, Sund S, Homsi EN, Challenger LF, Rameshwar P. A theoretical simulation of hematopoietic stem cells during oxygen fluctuations: prediction of bone marrow responses during hemorrhagic shock. Shock. 2004;22:415–422.

[135] Chow DC, Wenning LA, Miller WM, Papoutsakis ET. Modeling pO2 distributions in the bone marrow hematopoietic compartment II. Modified Kroghian models. Biophys J. 2001;81:685–696. doi:10.1016/S0006-3495(01)75733-5.

[136] Gordon DJ, Resio B, Pellman D. Causes and consequences of aneuploidy in cancer. Nat Rev Genet. 2012;13:189–203. doi:10.1038/nrg3123.

[137] Wang CY, Liu LN, Zhao ZB. The role of ROS toxicity in spontaneous aneuploidy in cultured cells. Tissue Cell. 2012;45:47–53. doi:10.1016/j.tice.2012.09.004.

[138] Barzilai A, Yamamoto K. DNA damage responses to oxidative stress. DNA Repair (Amst). 2004;3:1109–1115. doi:10.1016/j.dnarep.2004.03.002.

[139] Guachalla LM, Rudolph KL. ROS induced DNA damage and checkpoint responses: influences on aging? Cell Cycle. 2010;9:4058–4060. doi:10.4161/cc.9.20.13577.

[140] Treff NR, Su J, Taylor D, Scott RT. Telomere DNA deficiency is associated with development of human embryonic aneuploidy. PLoS Genetics. 2011;7:1–10. doi:10.1371/journal.pgen.1002161.

[141] Plentz RR, Schlegelberger B, Flemming P, Gebel M, Kreipe H, Manns MP, et al. Telomere shortening correlates with increasing aneuploidy of chromosome 8 in human hepatocellular carcinoma. Hepatology. 2005;42:522–526. doi:10.1002/hep.20847.

[142] LaBarge MA, Blau HM. Biological progression from adult bone marrow to mononucleate muscle stem cell to multinucleate muscle fiber in response to injury. Cell. 2002;111:589–601. doi:10.1016/S0092-8674(02)01078-4.

[143] Ankrum J, Karp JM. Mesenchymal stem cell therapy: two steps forward, one step back. Trends Mol Med. 2010;16:203–209. doi:10.1016/j.molmed.2010.02.005.

[144] Phinney DG, Prockop DJ. Concise review: mesenchymal stem/multipotent stromal cells: the state of trans differentiation and modes of tissue repair—current views. Stem Cells. 2007;25:2896–2902. doi:10.1634/stemcells.2007-0637.

[145] Jin J, Zhao Y, Tan X, Guo C, Yang Z, Miao D. An improved transplantation strategy for mouse mesenchymal stem cells in an acute myocardial infarction model. PLoS One. 2011;6:1–16. doi:10.1371/journal.pone.0021005.

[146] Leroux L, Descamps B, Tojais NF, Seguy B, Oses P, Moreau C, et al. Hypoxia preconditioned mesenchymal stem cells improve vascular and skeletal muscle fiber regeneration after ischemia through a wnt4-dependent pathway. Mol Ther. 2010;18:1545–1552. doi:10.1038/mt.2010.108.

[147] Liu H, Liu S, Li Y, Wang X, Xue W, Ge G, et al. The role of SDF-1-CXCR4/CXCR7 axis in the therapeutic effects of hypoxia-preconditioned mesenchymal stem cells for renal ischemia/reperfusion injury. PLoS One. 2012;7:1–13. doi:10.1371/journal.pone.0034608.

[148] Hung S-C, Pochampally RR, Hsu S-C, Sanchez C, Chen S-C, Spees J, et al. Short-term exposure of multipotent stromal cells to low oxygen increases their expression of CX3CR1 and CXCR4 and their engraftment *in vivo*. PLoS One. 2007;2:1–11. doi:10.1371/journal.pone.0000416.

[149] Lu G, Haider HK, Jiang S, Ashraf M. Sca-1þ stem cell survival and engraftment in the infarcted heart: dual role for preconditioning induced connexin-43. Circulation. 2009;119:2587–2596. doi:10.1161/CIRCULATIONAHA.108.827691.

[150] Huang WH, Chen HL, Huang PH, Yew TL, Lin MW, Lin SJ, et al. Hypoxic mesenchymal stem cells engraft and ameliorate limb ischaemia in allogeneic recipients. Cardiovasc Res. 2014;101:266–276. doi:10.1093/cvr/cvt250.

[151] Guest I, Ilic Z, Ma J, Grant D, Glinsky G, Sell S. Direct and indirect contribution of bone marrow-derived cells to cancer. Int J Cancer. 2010;126:2308–2318. doi:10.1002/ijc.24946.

[152] Tolar J, Nauta AJ, Osborn MJ, Panoskaltsis Mortari A, McElmurry RT, Bell S, et al. Sarcoma derived from cultured mesenchymal stem cells. Stem Cells. 2007;25:371–379. doi:10.1634/stemcells.2005-0620.

[153] Furlani D, Li W, Pittermann E, Klopsch C, Wang L, Knopp A, et al. A transformed cell population derived from cultured mesenchymal stem cells has no functional effect after transplantation into the injured heart. Cell Transplant. 2009;18:319–331. doi: 10.3727/096368909788534906.

[154] Tsubouchi M, Matsui S, Banno Y, Kurokawa K, Kawakami K. Overview of the clinical application of regenerative medicine products in Japan. Health Policy. 2008;88:62–72. doi:10.1016/j.healthpol.2008.02.011.

8

The Critical Role of Hypoxia in Tumor-Mediated Immunosuppression

Nassera Aouali, Manon Bosseler, Delphine Sauvage,

Kris Van Moer, Guy Berchem and Bassam Janji

Abstract

Underestimated for a long time, the involvement of the microenvironment has been proven essential for a better understanding of the cancer development. In keeping with this, the tumor is not considered anymore as a mass of malignant cells, but rather as an organ composed of various malignant and nonmalignant cell populations interacting with each other to create the tumor microenvironment. The tumor immune contexture plays a critical role in shaping the tumor immune response, and it is now well supported that such an immune response is impacted by the hypoxic stress within the tumor microenvironment. Tumor hypoxia is closely linked to tumor progression, metastasis, treatment failure, and escape from immune surveillance. Thus, hypoxia seems to be a key factor involved in creating an immune-suppressive tumor by multiple overlapping mechanisms, including the impairment of the function of cytotoxic immune cells, increasing the immunosuppressive properties of immunosuppressive cells, and activating resistance mechanism in the tumor cells. In this chapter, we review some recent findings describing how hypoxic stress in the tumor microenvironment hijacks the antitumor immune response.

Keywords: cancer, hypoxia, immune response, tumor microenvironment, autophagy, tumor plasticity, tumor heterogeneity

1. Introduction

Malignant cells are part of cellular and microenvironmental complexes which both define the initiation, progression, and maintenance of the malignant phenotype. In turn, malignant cells participate in creating a hostile microenvironment characterized by hypoxic areas within the tumors. Indeed, the oxygen level in the hypoxic tumor is usually lower than that of corresponding normal tissue. The oxygenation level of tumor is likely depending on (i) the initial oxygenation of the tissue; (ii) the degree of the tumor heterogeneity; (iii) the tumor size and stage. **Table 1** summarizes the percentage of oxygen level reported as a median in some healthy organs and their corresponding tumors, as defined by several studies.

Healthy tissue/corresponding cancer	% of oxygen (Median)
Brain/brain tumor	4.6/1.7
Breast/breast cancer	8.5/1.5
Cervix/cervical cancer	9.5/1.2
Kidney cortex/renal cancer	7.0/1.3
Liver/liver cancer	4.0–7.3/0.8
Lung/nonsmall cell lung carcinoma	5.6/2.2
Pancreas/pancreatic tumor	7.5/0.3
Rectal mucosa/rectal carcinoma	3.9/1.8

Table 1. Comparison of the percentage (%) of oxygen level in different healthy tissues and in their corresponding cancers.

It is now widely appreciated that hypoxia is one of the most relevant factor involved in the impairment of the antitumor immune response by damping the cytotoxic function of immune cells. There are numerous studies supporting that hypoxic stress leads to the establishment of immune tolerance of tumor cells by preventing the migration and the homing of immune effector cells into established tumors. Furthermore, hypoxia can also drive tumor cell plasticity and functional heterogeneity and, thus, favors the emergence of more aggressive tumors. Many strategies are emerging for targeting intratumor hypoxia in order to change the immunosuppressive properties of the tumor to a microenvironment able to support antitumor immunity.

2. Hypoxia is the major factor of the tumor microenvironment

The long-lasting tumor immunology research has validated the concept of tumor immuno-surveillance. The tumor immunosurveillance consists in the fact that cytotoxic immune cells recognize nascent transformed cells and destroy them before they become clinically apparent. Several types of immune cells are involved in the control of tumors such as immune effector and immune suppressor cells. Thus, cytotoxic T lymphocytes (CTL) belong to the adaptive immune system and they are able to recognize tumor antigens through the T-cell receptor (TCR) [1]. The antigens expressed exclusively by tumor cells are called tumor-specific anti-gens [2]. In addition to CTL, the tumor immune surveillance involves natural killer (NK) cells that belong to the innate immune system [1]. NK cells recognize tumor cells by mechanisms called "missing-self" and "induced-self" [3]. Briefly, NK cells are regulated by a balance of inhibitory and activating signals of surface receptors. Thus, NK cells can kill their target cell depending on the recognized ligand(s). The identification of activating or inhibitory ligands allows NK cells to distinguish between "self" versus "nonself" and "self" versus "altered self" by "missing-self" and "induced-self" recognitions. Indeed, the protection of normal cells from NK cell killing is achieved by balancing the stimulatory signals delivered by stimulatory ligands with inhibitory signals delivered by self MHC class I molecules. When the expression of self MHC class I molecules is lost following cell transformation or infection, the stimulatory signals delivered by the target cell remain unbalanced, leading to the activation of NK cells and lysis of target cells (known as missing-self recognition). Under some circumstances, transformed or infected cells overexpress stimulatory ligands that overcome the inhibitory signals leading to target cell lysis (known as induced-self recognition). It has been reported that both missing-self and induced-self recognition could operate simultaneously. In this case, NK cells display a high ability to discriminate between normal and transformed target cells [4].

In addition to cytotoxic immune cells, the tumor immune contexture contains immune suppressive cells such as myeloid-derived suppressor cells (MDSC) able to inhibit the function of immune effectors. Macrophages and neutrophil granulocytes are also involved in antitumor immunity [5]. These cells display tumor antigens and can stimulate other immune cells such as CTL, NK cells, or antigen-presenting cells (APC) [6]. Although both CTL and NK cells kill their target following the establishment of immunological synapse (IS) [7], the molecular mechanism by which they recognize their target tumor cells is fundamentally different. Two major pathways are used by CTL and NK cells to recognize and destroy tumor cells: (i) through the release by immune cells of cytotoxic granules containing perforin and granzymes and these cytotoxic granules are captured by tumor cells to induce cell death by apoptosis [8], and (ii) through tumor necrosis factor (TNF) superfamily-dependent mechanism [9].

It has been proposed that despite the powerful ability of the immune system to attack cancer cells, tumors can outmaneuver the immune effectors cells and escape the immune surveillance. It is now well documented that the ability of tumor cells to escape immune cell control is most likely resulted from the activation of several resistance mechanisms to evade effective and functional host immune response. Therefore, it stands to reason that established tumors, displaying multiple resistance mechanism, are likely not fully controlled by the immune system. In keeping with this, it is strongly believed that clinically detected cancers have most likely evaded effective antitumor immune responses. Recently, it has been reported that in addition to its role in protecting host against tumor development, the immune system can under certain circumstances sculpt the immunogenic phenotype of well-developed tumors. Such a mechanism favors the emergence of resistant tumor cell clones [10]. Accumulating experimental and clinical evidence suggest that the resistance mechanisms activated in tumor cells are multifactorial and that such resistance mechanisms are primarily evolved and activated in the tumor microenvironment [11]. It appears that hypoxia is the major tumor microenvironmental factor involved in the alteration of the transcriptome and the metabolome of tumor cells as well as their proliferation, survival, and invasion [12].

In this chapter, we summarize some recent findings describing how hypoxic stress in the tumor microenvironment regulates the antitumor immune response and leads to tumor escape from immunosurveillance. We focus on how hypoxia confers resistance to immune attack and impairs tumor cell killing mediated by CTL and NK cells.

2.1. Hypoxia and hypoxia-inducible factors (HIF) regulation

Tumor cells are able to adapt to hypoxic stress through the regulation of the hypoxia inducible factor family of transcription factors (HIFs) [13]. It has been reported for a large number of human cancers that HIFs were overexpressed and such overexpression is associated with poor response to treatment [14]. Moreover, evidence showed a clear positive correlation between enhanced hypoxic expression of HIFs and mortality [13]. Therefore, inhibition of HIFs could represent a novel approach to improve cancer therapies. Currently, efforts are being actively pursued to identify inhibitors of HIFs and to test their efficacy as anticancer therapeutics.

Three isoforms of HIF have been identified: HIF-1, HIF-2, and HIF-3. The hypoxia-inducible factor-1 (HIF-1) is the major factor mediating adaptive responses to changes in tissue oxygen level [15]. Indeed, HIF-1 is a heterodimer composed of a constitutively expressed HIF-1β subunit and an O_2-dependent regulated HIF-1α subunit. HIF-1α is a DNA-binding basic helix-loop helix of the PAS family [Per (period circadian protein); Arnt (aryl hydrocarbon receptor nuclear translocator protein); Sim (single-minded protein)] [16]. HIF-1α contains two oxygen-dependent degradation domains (ODDD), one in the N-terminal (N-ODDD) moiety and one in the C-terminal moiety (C-ODDD) [17, 18]. It also contains two transactivation domains (TADs), one N-terminal, which overlaps with the C-ODDD, and one C-terminal [19].

2.2. Regulation of HIF-1 level

The expression level of HIF-1α is determined by the rates of protein synthesis and protein degradation. While the synthesis of HIF-1α is regulated in an O_2-independent manner, its degradation is primarily regulated via an O_2-dependent mechanism. Thus, normoxic cells constantly synthesize HIF-1α protein and degrade it rapidly [17]. It has been shown that under normoxic conditions HIF-1α has a short half-life of less than 5 min [20]. However, under hypoxia or low oxygen level, the degradation of HIF-1α is blocked or dramatically decreased [21]. Under normoxia, HIF-1α is hydroxylated on proline residue 402 and/or 564 in the ODDD by prolyl hydroxylase domain protein 2 (PHD2) [17, 22]. Such oxygen-dependent hydroxylation of HIF-1α results in its binding to the von Hippel-Lindau tumor suppressor protein (pVHL). pVHL is the recognition component of an E3 ubiquitin-protein ligase complex that targets HIF-1α for proteolysis by the ubiquitin-proteasome pathway [23].

Enzymes regulating HIF-1α proteasomal degradation were first identified to be related to egl-9 in caenorhabditis elegans and to termed prolyl hydroxylase domain (PHD) enzymes (PHD1, PHD-2, and PHD3) [24, 25]. PHD2 uses oxygen as a substrate, and thus, its activity is inhibited under hypoxic conditions [25]. The inhibition of PHD2 leads to the inhibition of prolyl hydroxylation of HIF-1α and subsequently to the inhibition of HIF-1α-dependent proteasomal degradation. Consequently, HIF-1α rapidly accumulates in the cytoplasm, translocates to the nucleus and dimerizes with HIF-1β. The HIF-1α/HIF-1β heteromeric dimer binds to the hypoxia responsive element (HRE) in target genes, recruits coactivators and activates transcription [14] (**Figure 1A**).

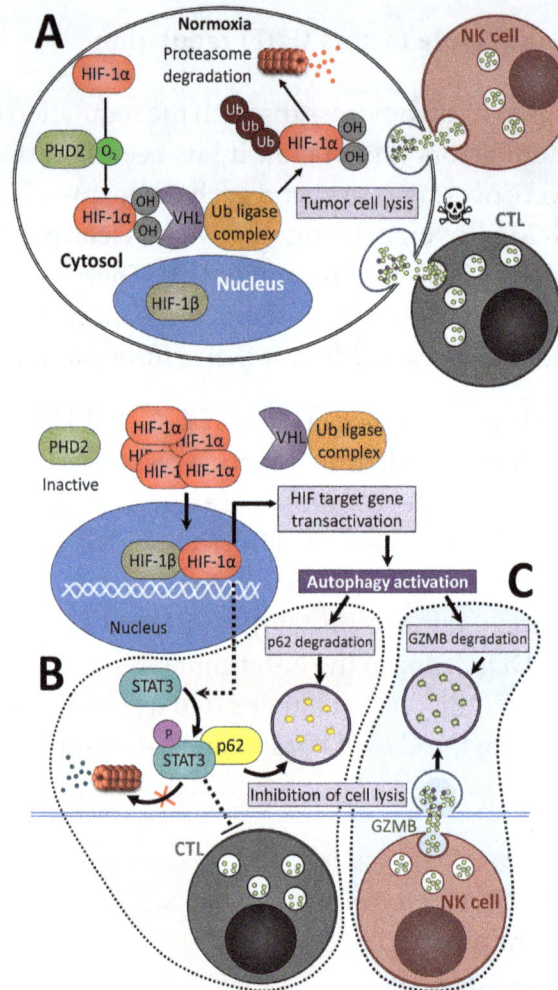

Figure 1. The role of hypoxic stress in the impairment CTL and NK-cell mediated lysis. (A) Under normoxia, the oxygen-sensitive prolyl hydroxylase domain protein 2 (PHD2) hydroxylates HIF-1α subunit. Hydroxylated HIF-1 interacted with Von Hippel-Lindau protein (VHL), subjected to ubiquitination and subsequently degraded by the ubiquitin-proteasome system. Under hypoxic stress, the function of PHD2 protein is blocked, HIF-1α is therefore stabilized and translocated to the nucleus to form heterodimeric complex with HIF-1β to transcriptionally induce the expression of HIF-target genes involved in several pathways such as autophagy. (B) Under hypoxia, STAT3 is phosphorylated at Ser-705 residue in a HIF-dependent manner by a mechanism which is not fully understood. (C) The hypoxia-dependent induction of autophagy leads to the degradation of the adaptor protein p62/SQSTM1, involved in targeting phospho-STAT3 to the ubiquitin proteasome system for degradation. Thus, targeting autophagy accumulated p62/SQSTM1 and therefore accelerated the degradation of phospho-STAT3. The degradation of phospho-STAT3 restores CTL-mediated lysis of tumor cells. In addition, the induction of autophagy in hypoxic tumor cells leads to the selective degradation of granzyme B (GZMB), a serine protease released by natural killer (NK) cells and contained in the cytotoxic granules. Such degradation inhibits NK-mediated lysis of tumor cells.

Using genomewide chromatin immunoprecipitation combined with DNA microarray (ChIP-chip) or DNA sequencing (ChIP-seq) analysis, it has been shown that more than 800 genes involved in several cell functions are direct targets of HIF [26, 27]. HIF-1 activates the expression of these genes by binding to a 50 base pair cis-acting HRE located in their enhancer and promoter regions [28]. The HREs of all these genes contain the core sequence 5′-[A/G]CGT-3′, which in most cases is ACGTG [29]. It has been reported that HIF transcription factors preferentially bind to specific bases in the 5′ and 3′ proximity of the core that has led to define the following HRE consensus sequence [T/G/C][A/G]CGTG[CGA][GTC][GTC][CTG] [29].

Similar to HIF-1α, the stabilization of HIF-2α is also regulated by oxygen-dependent hydroxylation [30]. This could be related to the fact that HIF-1α and HIF-2α displayed a similar structure of their DNA binding and dimerization domains. However, the major difference between the structure of HIF-1α and HIF-2α is in their transactivation domains [31]. In terms of genes expression, both HIF-1α and HIF-2α share overlapping target genes, and each one also regulates a set of unique targets [32].

In sharp contrast with HIF-1α and HIF-2α, HIF-3α lacks the transactivation domain and could function as an inhibitor of HIF-1α and HIF-2α. It has been reported that the expression of HIF-3α is regulated by HIF-1 [33]. In addition to the regulation of the expression of a large number of genes, HIF family members regulate hypoxia-related microRNAs (HRM) [34] and some chromatin modifying enzymes [35].

3. Intra-tumor hypoxia: a key feature that triggers several resistance mechanisms of tumor evasion from immune surveillance

It has been clearly established that the immune effector activity and the antitumor immune response are significantly regulated by hypoxia. Indeed, hypoxia, via HIF-1α, decreases the susceptibility of lung cancer cells to CTL-mediated killing. It appears that the resistance to CTL is related to the effect of HIF-1α to induce the phosphorylation of signal transducer and activator of transcription 3 (STAT3) in tumor cells by a mechanism involving the vascular endothelial growth factor (VEGF) secretion. These data suggest that following its translocation to the nucleus, HIF-1α cooperates with pSTAT3 to impair lung carcinoma cell susceptibility to CTL-mediated killing [36] (**Figure 1B**). More recently, it has been shown that the expression of the phosphorylated form of STAT3 at Ser-705 residue is tightly controlled by the induction of autophagy in hypoxic tumor cells as the accumulation of pSTAT3 was no longer observed when autophagy was targeted genetically in tumor cells [37]. Autophagy is a catabolic cell degradation process. Autophagy plays an essential role in preventing accumulation of altered cell components [38] and as an adaptive metabolic response to provide nutrients. Recently, an unexpected role of autophagy in shaping the antitumor immune response [39] and the acquisition of resistance to TNFα has been shown [40]. Autophagy is activated under stress conditions such as hypoxia, nutrient starvation, growth factor withdrawal, and endoplasmic reticulum stress. It has been reported that the molecular mechanism by which autophagy regulates the pSTAT3 level involves the protein p62/SQSTM1 the ubiquitin proteasome system [37, 41].

Another study showed that in addition to the mechanism described earlier, it has been shown that the stem cell self-renewal transcription factor NANOG is also involved in the regulation of CTL-mediated tumor cell lysis [42, 43]. Hypoxia regulates NANOG at both transcriptional and translational levels and targeting NANOG in hypoxic cells restored CTL-mediated tumor cell killing. Furthermore, NANOG depletion results in the inhibition of STAT3 phosphorylation and its nuclear translocation. The hypoxia-induced microRNA (miR)-210 is also involved in the regulation of CTL-mediated tumor cells lysis. In fact, HIF-1 induces the expression of miR-210 which subsequently targets nonreceptor protein tyrosine phosphatase type 1 (PTPN1), homeobox A1 (HOXA1), and tumor protein p53-inducible protein 11 (TP53I11), and thereby decreases tumor cell susceptibility to CTL [44]. In the context of NK-mediated tumor cell lysis, it has been described that hypoxia increases the shedding of the major histocompatibility complex (MHC) class I polypeptide-related sequence A (MICA), a ligand for the activating receptor natural killer group 2 member D (NKG2D), on the surface of prostate cancer cells leading to an impairment of NO signaling [45] and subsequent escape of tumor cells from NK- and CTL-mediated killing. MICA expression is also downregulated by HIF-1 in osteosarcoma cells resulting in tumor resistance to NK-mediated lysis [46]. Through the activation of autophagy, it has been recently reported that melanoma and breast tumor cells escape NK-mediated lysis and that targeting autophagy in hypoxic tumor cells was sufficient to restore NK-mediated lysis. In this study, it has been shown that the activation of autophagy under hypoxia was responsible for the degradation of NK-derived granzyme B making hypoxic tumor cells less sensitive to NK-mediated killing [39, 47, 48] (**Figure 1C**). In line with the studies described earlier, it is now well admitted that hypoxic stress in the tumor microenvironment is a key factor involved in the control of antitumor immune response. Beside its role in impairing the function of cytotoxic immune cells, the immunosuppressive effect of hypoxia contributes to the emergence of resistant tumor cells that compromise the effectiveness of the anti-tumor immune response [49].

4. Hypoxia and tumor cell heterogeneity and plasticity

Solid tumors frequently reveal pronounced tumor cell heterogeneity with regards to cell organization, cell morphology, cell size, and nuclei morphology [50]. The molecular mechanisms underlying the phenotypic heterogeneity involve genetic, epigenetic, and environmental factors. It is now well established that hypoxia is an important contributor to intra- and intertumor cell heterogeneity [15, 51] by altering the expression of specific genes involved in cellular phenotype. In this respect, it has been reported that neuroblastoma cells and breast cancer cells lose their differentiated gene expression patterns and develop stem cell-like phenotypes under hypoxic stress [52, 53]. As a low stage of differentiation in neuroblastoma and breast cancer is associated with poor prognosis, it is strongly believed that, in addition to its contribution to tumor heterogeneity, hypoxia-dependent induction of tumor cell dedifferentiation contributes to tumor cell plasticity and aggressiveness.

Several lines of evidence suggest that tumor microenvironment drives stem cell renewal and differentiation. Indeed, poorly vascularized tumors contain hypoxic regions with undifferentiated 'stem-like' tumor cells that survive under control of HIFs [54]. It has been reported that hypoxic stress in colon cancer inhibits the differentiation of tumor cells and maintains their stem-like phenotype [55]. In addition, myofibroblasts stromal cells secrete factors involved in maintaining cancer stem cells (CSC) population in colon cancer [56]. Furthermore, stromal cells drive a CSC phenotype on differentiated cancer cells, allowing a transient morphological heterogeneity observed in several cancers. In this regard, transient phenotypic changes from epithelial to mesenchymal (epithelial-mesenchymal transition (EMT)) or mesenchymal to epithelial (mesenchymal to epithelial transitions (MET)) phenotype, are initially considered as conversions facilitating cell plasticity but have recently gained appreciation as events involved in tumor heterogeneity [57]. In the context of tumor immunity, recent evidence revealed that tumor cell plasticity has serious implications in terms of immunological recognition and killing of the tumor, since such tumor cell plasticity may lead to the emergence of immunoresistant variants [58].

Although the role of the immune system in inhibiting early stages of tumor growth is well established, it is now strongly suggested that the immune system can also facilitate the advanced stages of tumor progression by sculpting the immunogenic phenotype of a developing tumor to favor the emergence of immune-resistant tumor cell variants. This has led to the concept of "immunoediting" which encompasses three phases: elimination, equilibrium, and escape. Thus, immunoediting allows tumors to evade immune destruction by becoming less immunogenic or more immunosuppressive [59]. Such adaptability, achieved through cell reprogramming, reflects an important property of tumors called immune-induced plasticity. While the molecular basis of immune-dependent induction of tumor cell plasticity and its effective contribution to the selection of tumor aggressive variants is still elusive, recent findings have revealed that activated CD8+ T cells can stimulate mammary epithelial tumor cells to undergo EMT and acquire the increased tumorigenic capability and therapy resistance of breast CSCs [60]. In this regard, it has been shown that reciprocal interactions between melanoma and immune cells enhances tumor cell plasticity and drives therapy resistance [61]. Based on these data, it is now well defined that targeting phenotypic plasticity should be considered for the development of novel therapeutic strategies with the ultimate goal to prevent the establishment of a more aggressive phenotype of cancer cells.

5. The clinical significance of targeting hypoxia

For many years, the major issue in the field of cancer immunity was to understand how cancer cells manage to evade immune surveillance despite the presence of a competent immune system. To address this issue, the major focus was on the mechanisms by which tumor cells escape cytotoxic immune cell recognition without considering the impact of the tumor microenvironment. This could partially explain why despite intense investigation, the gains provided by immunotherapy until recently are relatively modest. In addition, accumulating evidence suggests that tumor cell resistance mechanisms are likely evolved in the hypoxic tumor microenvironment. In keeping with this, it is therefore more accurate to consider cancer as a disease of the microenvironment rather than a disease of cells. Although remarkable progresses have been achieved over the past two decades regarding the impact of the tumor microenvironment in cancer biology and treatment, its contribution in the development of tumor resistance to immune cell killing remains fragmented.

Emerging data indicates that hypoxia stress within the tumor microenvironment is a key factor involved in the impairment of the antitumor immune response. [62] Therefore, a deep understanding of the molecular mechanism by which hypoxia induces tumor resistance may contribute to the development of more effective tumor immunotherapies.

Consistent with the fact that hypoxia-dependent overexpression of HIF-1α is associated with an increased patient mortality in several cancer types, it stands to reason that inhibition of HIF-1 activity in preclinical studies would have marked effects on tumor growth and survival. In keeping with this, efforts are underway to identify selective inhibitors of HIF-1 and to assess their efficacy as anticancer therapeutics. Currently, two main approaches are used to target hypoxia in tumors, namely bioreductive prodrugs, and inhibitors of molecular targets upon which hypoxic cell survival depends [63, 64]. However, several lines of evidence indicate that the HIF pathway is technically extremely challenging to target. Indeed, the first evidence is that transcription factors in general, including HIF, have long been considered "undruggable," and therefore, no specific inhibitor of HIF has been brought to the market so far. The second evidence is that multiple levels of regulation and signaling pathways converge on and emerge from HIF [65]. Nevertheless, based on the molecular mechanism of HIF-1 protein, it has been suggested that small molecules could be used to inhibit HIF-1 activity through a variety of mechanisms including inhibition of (i) HIF-1α protein synthesis; (ii) HIF-1α protein stabilization; (iii) HIF-1α/β dimerization, and (iv) HIF-1/DNA binding. Two comprehensive recent reviews summarize these mechanisms in detail and give fairly exhaustive lists of the small-molecule inhibitors for each level [15, 66].

Using a cell-based assay, several small-molecule inhibitors of HIF-1 activity have been identified. Briefly, topoisomerase I inhibitors block the expression of HIF-1α via an undefined mechanism [67]. The small molecule YC-1 (3-(5'-hydroxy-methyl-2'-furyl)-1-benzylindazole) was also shown to reduce the level of HIF-1α by a mechanism that has not been established but at least is known to work independently from its function as a stimulator of soluble guanylate-cyclase activity [68]. YC-1 is not in clinical use. The HSP90 inhibitor 17-allyl-aminogeldanamycin (17-AAG) has been reported to induce the degradation of HIF-1α in a VHL-independent manner [69–71]. PX-12 (thioredoxin-1 redox inhibitor) and PX-478 are both inhibitors of HIF-1α protein expression and HIF-1-mediated transactivation [72, 73]. Finally, the disruptor of microtubule polymerization 2-methoxyoestradiol (2ME2) is able to decrease the expression of HIF-1α. Currently, only topoisomerase I inhibitors, camptothecin and topotecan, are clinically approved agents, PX-478, 2ME2, and 17-AAG are under evaluation in clinical trials, whereas YC-1 and thioredoxin-1 inhibitors are not in clinical use.

Despite of the anticancer effects of these agents could be related, in part, to their inhibition of HIF-1, it seems that none of these drugs specifically targets HIF-1. Although such lack of selectivity does not disqualify these drugs as anticancer agents, it enhances the difficulty to correlate molecular and clinical responses in patients. Therefore, the identification of more selective HIF-1 inhibitors in the near future is required and more investigation needs to be done to identify novel potent and more specific inhibitors targeting clearly defined points in the HIF pathway.

Acknowledgements

This work was supported by grants from the Luxembourg Institute of Health (LECR 2013 11 05), Fondation Cancer (FC/2016/01) and Kriibskrank Kanner Foundation, Luxembourg.

Author details

Nassera Aouali[1], Manon Bosseler[1], Delphine Sauvage[1], Kris Van Moer[1], Guy Berchem[1,2] and Bassam Janji[1*]

*Address all correspondence to: bassam.janji@lih.lu

1 Laboratory of Experimental Cancer Research, Department of Oncology, Luxembourg Institute of Health, Luxembourg City, Luxembourg

2 Luxembourg Hospital Center, Department of Hemato-Oncology, Luxembourg City, Luxembourg

References

[1] Smyth, M.J., D.I. Godfrey, and J.A. Trapani. A fresh look at tumor immunosurveillance and immunotherapy. Nat Immunol, 2001. 2(4): p. 293-9.

[2] Rosenberg, S.A.. Progress in human tumour immunology and immunotherapy. Nature, 2001. 411(6835): p. 380-4.

[3] Watzl, C. and E.O. Long. Exposing tumor cells to killer cell attack. Nat Med, 2000. 6(8): p. 867-8.

[4] Raulet, D.H. and R.E. Vance. Self-tolerance of natural killer cells. Nat Rev Immunol, 2006. 6(7): p. 520-31.

[5] Di Carlo, E., G. Forni, P. Lollini, M.P. Colombo, A. Modesti, and P. Musiani. The intriguing role of polymorphonuclear neutrophils in antitumor reactions. Blood, 2001. 97(2): p. 339-45.

[6] Allavena, P., G. Germano, F. Marchesi, and A. Mantovani. Chemokines in cancer related inflammation. Exp Cell Res, 2011. 317(5): p. 664-73.

[7]   Grakoui, A., S.K. Bromley, C. Sumen, M.M. Davis, A.S. Shaw, P.M. Allen, and M.L. Dustin. The immunological synapse: a molecular machine controlling T cell activation. Science, 1999. 285(5425): p. 221-7.

[8]   Shresta, S., D.M. MacIvor, J.W. Heusel, J.H. Russell, and T.J. Ley. Natural killer and lymphokine-activated killer cells require granzyme B for the rapid induction of apoptosis in susceptible target cells. Proc Natl Acad Sci USA, 1995. 92(12): p. 5679-83.

[9]   Cullen, S.P., M. Brunet, and S.J. Martin. Granzymes in cancer and immunity. Cell Death Differ, 2010. 17(4): p. 616-23.

[10] Hamai, A., H. Benlalam, F. Meslin, M. Hasmim, T. Carre, I. Akalay, B. Janji, G. Berchem, M.Z. Noman, and S. Chouaib. Immune surveillance of human cancer: if the cytotoxic T-lymphocytes play the music, does the tumoral system call the tune? Tissue Antigens, 2010. 75(1): p. 1-8.

[11] Whiteside, T.L. The tumor microenvironment and its role in promoting tumor growth. Oncogene, 2008. 27(45): p. 5904-12.

[12] Majmundar, A.J., W.J. Wong, and M.C. Simon. Hypoxia-inducible factors and the response to hypoxic stress. Mol Cell, 2010. 40(2): p. 294-309.

[13] Semenza, G.L. Hypoxia-inducible factors: mediators of cancer progression and targets for cancer therapy. Trends Pharmacol Sci, 2012. 33(4): p. 207-14.

[14] Semenza, G.L. Defining the role of hypoxia-inducible factor 1 in cancer biology and therapeutics. Oncogene, 2010. 29(5): p. 625-34.

[15] Semenza, G.L. Targeting HIF-1 for cancer therapy. Nat Rev Cancer, 2003. 3(10): p. 721-32.

[16] Wang, G.L., B.H. Jiang, E.A. Rue, and G.L. Semenza. Hypoxia-inducible factor 1 is a basic-helix-loop-helix-PAS heterodimer regulated by cellular O_2 tension. Proc Natl Acad Sci USA, 1995. 92(12): p. 5510-4.

[17] Huang, L.E., J. Gu, M. Schau, and H.F. Bunn. Regulation of hypoxia-inducible factor 1alpha is mediated by an O_2-dependent degradation domain via the ubiquitin-proteasome pathway. Proc Natl Acad Sci USA, 1998. 95(14): p. 7987-92.

[18] Pugh, C.W., C.C. Tan, R.W. Jones, and P.J. Ratcliffe. Functional analysis of an oxygen-regulated transcriptional enhancer lying 3' to the mouse erythropoietin gene. Proc Natl Acad Sci USA, 1991. 88(23): p. 10553-7.

[19] Jiang, B.H., J.Z. Zheng, S.W. Leung, R. Roe, and G.L. Semenza. Transactivation and inhibitory domains of hypoxia-inducible factor 1alpha. Modulation of transcriptional activity by oxygen tension. J Biol Chem, 1997. 272(31): p. 19253-60.

[20] Jewell, U.R., I. Kvietikova, A. Scheid, C. Bauer, R.H. Wenger, and M. Gassmann. Induction of HIF-1alpha in response to hypoxia is instantaneous. FASEB J, 2001. 15(7): p. 1312-4.

[21] Jiang, B.H., G.L. Semenza, C. Bauer, and H.H. Marti. Hypoxia-inducible factor 1 levels vary exponentially over a physiologically relevant range of O_2 tension. Am J Physiol, 1996. 271(4 Pt 1): p. C1172-80.

[22] Ivan, M., K. Kondo, H. Yang, W. Kim, J. Valiando, M. Ohh, A. Salic, J.M. Asara, W.S. Lane, and W.G. Kaelin, Jr. HIFalpha targeted for VHL-mediated destruction by proline hydroxylation: implications for O_2 sensing. Science, 2001. 292(5516): p. 464-8.

[23] Salceda, S. and J. Caro. Hypoxia-inducible factor 1alpha (HIF-1alpha) protein is rapidly degraded by the ubiquitin-proteasome system under normoxic conditions. Its stabilization by hypoxia depends on redox-induced changes. J Biol Chem, 1997. 272(36): p. 22642-7.

[24] Bruick, R.K. and S.L. McKnight. A conserved family of prolyl-4-hydroxylases that modify HIF. Science, 2001. 294(5545): p. 1337-40.

[25] Epstein, A.C., J.M. Gleadle, L.A. McNeill, K.S. Hewitson, J. O'Rourke, D.R. Mole, M. Mukherji, E. Metzen, M.I. Wilson, A. Dhanda, Y.M. Tian, N. Masson, D.L. Hamilton, P. Jaakkola, R. Barstead, J. Hodgkin, P.H. Maxwell, C.W. Pugh, C.J. Schofield, and P.J. Ratcliffe. C. elegans EGL-9 and mammalian homologs define a family of dioxygenases that regulate HIF by prolyl hydroxylation. Cell, 2001. 107(1): p. 43-54.

[26] Schodel, J., S. Oikonomopoulos, J. Ragoussis, C.W. Pugh, P.J. Ratcliffe, and D.R. Mole. High-resolution genome-wide mapping of HIF-binding sites by ChIP-seq. Blood, 2011. 117(23): p. e207-17.

[27] Xia, X., M.E. Lemieux, W. Li, J.S. Carroll, M. Brown, X.S. Liu, and A.L. Kung. Integrative analysis of HIF binding and transactivation reveals its role in maintaining histone methylation homeostasis. Proc Natl Acad Sci U S A, 2009. 106(11): p. 4260-5.

[28] Semenza, G.L., M.K. Nejfelt, S.M. Chi, and S.E. Antonarakis. Hypoxia-inducible nuclear factors bind to an enhancer element located 3' to the human erythropoietin gene. Proc Natl Acad Sci U S A, 1991. 88(13): p. 5680-4.

[29] Wenger, R.H. and M. Gassmann. Oxygen(es) and the hypoxia-inducible factor-1. Biol Chem, 1997. 378(7): p. 609-16.

[30] Patel, S.A. and M.C. Simon. Biology of hypoxia-inducible factor-2alpha in development and disease. Cell Death Differ, 2008. 15(4): p. 628-34.

[31] Hu, C.J., A. Sataur, L. Wang, H. Chen, and M.C. Simon. The N-terminal transactivation domain confers target gene specificity of hypoxia-inducible factors HIF-1alpha and HIF-2alpha. Mol Biol Cell, 2007. 18(11): p. 4528-42.

[32] Lau, K.W., Y.M. Tian, R.R. Raval, P.J. Ratcliffe, and C.W. Pugh. Target gene selectivity of hypoxia-inducible factor-alpha in renal cancer cells is conveyed by post-DNA-binding mechanisms. Br J Cancer, 2007. 96(8): p. 1284-92.

[33] Makino, Y., R. Cao, K. Svensson, G. Bertilsson, M. Asman, H. Tanaka, Y. Cao, A. Berkenstam, and L. Poellinger. Inhibitory PAS domain protein is a negative regulator of hypoxia-inducible gene expression. Nature, 2001. 414(6863): p. 550-4.

[34] Kulshreshtha, R., R.V. Davuluri, G.A. Calin, and M. Ivan. A microRNA component of the hypoxic response. Cell Death Differ, 2008. 15(4): p. 667-71.

[35] Wu, M.Z., Y.P. Tsai, M.H. Yang, C.H. Huang, S.Y. Chang, C.C. Chang, S.C. Teng, and K.J. Wu. Interplay between HDAC3 and WDR5 is essential for hypoxia-induced epithelial-mesenchymal transition. Mol Cell, 2011. 43(5): p. 811-22.

[36] Noman, M.Z., S. Buart, J. Van Pelt, C. Richon, M. Hasmim, N. Leleu, W.M. Suchorska, A. Jalil, Y. Lecluse, F. El Hage, M. Giuliani, C. Pichon, B. Azzarone, N. Mazure, P. Romero, F. Mami-Chouaib, and S. Chouaib. The cooperative induction of hypoxia-inducible factor-1 alpha and STAT3 during hypoxia induced an impairment of tumor susceptibility to CTL-mediated cell lysis. J Immunol, 2009. 182(6): p. 3510-21.

[37] Noman, M.Z., B. Janji, B. Kaminska, K. Van Moer, S. Pierson, P. Przanowski, S. Buart, G. Berchem, P. Romero, F. Mami-Chouaib, and S. Chouaib. Blocking hypoxia-induced autophagy in tumors restores cytotoxic T-cell activity and promotes regression. Cancer Res, 2011. 71(18): p. 5976-86.

[38] Mathew, R. and E. White. Autophagy, stress, and cancer metabolism: what doesn't kill you makes you stronger. Cold Spring Harb Symp Quant Biol, 2011. 76: p. 389-96.

[39] Viry, E., J. Baginska, G. Berchem, M.Z. Noman, S. Medves, S. Chouaib, and B. Janji. Autophagic degradation of GZMB/granzyme B: a new mechanism of hypoxic tumor cell escape from natural killer cell-mediated lysis. Autophagy, 2014. 10(1): p. 173-5.

[40] Moussay, E., T. Kaoma, J. Baginska, A. Muller, K. Van Moer, N. Nicot, P.V. Nazarov, L. Vallar, S. Chouaib, G. Berchem, and B. Janji. The acquisition of resistance to TNFalpha in breast cancer cells is associated with constitutive activation of autophagy as revealed by a transcriptome analysis using a custom microarray. Autophagy, 2011. 7(7): p. 760-70.

[41] Noman, M.Z., B. Janji, G. Berchem, F. Mami-Chouaib, and S. Chouaib. Hypoxia-induced autophagy: a new player in cancer immunotherapy? Autophagy, 2012. 8(4): p. 704-6.

[42] Hasmim, M., M.Z. Noman, J. Lauriol, H. Benlalam, A. Mallavialle, F. Rosselli, F. Mami-Chouaib, C. Alcaide-Loridan, and S. Chouaib. Hypoxia-dependent inhibition of tumor cell susceptibility to CTL-mediated lysis involves NANOG induction in target cells. J Immunol, 2011. 187(8): p. 4031-9.

[43] Hasmim, M., M.Z. Noman, Y. Messai, D. Bordereaux, G. Gros, V. Baud, and S. Chouaib. Cutting edge: hypoxia-induced Nanog favors the intratumoral infiltration of regulatory T cells and macrophages via direct regulation of TGF-beta1. J Immunol, 2013. 191(12): p. 5802-6.

[44] Noman, M.Z., S. Buart, P. Romero, S. Ketari, B. Janji, B. Mari, F. Mami-Chouaib, and S. Chouaib. Hypoxia-inducible miR-210 regulates the susceptibility of tumor cells to lysis by cytotoxic T cells. Cancer Res, 2012. 72(18): p. 4629-41.

[45] Siemens, D.R., N. Hu, A.K. Sheikhi, E. Chung, L.J. Frederiksen, H. Pross, and C.H. Graham. Hypoxia increases tumor cell shedding of MHC class I chain-related molecule: role of nitric oxide. Cancer Res, 2008. 68(12): p. 4746-53.

[46] Yamada, N., K. Yamanegi, H. Ohyama, M. Hata, K. Nakasho, H. Futani, H. Okamura, and N. Terada. Hypoxia downregulates the expression of cell surface MICA without increasing soluble MICA in osteosarcoma cells in a HIF-1alpha-dependent manner. Int J Oncol, 2012. 41(6): p. 2005-12.

[47] Baginska, J., E. Viry, J. Paggetti, S. Medves, G. Berchem, E. Moussay, and B. Janji. The critical role of the tumor microenvironment in shaping natural killer cell-mediated anti-tumor immunity. Front Immunol, 2013. 4: p. 490.

[48] Viry, E., J. Paggetti, J. Baginska, T. Mgrditchian, G. Berchem, E. Moussay, and B. Janji. Autophagy: an adaptive metabolic response to stress shaping the antitumor immunity. Biochem Pharmacol, 2014. 92(1): p. 31-42.

[49] Baginska, J., E. Viry, G. Berchem, A. Poli, M.Z. Noman, K. van Moer, S. Medves, J. Zimmer, A. Oudin, S.P. Niclou, R.C. Bleackley, I.S. Goping, S. Chouaib, and B. Janji. Granzyme B degradation by autophagy decreases tumor cell susceptibility to natural killer-mediated lysis under hypoxia. Proc Natl Acad Sci USA, 2013. 110(43): p. 17450-5.

[50] Axelson, H., E. Fredlund, M. Ovenberger, G. Landberg, and S. Pahlman. Hypoxia-induced dedifferentiation of tumor cells—a mechanism behind heterogeneity and aggressiveness of solid tumors. Semin Cell Dev Biol, 2005. 16(4-5): p. 554-63.

[51] Harris, A.L. Hypoxia—a key regulatory factor in tumour growth. Nat Rev Cancer, 2002. 2(1): p. 38-47.

[52] Jogi, A., I. Ora, H. Nilsson, A. Lindeheim, Y. Makino, L. Poellinger, H. Axelson, and S. Pahlman. Hypoxia alters gene expression in human neuroblastoma cells toward an immature and neural crest-like phenotype. Proc Natl Acad Sci USA, 2002. 99(10): p. 7021-6.

[53] Helczynska, K., A. Kronblad, A. Jogi, E. Nilsson, S. Beckman, G. Landberg, and S. Pahlman. Hypoxia promotes a dedifferentiated phenotype in ductal breast carcinoma in situ. Cancer Res, 2003. 63(7): p. 1441-4.

[54] Kim, Y., Q. Lin, P.M. Glazer, and Z. Yun. Hypoxic tumor microenvironment and cancer cell differentiation. Curr Mol Med, 2009. 9(4): p. 425-34.

[55] Yeung, T.M., S.C. Gandhi, and W.F. Bodmer. Hypoxia and lineage specification of cell line-derived colorectal cancer stem cells. Proc Natl Acad Sci USA, 2011. 108(11): p. 4382-7.

[56] Vermeulen, L., E.M.F. De Sousa, M. van der Heijden, K. Cameron, J.H. de Jong, T. Borovski, J.B. Tuynman, M. Todaro, C. Merz, H. Rodermond, M.R. Sprick, K. Kemper, D.J. Richel, G. Stassi, and J.P. Medema. Wnt activity defines colon cancer stem cells and is regulated by the microenvironment. Nat Cell Biol, 2010. 12(5): p. 468-76.

[57] Zellmer, V.R. and S. Zhang. Evolving concepts of tumor heterogeneity. Cell Biosci, 2014. 4: p. 69.

[58] Holzel, M., A. Bovier, and T. Tuting. Plasticity of tumour and immune cells: a source of heterogeneity and a cause for therapy resistance? Nat Rev Cancer, 2013. 13(5): p. 365-76.

[59] Schreiber, R.D., L.J. Old, and M.J. Smyth. Cancer immunoediting: integrating immunity's roles in cancer suppression and promotion. Science, 2011. 331(6024): p. 1565-70.

[60] Santisteban, M., J.M. Reiman, M.K. Asiedu, M.D. Behrens, A. Nassar, K.R. Kalli, P. Haluska, J.N. Ingle, L.C. Hartmann, M.H. Manjili, D.C. Radisky, S. Ferrone, and K.L. Knutson. Immune-induced epithelial to mesenchymal transition in vivo generates breast cancer stem cells. Cancer Res, 2009. 69(7): p. 2887-95.

[61] Roesch, A., A. Paschen, J. Landsberg, I. Helfrich, J.C. Becker, and D. Schadendorf. Phenotypic tumour cell plasticity as a resistance mechanism and therapeutic target in melanoma. Eur J Cancer, 2016. 59: p. 109-12.

[62] Noman, M.Z., M. Hasmim, Y. Messai, S. Terry, C. Kieda, B. Janji, and S. Chouaib. Hypoxia: a key player in antitumor immune response. A review in the Theme: Cellular Responses to Hypoxia. Am J Physiol Cell Physiol, 2015. 309(9): p. C569-79.

[63] Guise, C.P., A.M. Mowday, A. Ashoorzadeh, R. Yuan, W.H. Lin, D.H. Wu, J.B. Smaill, A.V. Patterson, and K. Ding. Bioreductive prodrugs as cancer therapeutics: targeting tumor hypoxia. Chin J Cancer, 2014. 33(2): p. 80-6.

[64] Wilson, W.R. and M.P. Hay. Targeting hypoxia in cancer therapy. Nat Rev Cancer, 2011. 11(6): p. 393-410.

[65] Hoelder, S., P.A. Clarke, and P. Workman. Discovery of small molecule cancer drugs: successes, challenges and opportunities. Mol Oncol, 2012. 6(2): p. 155-76.

[66] Xia, Y., H.K. Choi, and K. Lee. Recent advances in hypoxia-inducible factor (HIF)-1 inhibitors. Eur J Med Chem, 2012. 49: p. 24-40.

[67] Rapisarda, A., B. Uranchimeg, D.A. Scudiero, M. Selby, E.A. Sausville, R.H. Shoemaker, and G. Melillo. Identification of small molecule inhibitors of hypoxia-inducible factor 1 transcriptional activation pathway. Cancer Res, 2002. 62(15): p. 4316-24.

[68] Yeo, E.J., Y.S. Chun, Y.S. Cho, J. Kim, J.C. Lee, M.S. Kim, and J.W. Park. YC-1: a potential anticancer drug targeting hypoxia-inducible factor 1. J Natl Cancer Inst, 2003. 95(7): p. 516-25.

[69] Isaacs, J.S., Y.J. Jung, E.G. Mimnaugh, A. Martinez, F. Cuttitta, and L.M. Neckers. Hsp90 regulates a von Hippel Lindau-independent hypoxia-inducible factor-1 alpha-degradative pathway. J Biol Chem, 2002. 277(33): p. 29936-44.

[70] Mabjeesh, N.J., D.E. Post, M.T. Willard, B. Kaur, E.G. Van Meir, J.W. Simons, and H. Zhong. Geldanamycin induces degradation of hypoxia-inducible factor 1alpha protein via the proteosome pathway in prostate cancer cells. Cancer Res, 2002. 62(9): p. 2478-82.

[71]   Zagzag, D., M. Nomura, D.R. Friedlander, C.Y. Blanco, J.P. Gagner, N. Nomura, and E.W. Newcomb. Geldanamycin inhibits migration of glioma cells in vitro: a potential role for hypoxia-inducible factor (HIF-1alpha) in glioma cell invasion. J Cell Physiol, 2003. 196(2): p. 394-402.

[72]   Welsh, S.J., R.R. Williams, A. Birmingham, D.J. Newman, D.L. Kirkpatrick, and G. Powis. The thioredoxin redox inhibitors 1-methylpropyl 2-imidazolyl disulfide and pleurotin inhibit hypoxia-induced factor 1alpha and vascular endothelial growth factor formation. Mol Cancer Ther, 2003. 2(3): p. 235-43.

[73]   Welsh, S., R. Williams, L. Kirkpatrick, G. Paine-Murrieta, and G. Powis. Antitumor activity and pharmacodynamic properties of PX-478, an inhibitor of hypoxia-inducible factor-1alpha. Mol Cancer Ther, 2004. 3(3): p. 233-44.

9

Vascular Smooth Muscle as an Oxygen Sensor: Role of Elevation of the $[Na^+]_i/[K^+]_i$

Sergei N. Orlov , Yulia G. Birulina ,

Liudmila V. Smaglii and Svetlana V. Gusakova

Abstract

The article presents a review of data from our own research and data obtained by other authors about the role of intracellular sodium (Na_i^+) and potassium (K_i^+) in transcriptomic changes in vascular smooth muscle cells (VSMC) during hypoxia. It was found that acute hypoxia suppressed $[K^+]_o$ and phenylephrine-induced contractions of aortic rings through voltage-gated as well as by Ca_i^{2+}- and ATP-sensitive K^+ channels; 24-h incubation of VSMC in ischemic conditions resulted in attenuation of ATP content, elevation of $[Na^+]_i$ and loss of $[K^+]_i$. Dissipation of Na^+ and K^+ gradients in low-Na^+, high-K^+ medium completely eliminated increment in Fos, Atf3, Ptgs2 and Per2 mRNAs and sharply diminished augmentation of Klf10, Edn1, Nr4a1 and Hes1 expression evoked by hypoxia. All these data suggest that Na_i^+/K_i^+-mediated signaling contribute to transcriptomic changes in VSMC subjected to sustained hypoxia.

Keywords: smooth muscle cells, hypoxia, intracellular $[Na^+]/[K^+]$ ratio, transcription, contraction

1. Introduction

Maintaining optimal oxygen tension level in cells promotes the metabolic and plastic processes that ensure their functional stability. To date, there are a lot of reports showing the high sensitivity of endothelium-denuded blood vessels to oxygen deficiency (hypoxia) [1–5]. These data allow considering vascular smooth muscle cells (VSMC) as an oxygen sensor involved in modulation of blood vessel tone and gene expression. Previously, using global gene expression profiling, we found that in several cell types including rat aortic VSMC Na^+, K^+-ATPase inhibition by ouabain or K^+-free medium led to the differential expression of dozens of genes whose altered expression was previously detected in cells subjected to hypoxia and ischemia/reperfusion [6, 7]. In view of this finding, we examined the relative impact of canonical hypoxia-inducible factor 1alpha (HIF-1α)- and Na_i^+/K_i^+-mediated signaling on transcriptomic changes evoked by hypoxia and glucose deprivation as well as its possible involvement in regulation of VSMC contraction.

2. Hypoxia affects excitation-contraction and excitation-transcription coupling: role of HIF-1α-mediated signaling

Blood vessels play a key role in the maintenance of a balanced supply of oxygen and nutrition in target tissues under acute and chronic hypoxic conditions. In systemic circulation, acute hypoxic conditions resulted in dilatation of vascular beds via direct actions of attenuated partial oxygen pressure (pO_2) on vascular smooth muscle cells (VSMC) as well as by ATP release from erythrocytes that, in turn, leads to activation of purinergic P2Y receptors and augmented production of nitric oxide by endothelial cells (for comprehensive reviews, see [1–3]).

Figure 1A shows that in the absence of erythrocytes, hypoxia attenuated by 20–30% the contraction of rat aortic strips triggered by agonist of α_1-adrenergic receptors phenylephrine. We found that inhibitory action of hypoxia was partially abolished by 4-aminopyridine (**Figure 1B**) and glibenclamide (**Figure 1C**), thus indicating activation of voltage-gated and ATP-sensitive K^+ channels, respectively. Recently, Gun et al. reported that hypoxic relaxation of mesenteric arteries is suppressed by a selective inhibitor of the large conductance Ca^{2+}-activated K^+ channels (BK_{Ca}) iberiotoxin [4].

Unlike systemic circulation, hypoxia results in augmented contraction of pulmonary arterial smooth muscle cells via inhibition of voltage-gated K^+ channels $K_v1.5$ and $K_v2.1$ and activation of nonselective cation channels TRPC1 (for reviews, see [5, 8]). It was shown that ATP release from erythrocytes triggered by shear stress and activation of cAMP-mediated signaling is sharply decreased in human with primary pulmonary hypertension [9]. To the best of our knowledge, the comparative analysis of hypoxia-induced ATP release from erythrocytes of normotensive and hypertensive patients and implication of purinergic receptors in regulation of vascular tone in systemic and pulmonary circulations have not yet been performed.

In addition, the regulation of vascular tone hypoxia leads to cell type-specific differential expression of hundreds of genes documented in global gene profiling studies [10–16]. It is generally accepted that these transcriptomic changes are mediated by hypoxia-inducible factor 1alpha (HIF-1α) involved in regulation of gene expression via interaction of HIF-1α/HIF-1β heterodimer with hypoxia-response elements (HREs) in promoter/enhancer regions of the target gene's DNA. In normoxia, oxygen-dependent prolyl hydroxylase hydroxylates HIF-1α and induces its proteasomal degradation. In contrast, under hypoxic conditions, HIF-1α is translocated to the nucleus, where it forms HIF-1α/HIF-1β complex [17–20]. The list of HIF-1-sensitive genes includes Hif-1α per se and others related to angiogenesis (vascular endothelial growth factor (Vegf) and its receptor Flt1), vasomotor control (endothelin-1, adrenomedullin, nitric oxide synthase-2), erythropoiesis and iron metabolism (transferrin, transferrin receptor, erythropoietin, ceruloplasmin), energy metabolism (phosphoenolpyruvate carboxylase, aldose, endolase, phosphoglucokinase-1, -L and -C, lactate dehydrogenase A, tyrosine hydroxylase and plasminogen activator inhibitor-1, glucose transporters Glut1-Glut3), and cell proliferation (Tgfb, Igf1, Igfbp1) [21]. Shimoda and coworkers reported that reduction in voltage-gated K^+ currents following hypoxia was absent in pulmonary arterial smooth muscle cells from heterozygous HIF-1α mice, thus suggesting and implicating this oxygen-sensing machinery in vascular bed-specific contractile responses [22].

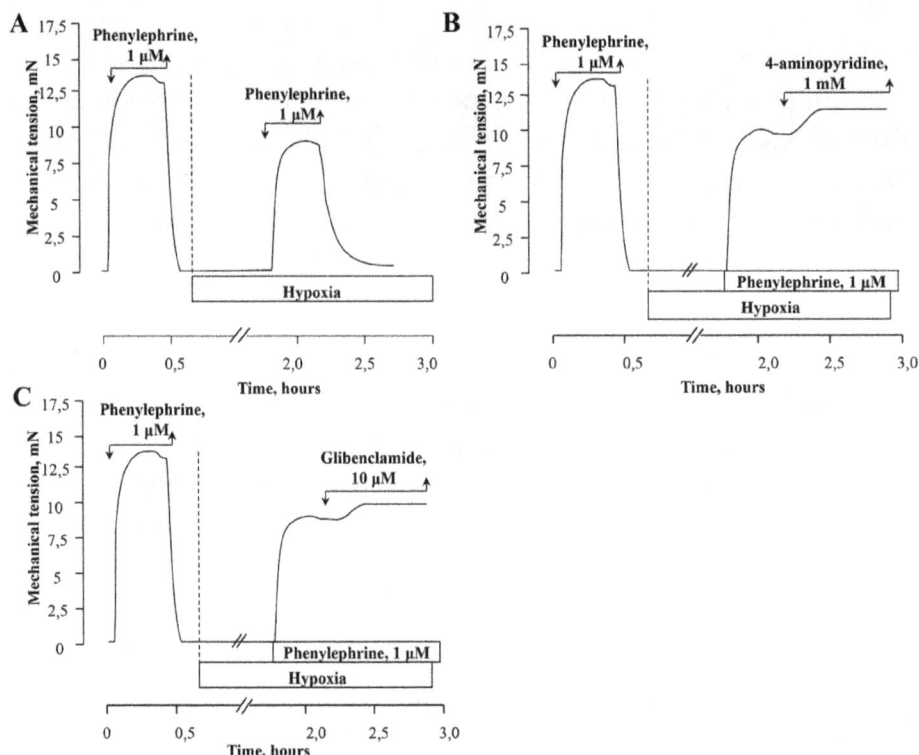

Figure 1. Hypoxia influences on phenylephrine (PE)-induced contraction of ring aortic segments from male Wistar rats. Aortic segments were incubated for 60 min in hypoxic Krebs solution ($pO_2 \sim 30$ mmHg) and then contacted with phenylephrine (1 μM). Registration of constrictive responses was performed by Myobath-2 Multi-Channel Tissue Bath System. Incubation in hypoxic solution decreased the amplitude of PE-induced constriction in comparison with contraction in normoxic solution (A). Both blocker of voltage-dependent potassium channel 4-aminopyridine (1 mM) (B) and blocker of ATP-dependent potassium channels glibenclamide (10 μM) (C) significantly decreased mechanical tension of aortic segments in comparison with PE-induced contraction in hypoxic solution ($p < 0.05$). X axis—time (h), Y axis—mechanical tension (mN). The arrows indicate the addition and removal of the respective solutions.

It should be noted that side-by-side with activation of HIF-1α-mediated signaling, attenuation of pO_2 and delivery of cell fuels resulted in decreased intracellular ATP content that, in turn, led to activation of AMP-sensitive protein kinase (AMPK) [23, 24], decline of ion transport ATPase activities and dissipation of electrochemical gradients of K^+, Na^+, Cl^- and Ca^{2+} [25]. Numerous research teams reported that $[Ca^{2+}]_i$ elevation triggers transcriptomic alterations via Ca^{2+}_i-sensitive transcriptional elements [26]. Importantly, along with the increment in $[Ca^{2+}]_i$, even transient ischemia increases $[Na^+]_i$ from 5–8 to 25–40 mM and causes reciprocal changes in $[K^+]_i$ [27]. These data motivate us to propose that Na_i^+/K_i^+-sensitive signaling pathways contribute to cellular responses triggered by sustained hypoxia [6, 28]. Investigations examining this hypothesis are considered below.

3. Intracellular monovalent cations as regulators of gene transcription

In the late 1990s, we observed that elevation of the $[Na^+]_i/[K^+]_i$ ratio protects rat aortic VSMC against apoptosis triggered by serum deprivation and staurosporine addition [29]. To further explore this antiapoptotic pathway, we treated cells with actinomycin D or cycloheximide. Both macromolecular synthesis inhibitors abolished protection against apoptosis by ouabain [30]. Later we employed proteomic technology and detected hundreds of differentially expressed protein spots in VSMC subjected to Na^+, K^+-ATPase inhibition by ouabain and other cardiotonic steroids (CTS) [30]. These data, together with augmented RNA synthesis observed in ouabain-treated VSMC [31], suggest that sharp transcriptomic changes seen in ouabain-treated cells are mediated by immediate response genes (IRG). Indeed, in both RASMC and HeLa cells, ouabain treatment resulted in augmentation of immunoreactive c-Fos and c-Jun by 10-fold and fourfold, respectively [32, 33]. Addition of ouabain induced a fourfold c-Fos mRNA increment accompanied by fivefold increment in $[Na^+]_i$ within 30 min. At the same time, we observed only 10–15% decrease in $[K^+]_i$ [32, 33]. Thus, we can assume that c-Fos expression is more sensitive to increase in $[Na^+]_i$ rather than $[K^+]_i$.

Recent studies have revealed that CTS may affect cells independently of suppression of Na^+, K^+-ATPase. Thus, ouabain induced interaction of α-subunit of the Na^+, K^+-ATPase with the membrane-associated nonreceptor tyrosine kinase Src, activation of Ras/Raf/ERK1,2, phosphatidylinositol 3-kinase (PI(3)K), PI(3)K-dependent protein kinase B, phospholipase C, $[Ca^{2+}]_i$ oscillations and increased production of the reactive oxygen species (for review, see [34–36]). Considering this, we employed K^+-free medium as an alternative approach for Na^+, K^+-ATPase inhibition. To identify Na_i^+, K_i^+-sensitive transcriptomes, both ubiquitous and cell type-specific, we compared the effect of ouabain and K^+-free medium on profiles of gene expression in rat VSMC, human umbilical vein endothelial cells (HUVEC) and the human carcinoma HeLa cell line [26]. Using Affymetrix-based technology, we found that expression of 684, 737 and 1839 transcripts in HeLa, HUVEC and RASMC, respectively, changes up to 60-fold. It is worth noting that there was a strong correlation in cells pretreated with ouabain or K^+-free medium for 3 h. We also found that 80 transcripts of examined Na_i^+/K_i^+-sensitive genes were common for all examined types of cells [26].

We found that genes involved in the regulation of transcription represents a half of ubiquitous Na_i^+, K_i^+-sensitive transcriptome. This amount was ~sevenfold higher than in the total human genome [37]. The group of ubiquitous Na_i^+/K_i^+-sensitive genes, whose expression was increased by more than threefold, included the transcription factor of the steroid-thyroid hormone-retinoid receptor superfamily Nr4a2, transcriptional regulator of C2H2-type zinc finger protein Egr-1, the basic helix-loop-helix transcription regulator Hes1, members of the superfamily of b-zip transcriptional factors possessing leucine-zipper dimerization motif and basic DNA-binding domain and forming heterodimeric activating protein AP-1 (Fos, FosB, Jun, JunB, Atf3) [26].

4. Evidence for Na_i^+/K_i^+-mediated, Ca_i^{2+}-independent excitation-transcription coupling

Because of the high electrochemical gradient, the opening of calcium channels resulted in rapid elevation of $[Ca^{2+}]_i$ from ~0.1 to 1 µM, its interaction with calmodulin and other $[Ca^{2+}]_i$ sensors, in turn, affects the expression of hundreds of genes, i.e., phenomenon termed excitation-transcription coupling [38]. Increase in $[Ca^{2+}]_i$ affects transcription via several signaling pathways. Thus, $[Ca^{2+}]_i$ elevation induces translocation of kappa-light-chain enhancer of nuclear factor (NFκB) of activated B cells from the cytosol to the nucleus. This process is triggered by activation of Ca^{2+}/calmodulin-sensitive protein kinase (CaMKI, II or III) and phosphorylated IkB kinase that phosphorylates the inhibitor of kB (IkB) [38]. $[Ca^{2+}]_i$ elevation also promotes translocation from cytosol to the nucleus; nuclear factor of activated T cells (NFAT) is evoked by its dephosphorylation by the (Ca^{2+}/calmodulin)-dependent phosphatase calcineurin [39]. In addition, increased cytosolic and nucleoplasmic Ca^{2+} concentrations lead to phosphorylation of cAMP response element-binding protein (CREB) by CaMKII and CaMKIV, respectively. Phosphorylated CREB regulates transcription via their binding to the (Ca^{2+}+cAMP)-response element (CRE) sequences of DNA [40].

Because the c-Fos promoter contains CRE, its augmented expression might be mediated by depolarization of ouabain-treated VSMC and the opening of voltage-gated Ca^{2+} channels. However, unlike high-K^+ medium, c-Fos expression in ouabain-treated cells was not affected by inhibition of L-type Ca^{2+} channels with nicardipine [41]. In additional experiments, we found that augmented c-Fos expression evoked by ouabain was preserved in Ca^{2+}-free medium and in the presence of extracellular (EGTA) and intracellular (BAPTA) Ca^{2+} chelators [30]. To study the role of Ca_i^{2+}-mediated and Na_i^+/K_i^+-independent signaling, we compared transcriptomic changes triggered by elevation of the $[Na^+]_i/[K^+]_i$ ratio in control and Ca^{2+}-depleted cells. Depletion of Ca^{2+} led to prevalent increase in Na_i^+/K_i^+-sensitive genes, both ubiquitous and cell-type specific [26]. For further investigation, we examined ubiquitous Ca_i^{2+}-sensitive genes whose expression is regulated by more than threefold independently of the presence of Ca^{2+} chelators and selected several transcription factors (Fos, Hes1, Nfkbia, Jun), protein phosphatase 1, dual specificity phosphatase Dusp8, interleukin-6, regulatory subunit, type 2 cyclooxygenase COX-2, cyclin L1 [41].

Considering these data, it is important to underline that Ca^{2+} chelators may affect cellular functions independently of Ca^{2+} depletion. Thus, we observed that the addition of EGTA increases permeability of VSMC for Na$^+$ [41]. It is also known that the affinity of EGTA for Mn^{2+}, Zn^{2+}, Cu^{2+}, Co^{2+}, Fe$^{2+/3+}$ is 10-fold to 10^7-fold higher than for Ca^{2+} [42–44]. These polyvalent cations are important in regulation of metaloenzymes activity and participate in protein-DNA and protein-protein interactions. Moreover, EGTA causes irreversible conformational transition and inactivation of transcriptional adaptor Zn^{2+}-binding domain that affects gene expression [45]. It is worth noting that in the human genome, the C2H2 zinc finger superfamily includes about half of all annotated transcription factors [46]. This implies that this and other chelators have Ca$_i^{2+}$-independent action on transcriptomic changes evoked by diverse stimuli. Keeping these data in mind, we compared the actions of Ca^{2+} chelators and Na$^+$, K$^+$-ATPase inhibitors on transcriptomic changes and concentration of monovalent cations in VSMC [47]. Our results show that transcriptomic changes seen in Ca^{2+}-depleted VSMC are at least partially caused by elevation of the [Na$^+$]$_i$/[K$^+$]$_i$ ratio and activation of Na$_i^+$/K$_i^+$-independent signaling pathways. This conclusion is supported by several observations. First, Ca^{2+} depletion led to a ~threefold elevation of [Na$^+$]$_i$ and a twofold attenuation of [K$^+$]$_i$. An increment in the [Na$^+$]$_i$/[K$^+$]$_i$ ratio seen in Ca^{2+}-depleted cells was caused by elevation of plasma membrane permeability for monovalent cations. Indeed, Ca^{2+} depletion resulted in almost threefold elevation of the rate of ^{22}Na and ^{86}Rb influx measured in the presence of inhibitors of Na$^+$, K$^+$-ATPase and Na$^+$, K$^+$, 2Cl$^-$ cotransport. Second, the list of genes whose mRNA content was increased in Ca^{2+}-depleted cells by more than fourfold includes a large number of genes whose expression was also attenuated by the Na$^+$, K$^+$-ATPase inhibition in K$^+$-free medium. Third, there was a strong positive correlation in mRNA content of 2071 genes whose expression was changed by more than 1.2-fold in cells subjected to Na$^+$, K$^+$-ATPase inhibition in K$^+$-free medium as well as in Ca^{2+}-depleted cells. Fourth, dissipation of transmembrane gradients of Na$^+$ and K$^+$ in high-K$^+$, low-Na$^+$ medium abolished the increment in the [Na$^+$]$_i$/[K$^+$]$_i$ ratio as well as sharp elevation of Atf3, Nr4a1 and Erg3 mRNA content triggered by 3-h incubation of VSMC in Ca^{2+}-free, EGTA-containing medium [47]. Thus, novel molecular biological and pharmacological approaches should be developed for precise identification of the relative impact of Ca^{2+}-mediated and Ca^{2+}-independent pathways on transcriptomic changes evoked by elevation of the [Na$^+$]$_i$/[K$^+$]$_i$ ratio.

5. Evidence for implication of [Na$^+$]$_i$/[K$^+$]$_i$-sensitive pathways in transcriptomic changes evoked by hypoxia

The crosstalk between transcriptomic changes and monovalent ion handling was initially supported by comparative analysis of Na$_i^+$/K$_i^+$-sensitive genes documented in our investigations [26] and data on genes whose expression in hypoxic conditions was changed in studies performed by other research groups [9, 11, 48–56]. Indeed, among genes whose augmented expression was detected both in vivo and in vitro models of ischemia/reperfusion, we found several ubiquitous Na$_i^+$/K$_i^+$-sensitive genes, including transcription factors EGR1, ATF3, NFKBIZ, HES1 as well as type 2 cyclooxygenase, IL6, thioredoxin-interacting protein TXNIP.

Moreover, using IPA-knowledge base data, we observed that ubiquitous Na^+_i, K^+_i-sensitive transcriptomes are highly significantly correlated with differential expression of genes in disorders triggered by kidney, liver and heart ischemia (**Figure 2**). These data allowed us to propose that transcriptomic changes in ischemic tissues are at least partially mediated by a novel Na^+_i, K^+_i-mediated excitation-transcription coupling [26, 27].

To examine this hypothesis, we compared the effect of ouabain and hypoxia on the content of monovalent ions and ATP in VSMC from the rat aorta. We observed that 24-h incubation of VSMC in hypoxia and glucose starvation decreased intracellular ATP content by ~three-fold, whereas ouabain attenuated this parameter by <20% (**Figure 3**). Ouabain led to almost 10-fold increase in $[Na^+]_i$ and similar decrease in $[K^+]_i$. Hypoxia also caused threefold increase in $[Na^+]_i$ and twofold decrease in $[K^+]_i$. At the same time, reduction in monovalent cations transmembrane gradients in low-Na^+, high-K^+ medium almost completely eliminated the actions of ouabain and hypoxia on the $[Na^+]_i/[K^+]_i$ ratio [57].

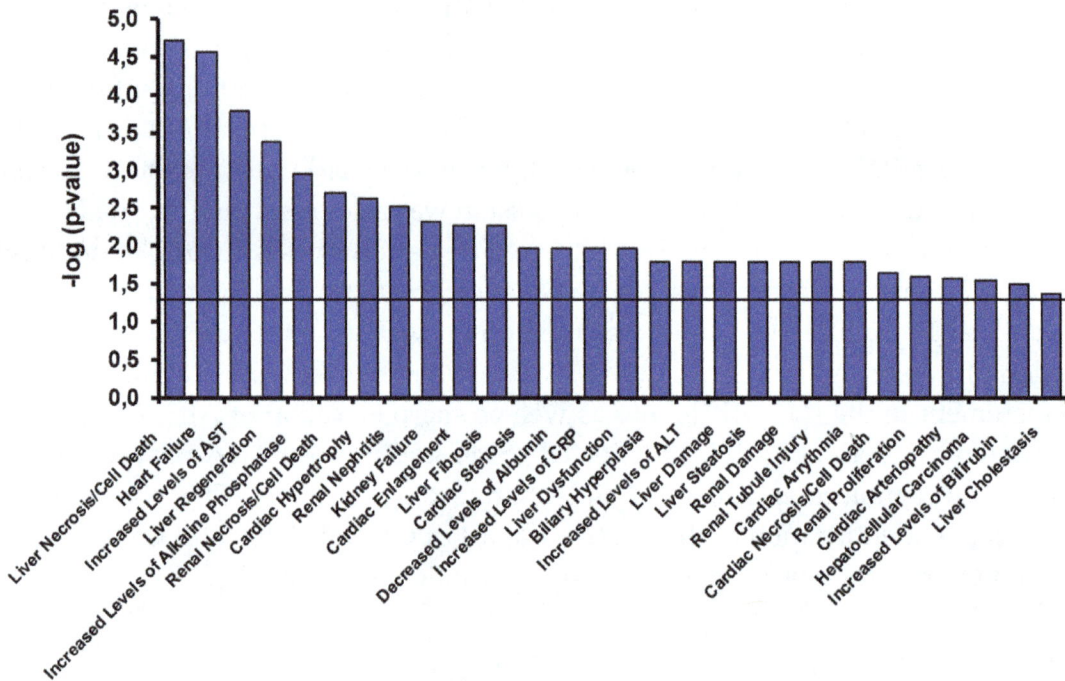

Figure 2. Disorders significantly associated with differential expression of genes whose expression was ubiquitously changed in VSMC from rat aorta, human umbilical vein endothelial cells and HeLa cell line subjected to Na^+, K^+-ATPase inhibition by both ouabain and K^+-free medium. The criteria with a threshold for significance of $p = 0.05$ (or 1.3 when expressed as $-\log(p$-value) are shown as straight line. Adopted with permission from [26].

We then identified the $[Na^+]_i/[K^+]_i$-sensitive transcriptome in rat VSMC. We found that 6-h inhibition of the Na^+, K^+-ATPase with ouabain or in K^+-free medium resulted in differential expression of 6412 transcripts exhibit highly significant ($p < 4 \times 10^{-9}$) and positive ($R^2 > 0.80$) correlation and classified as Ca^{2+}_i-sensitive genes [57]. To continue our studies, we selected genes whose participation in the pathogenesis of hypoxia was shown in previous studies combined with the property of the highest expression increments under sustained Na^+, K^+-

ATPase inhibition. These genes include Fos, Cyp1a1, Klf10, Atf3, Nr4a1, Hes1, Ptgs2 and Per2. Among these genes, Fos, Atf3 and JUN together form dimeric transcription factor AP-1 whose expression increased in all types of cells subjected to hypoxia [58]. Klf10 is a Kruppel-like zinc finger transcription factor family member involved in hypoxia-dependent angiogenesis via COX-1 activation [59]. Ptgs2 encodes an inducible isoform of cyclooxygenase-2 (COX-2) whose role in the pathophysiology of hypoxia is well documented [60]. Nur77 or Nr4a1, also known as nerve growth factor IB, is the nuclear receptor of transcription factors stabilizing HIF-1α which increases its transcriptional activity [61]. Hes1 is the main helix-loop-helix transcription factor that enhances the expression after ischemic renal failure [52]. Clock, Bmal1, Per1, Per2, Cry1 and Cry2 are the positive (Clock and Bmal1) and negative (others) regulators of a transcription-translation feedback loop forming the core circadian oscillator [62]. Cyp1a1 encodes a cytochrome P450 family member and its expression is mediated by HIF-1β [63, 64]. Per2 promotes circadian stabilization of HIF-1α activity that is critical for myocardial adaptation to ischemia. The positive controls for canonical HIF-1α-sensitive genes are endothelin (Edn1) and vascular endothelial growth factor (Vegfa).

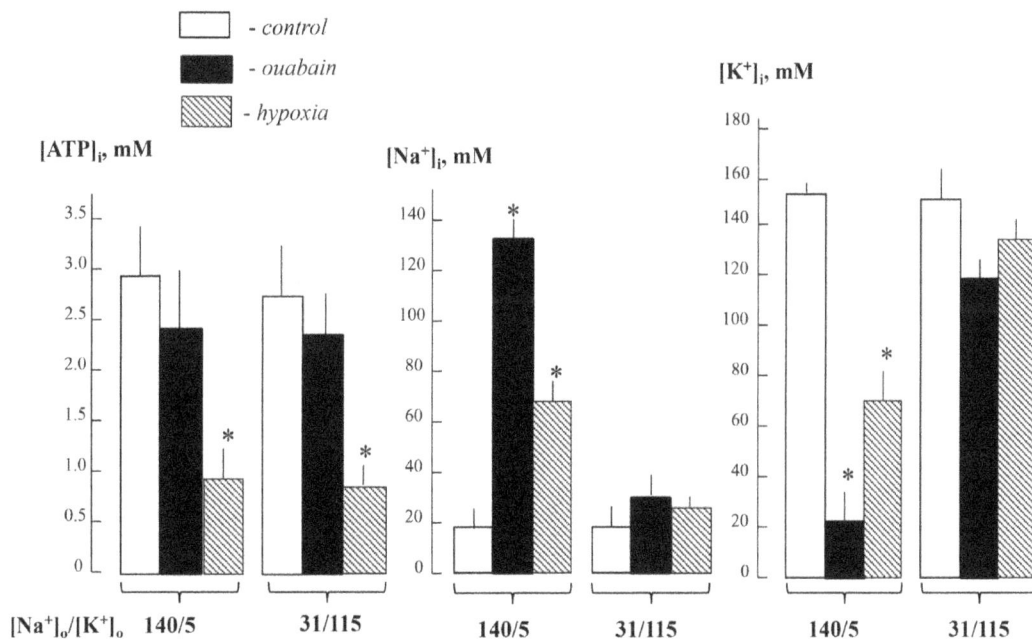

Figure 3. Effect of ouabain and hypoxia on intracellular Na$^+$, K$^+$ and ATP concentrations in VSMC from the rat aorta. Cells were exposed to normal oxygen partial pressure (5% CO_2/air—control) ±3 μM ouabain or exposure to hypoxia (5% CO_2/95% N_2)/glucose deprivation for 24 h in normal high-Na$^+$, low-K$^+$ ([Na$^+$]/[K$^+$] = 140/5) or in low-Na$^+$, high-K$^+$ DMEM-like medium ([Na$^+$]/[K$^+$] = 131/115). Intracellular K$^+$ and Na$^+$ Cl$^-$ content was measured as the steady-state distribution of extra- and intracellular ^{86}Rb and ^{22}Na, respectively. Intracellular ATP content was measured by assaying luciferase-dependent luminescence with ATP bioluminescent assay kit. Means ± S.E. from three independent experiments performed in quadruplicate are shown. *$p < 0.05$ compared to the controls. Adopted with permission from [57].

To assess the role of [Na$^+$]$_i$/[K$^+$]$_i$-dependent and HIF-1α-mediated signaling, we compared expression of the above-listed selected genes in hypoxic conditions and under the action of ouabain in control high-Na$^+$, low-K$^+$ medium and in high-K$^+$, low-Na$^+$ medium with dissipated transmembrane gradients of monovalent cations and after cells transfection with Hif-1a siRNA

[57]. As demonstrated in other cell types [65, 66], hypoxia slightly enhanced Hif-1a mRNA (**Figure 4**) but increased immunoreactive HIF-1α protein content by ~fivefold (**Figure 5**).

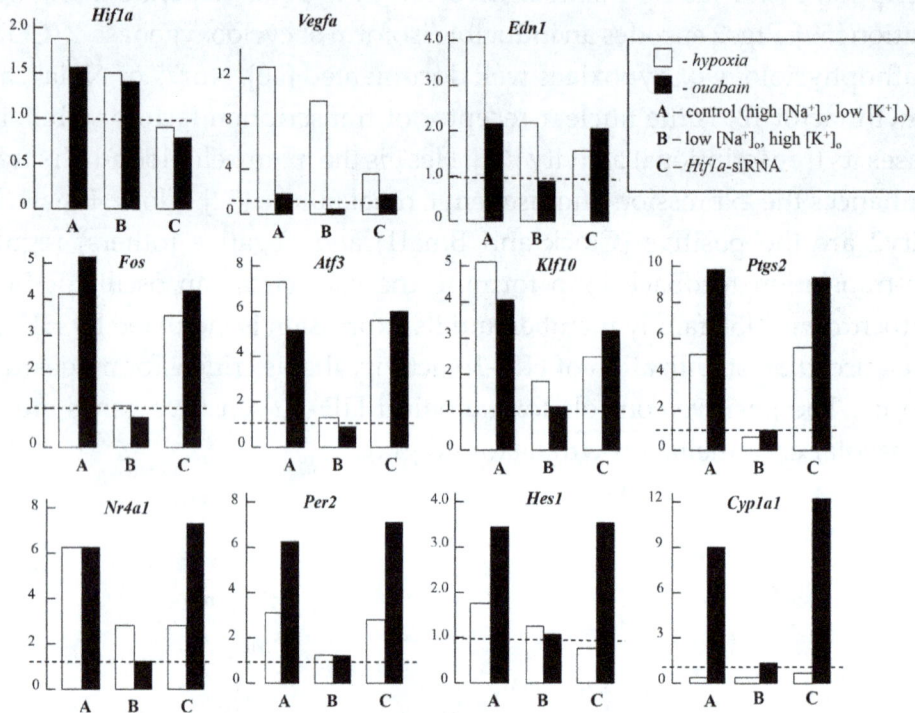

Figure 4. Effect of hypoxia and ouabain on gene expression in VSMC from the rat aorta. Cells were incubated for 24 h under normoxia, hypoxia/glucose deprivation or 3 mM ouabain in control high-Na⁺, low-K⁺ medium (A, C), or high-K⁺, low-Na⁺ medium (B). In some experiments, RASMC were transfected with Hif-1α siRNA (C). The content of mRNA in normoxia was taken as 1.00 and shown as broken lines. Adopted with permission from [57].

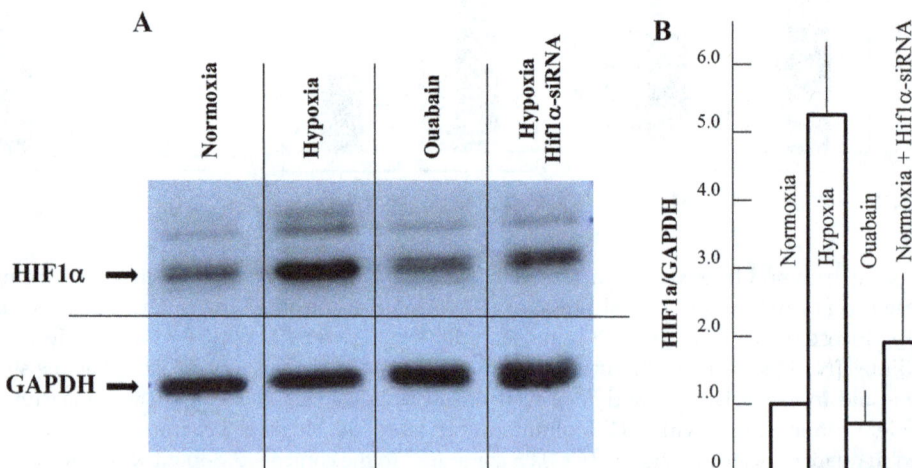

Figure 5. (A). Representative Western blots of GAPDH and HIF-1α in VSMC incubated for 24 h under control conditions (normoxia), hypoxia/glucose deprivation, 3 mM ouabain or hypoxia/glucose deprivation in cells transfected with Hif-1α siRNA. (B). Hypoxia/glucose deprivation and ouabain influence on HIF-1α protein relative content in RASMC. The HIF-1α/GAPDH ratio in control conditions was taken as 1.00. Data obtained in three independent experiments are reported as means ± S.E. Adopted with permission from [57].

Transfection of rat VSMC with Hif-1α siRNA but not with scrambled siRNA led to ~threefold expression reduction in Hif-1a and lowered hypoxia-induced HIF-1a protein gain (**Figure 5**). Pretreatment with ouabain slightly changed HIF-1α protein content (**Figure 5**) and amplified baseline Hif-1a mRNA by ~50% (**Figure 4**). Hypoxia causes fourfold and 12-fold increase in Edn1 and Vegfa mRNA content, respectively, (**Figure 4**), which is consistent with earlier observations [19]. Hypoxia-dependent increase in Edn1 and Vegfa mRNA was attenuated after transfection with Hif-1a siRNA by ~twofold and fourfold, respectively. At the same time, ouabain augmented Edn1 mRNA by 2.5-fold but did not significantly impair Vegfa. Similarly, low-Na$^+$, high-K$^+$ medium that is characterized with dissipation of the transmembrane gradients of monovalent cations also did not affect hypoxia-induced expression of Vegfa and reduced Edn1 mRNA by twofold. All these data strongly support the efficacy of Hif1α-siRNA function [57].

In hypoxic conditions, dissipation of monovalent cations transmembrane gradients completely suppressed increments in Fos, Atf3, Ptgs2 and Per2 mRNA and diminished increase in Klf10, Edn1, Nr4a1 and Hes1 expression (**Figure 4**). Hypoxia caused from twofold to sixfold aug-mentation of Atf3, Fos, Ptgs2, Klf10, Nr4a2, Hes1 and Per2 expression (**Figure 4**). These data 17 are consistent with the observations obtained in other cell types, including human VSMC [67, 68]. Transfection with Hif-1a siRNA led to twofold attenuation of hypoxia-induced increase in Nr4a and Klf10 mRNA without significant influence on expression of Fos, Atf3, Ptgs2 and Per2 evoked by hypoxia. At the same time, hypoxic conditions led to twofold decrease in Cyp1a1 mRNA and attenuated expression of Cyp1a1 obtained from human microvasculature [69]. Ouabain enhanced the expression of all eight tested genes from threefold to 10-fold that were completely abolished in low-Na$^+$, high-K$^+$ medium characterized with dissipation of the transmembrane gradients of monovalent cations [57]. However, in ouabain-treated RASMC, the expression of these genes was not affected by transfection with Hif-1a siRNA, but decrease in monovalent cations transmembrane gradient sharply decreased elevation of Edn1, Klf10, Hes1 and Nr4a1 expression seen in hypoxic conditions and com-pletely abolished increase in Atf3, Fos, Ptgs2 and Per2 mRNA (**Figure 4**).

6. Unresolved issues and future directions

Viewed collectively, our results demonstrate a key role of [Na$^+$]$_i$/[K$^+$]$_i$-mediated excitation-transcription coupling in overall transcriptomic changes triggered by sustained ischemia. The molecular organization of sensors for monovalent cation is still unclear in contrast to rapid progress in the identification of Ca$_i^{2+}$ sensors. Initially, such sensors were identified in parval-bumin and calmodulin. These high-affinity binding sites (the so-called EF-hand domains) are formed by a highly conservative linear amino acid sequence consisting of 14 amino acid residues. Further screening of cDNA libraries allowed to identify more than 30 other Ca$_i^{2+}$ [70].

Moreover, high-affinity sensors for Na$_i^+$ are almost completely saturated at [Ca^{2+}]$_i$ of 1 μM. This allows identifying amino acid residues using ^{45}Ca binding assay. In contrast, molecular sensors for monovalent ion may be presented by 3D protein structures formed with space-separated amino acid residues [27, 71]. Besides this, cellular functions are affected by monovalent cations when they act in the millimolar concentrations that make their detection with radioisotopes more complicate. As it was shown by Ono and coworkers, Na^+ may interact with calpain Ca^{2+}-binding sites at the baseline level of $[Ca^{2+}]_i$ (~100 nM). Thus, calpain functions as Ca_i^{2+}-dependent protease with $K_{0.5}$ of 15 mM for Na^+ [72]. Additional experiments should be performed to examine the role of Ca^{2+}-binding proteins as $[Na^+]_i$ sensors involved in cellular responses evoked by hypoxia.

It is generally accepted that transcription is under the control of proteins interacting with specific response elements within 5'- and 3'-untranslated region (UTR). Considering this, we tried to find Na^+ response element (NaRE) within c-Fos promoter. With the CRE and all other known c-Fos promoter transcription elements, we observed massive accumulation of endogenous c-Fos mRNA and immunoreactive protein in HeLa cells subjected to 6-h inhibition of Na^+, K^+-ATPase, but we did not find any significant increase in luciferase expression in ouabain-treated HeLa cells [33]. Negative results obtained in this study may be explained by the following hypotheses: (i) NaRE is located within the c-Fos 3'-UTR and/or introns. (ii) Elevation of $[Na^+]_i/[K^+]_i$ ratio influences on gene expression through epigenetic modification of regulatory mechanism having a significant impact on various cellular functions, such the DNA, histones or nucleosome remodeling [73]. Importantly, the epigenetic mechanism of gene expression does not contribute to the regulation of L-luc transcription in the plasmid employed in our experiments [33]. (iii) More evidence indicates that gene activation or silencing is under the complex control of three-dimensional (3D) positioning of genetic materials and chromatin in the nuclear space (for review, see [74]). It may be proposed that gene transcription is affected by increased $[Na^+]_i/[K^+]_i$ ratio through changing of the 3D organization of DNA-chromatin complex. These hypotheses will be verified in forthcoming studies.

Some studies have shown that epigenetic modulatory mechanism of histone methylation is a key process that helps cells to adapt to hypoxia [75]. Growing evidence shows that along with the 5'-UTR regulation by transcription factors, gene activation or silencing is controlled by 3D positioning of genetic materials and chromatin in nuclear spaces [74, 76]. The epigenetic regulation of 3D genome organization with considering the $[Na^+]_i/[K^+]_i$ ratio and its role in gene silencing and activation is currently being examined in our laboratory.

Matrix metalloproteinases play an important role in pathophysiology of hypoxic chronic venous disease via their implication in the regulation of migration, proliferation and endothelium-dependent VSMC contraction [77]. We found that sustained elevation of the $[Na^+]_i/[K^+]_i$ ratio resulted in ~fivefold elevation of Mmp28 metalloproteinase expression in rat VSMC [57]. The same procedure resulted in sevenfold elevation of the content of Nccp mRNA encoding natriuretic peptide precursor C [57]. NCCP is proteolytically processed to C-type natriuretic peptide (CNP), i.e., a selective agonist for the B-type natriuretic receptor whose role in cGMP-mediated vasorelaxation is well documented. We noted that in endothelial cells, modest long-term inhibition of the Na^+,K^+-ATPse causes ~sevenfold attenuation of expression of Edn encoding preproendothelin-1 that is proteolytically processed to the most powerful endothelium-derived vasoconstrictor endothelin-1. We also observed ~10-fold elevation of the content of mRNA encoding ubiquitously derived vasodilator adrenomedullin (unpublished results). Do these $[Na^+]_i/[K^+]_i$-mediated transcriptomic changes contribute to the pathophysiology of hypoxic vascular disorders? Does partial dissipation of electrochemical gradients of monovalent cations seen in VSMC subjected to ischemia and glucose deprivation have an impact on the distinct regulation of systemic and pulmonary circulation under hypoxic conditions? We will address these questions to forthcoming studies.

Acknowledgements

This work was supported by Grants from the Russian Foundation for Basic Research #15-04-00101 and the Russian Science Foundation #14-15-00006 and #16-15-10026.

Author details

Sergei N. Orlov[1,2*], Yulia G. Birulina[1], Liudmila V. Smaglii[1] and Svetlana V. Gusakova[1]

*Address all correspondence to: sergei.n.orlov@yandex.ru

1 Siberian State Medical University, Tomsk, Russia

2 MV Lomonosov Moscow State University, Moscow, Russia

References

[1] Ellsworth ML, Ellis CG, Goldman D, Stephenson AH, Dietrich HH, Sprague RS. Erythrocytes: oxygen sensors and modulators of vascular tone. Physiology. 2008; 24: 107–116.

[2] Ralevic V, Dunn WR. Purinergic transmission in blood vessels. Auton Neurosci Basic Clin. 2015; 191: 48–66.

[3] Luneva OG, Sidorenko SV, Maksimov GV, Grygorczyk R, Orlov SN. Erythrocytes as regulators of blood vessel tone. Biochem (Moscow) Suppl Ser A Membr Cell Biol. 2015; 9: 161–171.

[4] Guan Y, Li N, Tian Y-M, Zhang L, Ma H-L, Maslov LN, et al. Chronic intermittent hypobaric hypoxia antagonizes renal vascular hypertension by enhancement of vasorelaxation via activating of BKCa. Life Sci. 2016; 157: 74–81.

[5] Sylvester JT, Shimoda LA, Aaronson PI, Ward JP. Hypoxic pulmonary vasoconstriction. Physiol Rev. 2012; 92: 367–520.

[6]   Koltsova SV, Trushina Y, Haloui M, Akimova OA, Tremblay J, Hamet P, Orlov SN. Ubiquitous $[Na^+]_i/[K^+]_i$-sensitive transcriptome in mammalian cells: evidence for Nai+,Ki+-independent excitation-transcription coupling. PLoS One. 2012; 7: e38032.

[7]   Taurin S, Seyrantepe V, Orlov SN, Tremblay T-L, Thibaut P, Bennett MR, et al. Proteome analysis and functional expression identify mortalin as an anti-apoptotic gene induced by elevation of $[Na^+]_i/[K^+]_i$ ratio in cultured vascular smooth muscle cells. Circ Res. 2002; 91: 915–922.

[8]   Veith C, Schermuly RT, Brandes RP, Weissmann N. Molecular mechanisms of hypoxia-inducible factor-induced pulmonary arterial smooth muscle cell alterations in pulmonary hypertension. J Physiol. 2016; 594: 1167–1177.

[9]   Sprague RS, Stephenson AH, Ellsworth ML, Keller C, Lonigro AJ. Impaired release of ATP from red blood cells of humans with primary pulmonary hypertension. Exp Biol Med. 2001; 226: 434–439.

[10] Mazzatti D, Lim F-L, O'Hara A, Wood IS, Trayhurn P. A microarray analysis of the hypoxia-induced modulation of gene expression in human adipocytes. Arch Physiol Biochem. 2012; 118: 112–120.

[11] Lu A, Tang Y, Ran R, Clark JF, Aronow BJ, Sharp FR. Genomics of the periinfarction cortex after focal cerebral ischemia. J Cereb Blood Flow Metab. 2003; 23: 786–810.

[12] Kamphuis W, Dijk F, van Soest S, Bergen AAB. Global gene expression profiling of ischemic preconditioning in the rat retina. Mol Vision. 2007; 13: 1020–1030.

[13] Tang Y, Pacary E, Freret T, Divoux D, Petit E, Schumann-Bard P, Bernaudin M. Effect of hypoxic preconditioning on brain genomic response before and following ischemia in the adult mouse: identification of potential neuroprotective candidate for stroke. Neurobiol Dis. 2006; 21: 18–28.

[14] Ong LL, Oldigs JK, Kaminski A, Gerstmayer B, Piechaczek C, Wagner W, et al. Hypoxic/normoxic preconditioning increases endothelial differentiation potential of human bone marrow CD133+ cells. Tissue End Part C Methods. 2010; 16: 1069–1081.

[15] Manalo DJ, Rowan S, Lavoie T, Natarajan L, Kelly BD, Ye SQ, et al. Transcription regulation of vascular endothelial cell responses to hypoxia by HIF-1. Blood. 2005; 105: 659–669.

[16] Leonard MO, Cottell DC, Godson C, Brady HR, Taylor CT. The role of HIF-1a in transcriptional regulation of the proximal tubular epithelial cell response to hypoxia. J Biol Chem. 2003; 278: 40296–40304.

[17] Forsythe JA, Jiang BH, Iber NV, Agani F, leung SW, Koos RD, Semenza GL. Activation

of vascular endothelial growth factor gene transcription by hypoxia-inducible factor 1. Mol Cell Biol. 1996; 16: 4604–4613.

[18] Maxwell PH, Wiesener MS, Chang GW, Clifford SC, Vaux EC, Cockman ME, et al. The tumor suppressor protein VHL targets hypoxia-inducible factor for oxygen-dependent proteolysis. Nature. 1999; 399: 271–275.

[19] Kallio PJ, Pongratz I, Gradin K, McGuire J, Poellinger L. Activation of hypoxia-inducible factor 1a: posttranslational regulation and conformational change by recruitment of the Arnt transcription factor. Proc Natl Acad Sci USA. 1997; 94: 5667–5672.

[20] Semenza GL, Jiang BH, leung SW, Passantino R, Concordet JP, Maire P, Giallongo A. Hypoxia response elements in the aldolase A, enolase 1, and lactate dehydrogenase A gene promoters contain essential binding sites for hypoxia-inducible factor 1. J Biol Chem. 1996; 271: 32529–32537.

[21] Sharp FR, Ran R, Lu A, Tang Y, Strauss KI, Glass T, et al. Hypoxic preconditioning protects against ischemic brain injury. NeuroEx. 2004; 1: 26–35.

[22] Shimoda LA, Manalo DJ, Sham JS, Semenza GL, Sylvester JT. Partial HIF-1a deficiency impairs pulmonary arterial myocyte electrophysiological responses to hypoxia. Am J Physiol Lung Cell Mol Physiol. 2001; 291: L202–L208.

[23] Kahn BB, Alquier T, Carling D, Hardie DG. AMP-activated protein kinase: ancient energy gauge provides clues to modern understanding of metabolism. Cell Metab. 2005; 1: 15–25.

[24] Evans AM, Lewis SA, Ogunbayo OA, Moral-Sanz J. Modulation of the LKB1-AMPK signaling pathways underpins hypoxic pulmonary vasoconstriction and pulmonary hypertension. Adv Exp Med Biol. 2015; 860: 88–99.

[25] Williams RS, Benjamin IJ. Protective responses in the ischemic myocardium. J Clin Invest. 2000; 106: 813–818.

[26] Coulon V, Blanchard J-M. Flux calciques et expression günigue. Mйdicine Sciences. 2001; 17: 969–978.

[27] Murphy E, Eisner DA. Regulation of intracellular and mitochondrial sodium in health and disease. Circ Res. 2009; 104: 292–303.

[28] Orlov SN, Hamet P. Salt and gene expression: evidence for Na_i^+,K_i^+-mediated signaling pathways. Pflugers Arch Eur J Physiol. 2015; 467: 489–498.

[29] Orlov SN, Thorin-Trescases N, Kotelevtsev SV, Tremblay J, Hamet P. Inversion of the intracellular Na^+/K^+ ratio blocks apoptosis in vascular smooth muscle at a site upstream of caspase-3. J Biol Chem. 1999; 274: 16545–16552.

[30] Orlov SN, Taurin S, Thorin-Trescases N, Dulin NO, Tremblay J, Hamet P. Inversion of the intracellular Na^+/K^+ ratio blocks apoptosis in vascular smooth muscle cells by induction of RNA synthesis. Hypertension. 2000; 35: 1062–1068.

[31] Orlov SN, Taurin S, Tremblay J, Hamet P. Inhibition of Na^+,K^+ pump affects nucleic acid synthesis and smooth muscle cell proliferation via elevation of the $[Na^+]_i/[K^+]_i$ ratio: possible implication in vascular remodeling. J Hypertens. 2001; 19: 1559–1565.

[32] Taurin S, Dulin NO, Pchejetski D, Grygorczyk R, Tremblay J, Hamet P, Orlov SN. c-Fos expression in ouabain-treated vascular smooth muscle cells from rat aorta: evidence for an intracellular-sodium-mediated, calcium-independent mechanism. J Physiol. 2002; 543: 835–847.

[33] Haloui M, Taurin S, Akimova OA, Guo D-F, Tremblay J, Dulin NO, et al. Nai+-induced c-Fos expression is not mediated by activation of the 5'-promoter containing known transcriptional elements. FEBS J. 2007; 274: 3257–3267.

[34] Aperia A. New roles for an old Na,K-ATPase emerges as an interesting drug target. J Intern Med. 2007; 261: 44–52.

[35] Schoner W, Scheiner-Bobis G. Endogenous and exogenous cardiac glycosides: their role in hypertension, salt metabolism, and cell growth. Am J Physiol Cell Physiol. 2007; 293: C509–C536.

[36] Liu J, Xie Z. The sodium pump and cardiotonic steroids-induced signal transduction protein kinases and calcium-signaling microdomain in regulation of transporter trafficking. Biochim Biophys Acta. 2010; 1802: 1237–1245.

[37] Tupler R, Perini G, Green MR. Expressing the human genome. Nature. 2001; 409: 832–833.

[38] Santana LF. NFAT-dependent excitation-transcription coupling in heart. Circ Res. 2008; 103: 681–683.

[39] McDonald TF, Pelzer S, Trautwein W, Pelzer DJ. Regulation and modulation of calcium channels in cardiac, skeletal, and smooth muscle cells. Physiol Rev. 1994; 74: 365–512.

[40] Hardingham GE, Chawla S, Johnson CM, Bading H. Distinct functions of nuclear and cytoplasmic calcium in the control of gene expression. Nature. 1997; 385: 260–265.

[41] Orlov SN, Aksentsev SL, Kotelevtsev SV. Extracellular calcium is required for the maintenance of plasma membrane integrity in nucleated cells. Cell Calcium. 2005; 38: 53–57.

[42] Martell AE, Smith RM. Critical stability constants. 1974. New York, Plenum Press.

[43] Bartfai T. Preparation of metal-chelate complexes and the design of steady-state kinetic experiments involving metal nucleotide complexes. Adv Cyclic Nucl Res. 1979; 10: 219–242.

[44] Orlov SN, Grygorczyk R, Kotelevtsev SV. Do we know the absolute values of intracellular free calcium concentration? Cell Calcium. 2003; 34: 511–515.

[45] Matt T, Martinez-Yamout MA, Dyson HJ, Wright PE. The CBP/p300 XAZ1 domain in its native state is not a binding partner of MDM2. Biochem J. 2004; 381: 685–691.

[46] Emerson RO, Thomas JH. Adaptive evolution in zinc finger transcription factors. PLoS Genetics. 2009; 5: e1000325.

[47] Koltsova SV, Tremblay J, Hamet P, Orlov SN. Transcriptomic changes in Ca^{2+}-depleted cells: role of elevated intracellular $[Na^+]/[K^+]$ ratio. Cell Calcium. 2015; 58: 317–324.

[48] Beck H, Semisch M, Culmsee C, Plesnila N, Hatzopoulos AK. Egr-1 regulates expression of the glial scar component phosphacan in astrocytes after experimental stroke. Am J Pathol. 2008; 173: 77–92.

[49] Suzuki S, Tanaka K, Nogawa S, Nagata E, Ito D, Dembo T, Fukuuchi Y. Temporal profile and cellular localization of interleukin-6 protein after focal cerebral ischemia in rats. J Cereb Blood Flow Metab. 1999; 19: 1256–1262.

[50] Yuen PST, Jo S-K, Holly MK, Hu X, Star RA. Ischemic and nephrotoxic acute renal failure are distinguished by their broad transcriptomic responses. Physiol Genomics. 2006; 25: 375–386.

[51] Li HF, Cheng CF, Liao WJ, Lin H, Yang RB. ATF3-mediated epigenetic regulation protects against acute kidney injury. J Am Soc Nephrol. 2010; 21: 1003–1013.

[52] Kobayashi T, Terada Y, Kuwana H, Tanaka H, Okada T, Kuwahara M, et al. Expression and function of the Delta-1/NOtch-2/Hes-1 pathway during experimental acute kidney injury. Kidney Int. 2008; 73: 1240–1250.

[53] Bolli R, Shinmura K, Tang XL, Kodani E, Xuan YT, Guo Y, Dawn B. Discovery of a new function of cyclooxygenase (COX)-2: COX-2 is a cardioprotective protein that alleviates ischemia/reperfusion injury and mediates the late phase of cardioprotection. Cardio-vasc Res. 2002; 15: 506–519.

[54] Corss AK, Haddock G, Stock CJ, Allan S, surr J, Bunning BR, et al. ADAMTS-1 and -4 are up-regulated following transient middle cerebral artery occlusion in the rat and their expression is modulated by TNF in cultured astrocytes. Brain Res. 2006; 1088: 19–30.

[55] Cheng O, Ostrowski RP, Wu B, Liu W, Chen C, Zhang JH. Cyclooxygenase-2 mediates hyperbaric oxygen preconditioning in the rat model of transient global cerebral ischemia. Stroke. 2011; 42: 484–490.

[56] Wood IS, Perez de Heredia F, Wang B, Trayhurn P. Cellular hypoxia and adipose tissue dysfunction in obesity. Proc Nutr Soc. 2009; 68: 370–377.

[57] Koltsova SV, Shilov B, Birulina JG, Akimova OA, Haloui M, Kapilevich LV, et al. Transcriptomic changes triggered by hypoxia: evidence for HIF-1a -independent, $[Na^+]_i/[K^+]_i$-mediated excitation-transcription coupling. PLoS One. 2014; 9: e110597.

[58]   Cummins EP, Taylor CT. Hypoxia-responsive transcription factors. Pfluger Arch Eur J Physiol. 2005; 450: 363–371.

[59]   Yang DH, Hsu CF, Lin CY, Guo JY, Yu WC, Chang VH. Kruppel-like factor 10 upregulates the expression of cyclooxygenase 1 and further modulates angiogenesis in endothelial cell and platelet aggregation in gene-deficient mice. Int J Biochem Cell Biol. 2013; 45: 419–428.

[60]   Phillis JW, Horrocks LA, Farooqui AA. Cyclooxygenases, lipoxygenases, and epoxygenases in CNS: their role and involvement in neurological disorders. Brain Res. 2006; 52: 201–243.

[61]   Kim B-J, Kim H, Cho E-J, Youn H-D. Nur77 upregulates HIF-a by inhibiting pVHL-mediated degradation. Exp Mol Med. 2008; 40: 71–83.

[62]   Hamet P, Tremblay J. Genetics of the sleep-wake cycle and its disorders. Metabolism Clin Exp. 2006; 55: S7–S12.

[63]   Koyanagi S, Kuramoto Y, Nakagawa H, Aramaki H, Ohdo S, Soeda S, Shimeno H. A molecular mechanism regulating circadian expression of vascular endothelial growth factor in tumor cells. Cancer Res. 2003; 63: 7277–7283.

[64]   Eckle T, Hartmann K, Bonney S, Reithel S, Mittelbronn M, Walker LA, et al. Adora2b-elicited Per2 stabilization promotes a HIF-dependent metabolic switch critical for myocardial adaptation to ischemia. Nature Med. 2012; 18: 774–782.

[65]   Ke Q, Costa M. Hypoxia-inducible factor-1 (HIF-1). Mol Pharmacol. 2006; 70: 1469–1480.

[66]   Zhang H, Qian DZ, Tan YS, Lee K, Gao P, Ren YR, et al. Digoxin and other cardiac glycosides inhibit HIF-1a synthesis and block tumor growth. Proc Natl Acad Sci USA. 2008; 105: 19579–19586.

[67]   Zuloaga KL, Gonzales RJ. Dihydrotestosterone attenuates hypoxia inducible factor-1a and cycloxygenase-2 in cerebral arteries during hypoxia with glucose deprivation. Am J Physiol Heart Circ Physiol. 2011; 301: H1882–H1890.

[68]   Camacho M, Rodriguez C, Guadall A, Alcolea S, Orriols M, Escudero J-R, et al. Hypoxia upregulates PGI-synthase and increases PGI2 release in human vascular cells exposed to inflammatory stimuli. J Lipid Res. 2011; 52: 720–731.

[69]   Zhang N, Walker MK. Crosstalk between the aryl hydrocarbon receptor and hypoxia on the constitutive expression of cytochrome P4501A1 mRNA. Cardiovasc Toxicol. 2007; 7: 282–290.

[70]   Heizmann CW, Hunziker W. Intracellular calcium-binding proteins: more sites than insights. TiBS. 1991; 16: 98–103.

[71] Orlov SN, Hamet P. Intracellular monovalent ions as second messengers. J Membr Biol. 2006; 210: 161–172.

[72] Ono Y, Ojimam K, Torii F, Takaya E, Doi N, Nakagawa K, et al. Skeletal muscle-specific calpain is an intracellular Na^+-dependent protease. J Biol Chem. 2010; 285: 22986–22998.

[73] Graff J, Kim D, Dobbin MM, Tsai L-H. Epigenetic regulation of gene expression in physiological and pathological brain processes. Physiol Rev. 2011; 91: 603–649.

[74] Lanctot C, Cheutin T, Cremer M, Cavalli G, Cremer T. Dynamic genome architecture in the nuclear space: regulation of gene expression in three dimensions. Nature Rev Genet. 2007; 8: 104–115.

[75] Johnson AB, Denko N, Barton MC. Hypoxia induces a novel signature of chromatin modifications and global repression of transcription. Mutat Res. 2008; 640: 174–179.

[76] Gibcus JH, Dekker J. The hierarchy of the 3D genome. Mol Cell. 2013; 49: 773–782.

[77] MacColl E, Khalil RA. Matrix metalloproteinases as regulator of vein structure and function: implications in chronic venous disease. J Pharmacol Exp Ther. 2015; 355: 410–420.

10

Hypothermia in Stroke Therapy: Systemic versus Local Application

Mitchell Huber, Hong Lian Duan, Ankush Chandra,
Fengwu Li, Longfei Wu, Longfei Guan,
Xiaokun Geng and Yuchuan Ding

Abstract

Presently, there are no effective, widely applicable therapies for ischemic stroke. There is strong clinical evidence for the neuroprotective benefits of hypothermia, and surface-cooling methods have been utilized for decades in the treatment of cerebral ischemia during cardiac arrest, but complications with hypothermia induction have hindered its clinical acceptance in ischemic stroke therapy. Recently, the microcatheter-based local endovascular infusion (LEVI) of cold saline directly to the infarct site has been proposed as a solution to the drawbacks of surface cooling. The safety and efficacy of LEVI in rat models have been established, and implementation in larger animals has been similarly encouraging. A recent pilot study even established the safety of LEVI in humans. This review seeks to outline the major research on LEVI, discusses the mechanisms that mediate its superior neuroprotection over surface and systemic cooling, and identifies areas that warrant further investigation. While LEVI features improvements on surface cooling, its core mechanisms of neuroprotection are still largely shared with therapeutic hypothermia in general. As such, the mechanisms of hypothermia-based neuroprotection are discussed as well.

Keywords: local endovascular infusion, therapeutic hypothermia, ischemic stroke therapy, neuroprotection, microcatheter

1. Introduction

Ischemic stroke is the leading cause of death and disability worldwide, yet effective treatment is limited. Despite considerable research efforts, intravenous (IV) thrombolysis with recombinant tissue plasminogen activator (rt-PA) within the first 4.5 h of symptom onset remains the only proven acute therapy for ischemic stroke [1]. Outside of the treatment window, rt-PA fails to be an option, and given that only 25.4% of stroke patients arrive to the hospital within 3 h of symptom onset, a significant minority of patients are even eligible to receive rt-PA [2]. Thus, alternative treatment strategies for ischemic stroke are urgently needed. Although over a thousand drugs and nonpharmacological strategies have been tested for neuroprotective ability in acute stroke as of 2003, none have proven effective and applicable enough for widespread clinical acceptance [3]. However, hypothermia has prevailed as a promising therapeutic option for stroke patients. In fact, hypothermia is the only neuroprotective approach found thus far whose efficacy has been experimentally demonstrated in a randomized controlled clinical trial [4]. The neuroprotective benefits of hypothermia have been utilized for decades in the treatment of global cerebral ischemia following cardiac arrest and for hypoxic-ischemic encephalopathy in newborns, but its use in stroke therapy has garnered attention only in recent years [4, 5].

Hypothermia has been consistently shown to reduce infarct volumes and improve functional outcomes in animal models of focal cerebral ischemia. In a meta-analysis, the use of hypothermia in animal models of ischemic stroke was shown to reduce infarct volumes by 44% on average [6]. Given the robust neuroprotective effects of therapeutic hypothermia (TH) in animal models of temporary artery occlusion, studies are being conducted at an increasing rate to empirically establish hypothermia as a high-yield front-line stroke therapy.

1.1. Degrees of hypothermia

Therapeutic hypothermia is defined as the deliberate reduction of core body temperature for therapeutic benefit [7]. While there is no exact consensus on the optimal degree of cooling, several studies have found cooling at 33°C to be most effective [7–10]. The vast majority of investigations on the topic feature a mild to moderate degree of cooling, with very few venturing into moderate-deep to deep hypothermia (**Table 1**). In fact, temperature depressions to such an extent have been reported to primarily provide negative consequences [9]. For this review, therapeutic hypothermia refers to mild-moderate hypothermia, unless otherwise specified.

Degree of hypothermia	Mild	Moderate	Moderate-deep	Deep
Body temperature (°C)	35.9–34	33.9–32	31.9–30	<30

Table 1. Terms for degrees of hypothermia by body temperature.

2. Systemic hypothermia

The majority of studies on the induction of TH in acute ischemic stroke therapy have applied whole-body cooling. Therapeutic cerebral hypothermia can be most easily established by either surface cooling or systemic endovascular infusion cold saline [11, 12]. In clinical stroke cases, surface and endovascular cooling have both been used for successful whole-body hypothermia induction and maintenance.

The sentinel study on therapeutic hypothermia exclusively considered "surface cooling," cooling with ice packs or air-circulating cooling blankets/mattresses. This study demonstrated improved survival outcomes in cardiac arrest patients with therapeutic hypothermia [5, 12]. The Cooling for Acute Ischemic Brain Damage (COOL AID) study additionally showed that moderate therapeutic hypothermia (target temperature 32°C by surface cooling) in patients with acute ischemic stroke is feasible and can be accomplished safely by surface cooling [13]. Surface-cooling methods are easy to use and permit early treatment initiation, which makes them an attractive option. However, there are numerous logistical problems associated with surface cooling that outweigh its benefit.

Systemic endovascular infusion methods reduce body temperature invasively using intravenously placed cooling catheters or intravenous cold infusions of isotonic saline into a major systemic blood vessel. The safety of endovascular cooling in patients with acute ischemic stroke was assessed in both the COOL AID II study [14] and the Intravascular Cooling in the Treatment of Stroke (ICTuS) study [15]. The approach was shown in both cases to reduce body temperature more rapidly than surface cooling could accomplish, and since a temperature probe is embedded in the catheter, precise temperature monitoring and regulation was far superior to surface-cooling methods. The disadvantages of systemic endovascular hypothermia induction stem from its invasive nature; the method carries a much higher risk of deep venous thrombosis (DVT), bacteremia, and sepsis than surface cooling [16, 17]. Additionally, the Intravascular Cooling in the Treatment of Stroke-Longer tPA Window (ICTuS-L) study results showed a statistically significant increase in the occurrence of pneumonias in patients receiving systemic endovascular TH [18].

Unfortunately, whole-body cooling by either method creates a number of serious complications. Chiefly, whole-body cooling frequently causes shivering and dermal vasoconstriction, which can complicate effective progression to optimal cooling ranges; whole-body cooling frequently requires 3–7 h to reach target temperatures [19]. Shivering also raises intracranial pressure (ICP) and requires the use of several pharmacological agents to inhibit these effects along with skin warming to address physical discomfort [20, 21]. Another side effect of whole-body cooling is the risk of shear-induced platelet aggregation, which can develop as blood viscosity increases at low temperatures [22]. Even a minor amount of coagulation can cause a blockage of the microcirculation of the brain and heart, which ironically creates the exact problem that hypothermia attempts to treat [21]. Furthermore, whole-body cooling increases the likelihood of ventricular fibrillations, bradycardia, reduced cardiac output, hemostatic or hemorrhagic changes, decreased urine output, and metabolic dysfunction [14, 23, 24]. With this extensive list of severe complications, a more graceful therapeutic modality is urgently needed.

3. Hypothermia via local endovascular infusion

Recently, the selective induction of hypothermia into the ischemic region using an endovascular microcatheter has garnered attention as a novel strategy to optimize the neuroprotective benefits of therapeutic hypothermia with the myriad of comorbidities accompanying full-body cooling. In contrast to other cooling methods, which require hypothermia to slowly spread into the ischemic region, local endovascular infusion (LEVI) reduces infarct temperatures effectively by perfusing ice-cold saline directly to the ischemic region. This allows for more rapid achievement of target temperatures and permits greater specificity of hypothermia while avoiding the side effects of systemic cooling. During these procedures, an infusion microcatheter, guided to the site of the lesion via the guide catheter over a microguidewire, is advanced distally to the site of occlusion, and cold saline is perfused [25] for a variable length of time, usually from 5 to 30 min. The logistics of actually performing LEVI in humans are relatively simple, as this is a normal part of performing endovascular interventions for many neuroendovascular surgeons [26]. Therefore, it is expected that this new therapy could easily be added to an angiography suite [27].

LEVI has been tested in animal models of stroke both before and after reperfusion. Pre-reperfusion flushing was first proposed by Ding et al. [28], when the technique was used in a transient middle cerebral artery occlusion (MCAO) rat model. The study produced a 65% reduction in infarct volumes and 61% reduction in leukocyte infiltration when resolution of a 2-h middle cerebral artery occlusion was preceded by LEVI (23°C saline infused at 2 mL/min for 3–4 min) [28]. Pre-reperfusion LEVI has since been shown to reduce infarct volumes by 75 [29] to 90% [30] and significantly conserve motor function both hours and weeks after stroke [29, 30]. Post-reperfusion LEVI has also been considered in some studies, in which a catheter was introduced into the internal carotid artery after blood flow to the ischemic territory had been reestablished [31, 32]. Significant improvements in both infarct volume and functional recovery were observed in every post-reperfusion LEVI trial tested, but these improvements were not as pronounced as those from pre-reperfusion LEVI.

Although the majority of current experimental data on LEVI in stroke are based on rat models, a few large animal studies that have been conducted are equally encouraging. A recent investigation using swine showed that LEVI significantly reduced infarct volumes following 4–4.5-h MCAO (the longest delay of hypothermia in any LEVI large animal study) [33]. The credibility [34], safety, and efficacy of LEVI in Rhesus monkeys were also confirmed, as infusion of cold-lactated Ringer's solution was used to achieve statistically significant degrees of peri-infarct cooling without apparent vasogenic edema or other comorbidities [35]. Additionally, the safety and feasibility of LEVI was recently verified in humans [36]. In nine human patients with partially or completely treated cerebrovascular diseases undergoing diagnostic cerebral angiogram, 7°C LEVI at ~33 mL/min for 10–13 min was able to reduce jugular venous blood temperature (a proxy for brain temperature) by 0.84°C while reducing rectal temperature by 0.15°C and having no significant effects on vital signs. LEVI was also recently implemented in patients actively undergoing ischemic stroke (within 8 h of symptom onset), which confirmed the safety and feasibility of the procedure [25]. The neuroprotective efficacy of LEVI, however, remains to be established in a clinical setting.

Despite recent milestones in LEVI testing, several systematic obstacles have hindered widespread acceptance. Chief among these obstacles is heterogeneity of experimental designs. Since TH is only widely used for cardiac arrest, the majority of studies utilize a global ischemia model, which has been found to unfaithfully simulate the physiological conditions of focal ischemia [37]. Hypothermia-based investigations also vary in animal model, animal age, duration of ischemia, duration of hypothermia, depth of hypothermia, method of hypothermia induction, and rate of cooling, all of which have consistently been shown to play critical roles in the efficacy of TH treatments. Additionally, current animal models have failed to adequately simulate the reaction of a human to such an intervention. While the majority of LEVI studies have used rat models, rats have been widely criticized for their poor translatability to clinical practice [38]. There even exists heterogeneity among the species; rats of similar strains from different suppliers have been found to show variations in response to ischemia [12]. Given that stroke accounts for 9% of deaths worldwide and ~25% of stroke survivors are permanently disabled [39], such a promising therapy is in serious need of further exploration.

3.1. Benefits of LEVI over systemic infusion

LEVI is an optimized version of general TH. As such, its mechanisms of neuroprotection are predominately the same as those of full-body cooling. However, LEVI retains a few unique features that make it considerably more effective than global cooling. These features are summarized in the present section.

3.1.1. Maximized rate of cooling

Although there is no consensus on the exact treatment window for therapeutic hypothermia, it would be difficult to dispute the time-sensitive nature of hypothermia induction [31, 40]. While one author found that TH is ineffective after 45 min of ischemia [41] and most others have found neuroprotective efficacy when induction follows 2–3 h of ischemia [30, 42], there is a strong consensus that this efficacy diminishes over the course of hours. Considering that surface-cooling methods frequently take 3–7 h to reach target temperatures [19], it would be impossible for any stroke patient to fall within an optimal treatment window. By contrast, LEVI can establish target temperatures in a matter of minutes [36]; in a 300-g localized cerebral infarct, LEVI attained target temperatures 30 times faster than classic surface cooling and 10–20 times faster than systemic infusion of cold saline into the inferior vena cava [27]. The time saved by using LEVI translates to superior degrees of neuroprotection and an improved quality of life for ischemic stroke patients.

3.1.2. Metabolite washout and attenuated hyper- or hypoperfusion

One mechanism by which ischemic stroke damages the brain is through postischemic hyperperfusion. Under ischemic conditions, brain cells are forced to conduct anaerobic respiration, the byproducts of which (lactate, prostaglandins, and carbon dioxide) are vasodilatory at elevated levels [43]. In the absence of adequate perfusion, these vasodilatory metabolites accumulate in the ischemic region and trigger an excessive vasodilation once perfusion is restored. Literature on postischemic hyperperfusion has been discrepant, but suggests that the phenomenon is associated with larger infarcts and early death [44, 45]. This "luxury reperfusion" has been implicated in post-reperfusion edema formation, the primary cause of death within 1 month of ischemic stroke [45, 46]. While hypothermia prevents intracranial-pressure elevations by itself, LEVI provides an additional protective mechanism by washing out vasodilatory metabolites built up during the ischemic period, which minimizes the extent of hyperperfusion-related injury [29, 47]. As evidence of this mechanism, fast warm (37°C)-saline LEVI has been shown to significantly reduce infarct volumes and improve functional recoveries compared to systemic infusion of warm saline [28].

Pre-reperfusion flushing also significantly reduces leukocyte infiltration and ICAM-1 expression in the peri-infarct vasculature [28, 48], leading to improved postischemic perfusion. Luan et al. showed that LEVI was able to reduce cerebral poststroke ICAM-1 expression and leukocyte infiltration to a significantly greater degree than that of local warm-saline infusion or systemic cold-saline infusion were able to [48]. Other studies have reported similar reductions in ICAM-1 expression and infiltration/activation of PMN leukocytes and microglia [49]. These data imply that the neuroprotective advantages of LEVI over systemic infusion rely partially on its metabolite-washout ability and subsequent improved perfusion.

3.1.3. Drug delivery into ischemic territory through LEVI

In addition to the hypothermia-associated benefits of cold-saline infusion, LEVI allows for coadministration of neuroprotective drugs directly into the ischemic region along with hypothermic fluids, which maximizes local drug concentrations while minimizing systemic drug concentrations, thereby circumventing dose-dependent systemic side effects [50]. Preliminary studies using LEVI with neuroprotective drugs have shown exceptional promise; a 2012 study by Song et al. found that LEVI of a magnesium sulfate solution at 15°C caused a 65% reduction in infarct volumes compared to a 48% reduction from LEVI alone [51]. Similar results were found following LEVI of a 20% human albumin solution cooled to 0°C [52]. Normothermic local infusion of drugs has shown potential as well, as LEVI of erythropoietin at room temperature reduced infarct volumes by 21% (significant compared to control), decreased apoptosis in the ischemic core and penumbra, and significantly preserved neurological scores [53].

LEVI can also aid in drug permeation into the brain parenchyma. Blood-brain barrier (BBB) impermeability has been described as the most important factor limiting the growth of neurotherapeutic drugs [54] and remains a challenging issue today. However, BBB breakdown is a natural product of cerebral ischemia, which allows for the perfusion of drugs into the brain parenchyma that would otherwise be prevented from reaching their target [50]. When coupled with LEVI-based drug administration, BBB breakdown can be capitalized on to provide benefits for stroke therapy. This hypothesis was confirmed experimentally in a 2007 study by Woitzik et al. in which microcatheter-based infusion of MK-801 (an NMDA receptor antagonist) into the ischemic region resulted in 30% smaller infarct volumes at 24 h after infusion than when MK-801 was infused systemically [50]. MK-801 has shown significant neuroprotective potential, but has not attained clinical acceptance due to significant side effects when administered at high enough doses to be effective when infused systemically [55], a problem nullified by LEVI-based administration. While LEVI with neuroprotective drugs has never been tested in a clinical setting, it is possible that the combination could open the door for the use of neuroprotective pharmacotherapies that would otherwise be prohibited from reaching target tissues [50, 56].

4. Mechanisms underlying hypothermia-induced neuroprotection

In addition to LEVI-specific neuroprotective mechanisms, LEVI benefits from neuroprotective mechanisms of therapeutic hypothermia in general. These mechanisms exhibit significant redundancy, as they affect multiple steps in several parallel pathways of hypoxia-induced brain injury. Hypothermia primarily exerts its neuroprotective effects by slowing essential metabolic processes while preserving life, which subsequently attenuates pathways involved in excitotoxicity, free radical production, inflammation, edema, and apoptosis [12, 37, 57, 58]. However, a common theme in literature on the topic is consensus on effects and uncertainty of mechanisms. While virtually every paper finds TH administration to be neuroprotective, there is very little agreement on how this works. This is due, in part, to the correlative goal of most studies. The majority of work on the topic identifies alterations in the levels of one indicator or another when TH is implemented, but fails to elucidate exactly where TH exerts its neuroprotective effects. While this is valuable information, without a causative component, these studies always leave the door open for the participation of a third variable. In light of frequently conflicting findings, this section features few concrete lessons from the literature. Rather, we attempt to discuss the pathways that TH acts on, and consider the most likely points at which TH exerts its neuroprotective effects.

4.1. Metabolic crisis

The primary culprit of ischemia-induced brain damage is oxygen-supply cessation, which initiates a cascade of secondary problems. In the absence of oxygen, neurons are unable to generate high-energy metabolites, which prohibit effective maintenance of ion gradients. Ion-gradient breakdown leads to involuntary depolarization, which allows for excessive glutamate release. This wave of glutamate then stimulates NMDA and AMPA receptors, which results in increased intracellular calcium levels and ultimately leads to excitotoxicity, a phenomenon characterized by mitochondrial membrane depolarization, caspase activation, production of reactive oxygen and nitrogen species, and apoptosis [37, 59]. In addition to excitotoxicity, ion-gradient breakdown causes Na^+ to build up in brain cells and in particular astrocytes. This establishes an osmotic gradient favoring the movement of water into astrocytes (and to a lesser extent, all other brain cells), thereby creating cytotoxic edema [60]. The edema increases intracranial pressure and ultimately exacerbates brain damage (**Figure 1**).

Hypothermia combats this cascade at several points (**Figure 1**). Reduced brain temperatures have been shown to lower cerebral metabolic rate by 5% for every 1°C reduction in body temperature, allowing for prolonged maintenance of ion gradients (preventing excitotoxicity) and minimized need to conduct anaerobic respiration, thereby diminishing the extent of reperfusion injury [58]. In patients with traumatic brain injury who received therapeutic hypothermia to 32–33°C, cerebral oxygen consumption was reduced to 27% after 24 h of hypothermia [61]. Hypothermia has also been shown to reduce the production of glycolytic intermediates by an average of 30% and tricarboxylic acid (TCA) cycle intermediates by 30–70% [62]. Alternatively, ratios of phosphocreatinine:inorganic phosphate and adenosine triphosphate (ATP):inorganic phosphate seem to increase slightly during transient hypothermia, implying that the real energy conservation mechanism at play is one of the slowing energy-consuming reactions, rather than slowing glycolytic flux [62]. Hypothermia has also been routinely reported to improve ATP recovery after reperfusion [37]; mild hypothermia has led to a 10–20% increase in the rate of metabolic recovery in the first 10–25 min after reperfusion compared to normothermic animals [63], a finding echoed in other studies [62, 64]. It is possible, then, that the primary energy conservation mechanism that underlies TH is that of accelerated energy recovery after reperfusion rather than energy preservation during hypoxia. However, while metabolic depression during hypothermia has been well documented as a phenomenon, its underlying mechanism is still poorly understood. Thus, the points at which hypothermia exerts its neuroprotective effects are unclear, and whether its main mechanism of neuroprotection involves cellular respiration at all remains to be elucidated.

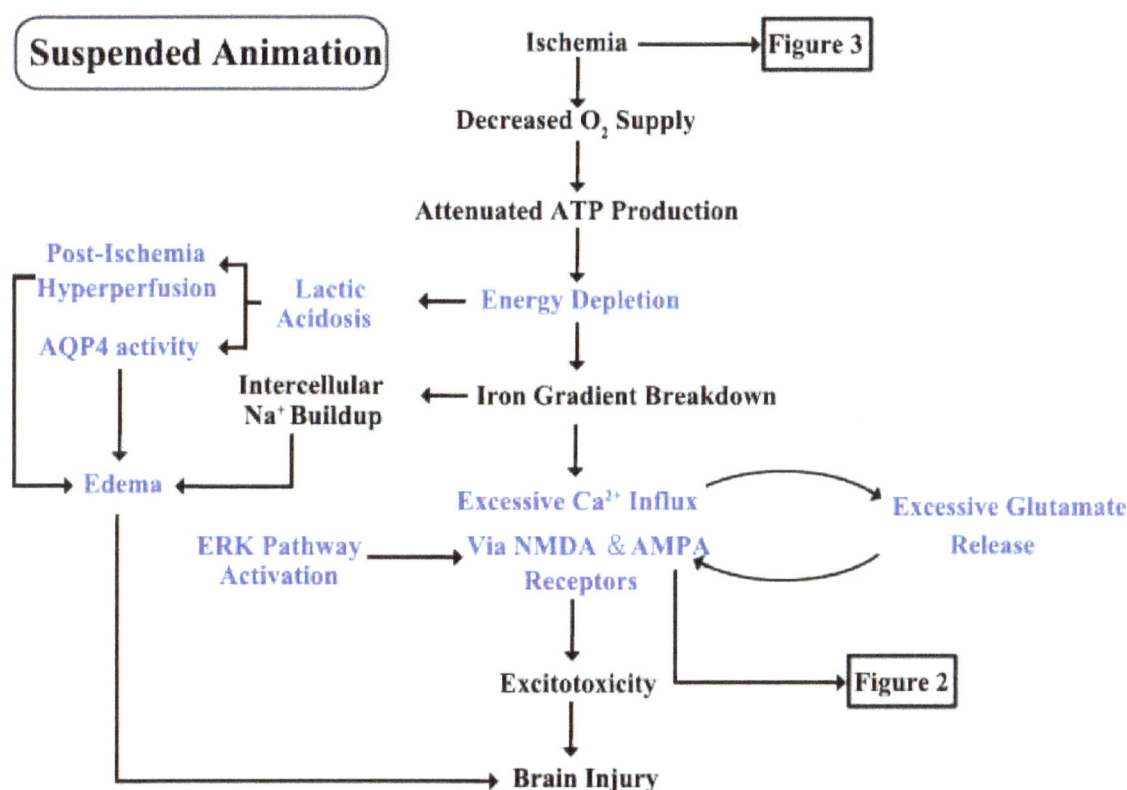

Figure 1. The figure describes the pathogenesis of stroke as it relates to ischemia-induced metabolic crisis. The points at which hypothermia exerts its neuroprotective effects remain largely unclear. Studies have shown that TH attenuates a multitude of steps in the cascade of ischemia-induced brain damage compared to stroke without hypothermia, but whether the observed attenuations are direct effects of TH or byproducts of upstream attenuations has yet to be elucidated. As such, blue font indicates steps discussed in the present review that hypothermia has been shown to attenuate. Black font indicates steps that we have not discussed in the present review, but does not necessarily indicate that these steps are unaffected by hypothermia.

Hypothermia has also been shown to prevent anoxic depolarization. In an aged rat model, mild hypothermia was shown to completely inhibit the efflux of excitatory amino acids (glutamate and aspartate) while significantly increasing the release of the inhibitory amino acid taurine [65]. While no mechanism has been firmly tied to this phenomenon, several have been speculated. TH has been reported to prevent activation of protein kinase C (PKC) and calcium-calmodulin kinase II during ischemia, both of which are associated with neurotransmitter release [65]. Therapeutic cooling also attenuates ischemia-induced downregulation of the GluR2 (glutamate receptor 2) CA1 subunit, which is responsible for limiting Ca^{2+} influx through AMPA receptors in a global cerebral ischemia model [66]. It is also possible that this facet of hypothermic neuroprotection is accomplished by the preservation of ion gradients due to metabolic downregulation. However, some reports have suggested that hypothermia simply delays anoxic depolarization rather than preventing it [67]. In light of conflicting research on the topic, it is likely that multiple mechanisms are at play, culminating in the robust excitation prevention associated with therapeutic hypothermia.

Hypothermia has also been found to combat cytotoxic edema after ischemic stroke (**Figure 1**). This edema is largely mediated by aquaporin 4 (AQP4), which is expressed in the glial-limiting membranes, ependyma, and pericapillary foot processes of astrocytes [68]. In mice, AQP4 knockout has been associated with reduced infarct sizes, decreased brain water content, and improved neurological and survival outcomes [60]. While the brain naturally downregulates AQP4 expression following hypoxia [60], hypothermia has been shown to augment this downregulation [60, 69, 70]. It is possible that this downregulation is a downstream effect of TH. In experimental models, AQP4 levels in astrocyte cell membranes were increased by increased lactic acid concentration, but AQP4 mRNA levels were unchanged, which implies that the observed increases in membrane-bound AQP4 came as the result of redistribution or posttranslational modification, rather than increased expression [71]. Several other mechanisms have also been proposed for this upregulation [72]; thus, the specifics of ischemia-induced aquaporin modulation have still yet to be fully elucidated.

At the molecular level, several studies have implicated immediate induction of early gene expression (miRNAs) and cellular stress response (heat-shock proteins, HSPs) activation in hypothermia-induced neuroprotection. Hypothermia has been shown to suppress transcription of some pro-inflammatory molecules (interleukin (IL)-1β and osteopontin) and enhance transcription of anti-inflammatory substances (HSP70) [73]. The duration of post-reperfusion hypothermia seems to play a role in the modulation of transcriptional rate, as the expression of numerous genes differs when hypothermia is sustained for 8 h compared to 4 h. One such gene is early growth response-1 (Egr-1), which is an early regulator of other pro-inflammatory mediators (IL-1β MCK-1, and MIP-2) [73]. This is consistent with other reports on the topic, which suggests that Egr-1 is the key component modulated by TH. However, information regarding early cellular response to ischemia and hypothermia has largely been conflicting, leaving the specifics of its involvement unclear [38] and inconsistent [31, 32].

While there exists a general consensus that TH is neuroprotective, the precise mechanisms of this effect are still very much theoretical. Additionally, if TH attenuated metabolic crisis alone, it would not be able to accomplish such a robust degree of neuroprotection [74]. It comes as no surprise, then, that suspended animation is just the appetizer in the multicourse meal that is TH-mediated neuroprotection.

4.2. Inflammation and blood-brain barrier breakdown

In stroke therapy, the restoration of blood flow is of chief concern. Surprisingly, however, recanalization is not exclusively beneficial. Reperfusion often initiates a detrimental cascade, collectively termed ischemia/reperfusion injury, which can be disastrous; in some animal models, reperfusion after an extended period of ischemia caused larger infarct volumes than if the occlusion had been left permanently [45]. Reperfusion injury is a complex, multifaceted injury cascade initiated by sterile inflammation from anoxic tissue damage, and propagated by both the innate and adaptive immune systems and complement system [75, 76].

Mechanistically, ischemia/reperfusion injury is initiated by the aberrant Ca^{2+} influx characteristic of ischemic stroke, which activates phospholipases and eventually results in the production of pro-inflammatory mediators from microglia, including proteases, leukotrienes, IL-1β IL-6, NO, and tumor necrosis factor (TNF)-a [77]. These mediators contribute to post-reperfusion insult directly, by increasing vascular permeability, and indirectly, by increasing endothelial ICAM-1 expression and serving as potent chemotactic agents for polymorphonuclear leukocytes, both of which increase leukocyte extravasation into the brain parenchyma [46, 78]. The pro-inflammatory transcription factor nuclear factor kappa B (NF-κB) is likely the cause of this upregulation, as it is responsible for inducing the expression of IL-1β IL-6, TNF-α, and ICAM-1 [78]. In addition to recruiting leukocytes to the infarct site, IL-1β and TNF-α have also been found to increase the production of matrix metalloproteinases (MMPs) [79]. MMP-2 and MMP-9 have been shown to contribute to vasogenic edema by degrading extracellular matrix components during ischemic stroke, and MMP-9 knockout mice experience reduced infarct volumes and less severe motor deficits than wild-type mice [79]. The effect of MMPs ultimately perpetuates the development of inflammation and edema, which further encourages leukocyte extravasation. Once leukocytes enter the brain tissue, they produce ROS and pro-inflammatory factors of their own, thereby creating a viscous cycle of brain injury, inflammation, and blood-brain barrier (BBB) breakdown (**Figure 2**).

A common effect of reperfusion injury mechanisms is BBB disruption. Reperfusion activates matrix-degrading proteases within hours, which makes the vessels particularly leaky and allows for migration of albumin and other blood proteins into the brain parenchyma within 4–6 h of BBB disruption [72]. Water osmotically follows these proteins, thereby creating vasogenic edema, which may increase brain water content by more than 100% in poorly perfused regions [72, 80]. Vasogenic edema is the primary cause of death within the first month of an ischemic stroke [46], as it increases intracranial pressure (ICP) and compresses cerebrovasculature within the inflexible confines of the skull, causing further ischemia and eventually brain herniation [56].

Therapeutic hypothermia is able to confer anti-inflammatory neuroprotection by reducing the secretion of pro-inflammatory cytokines (IL-1β TNF-α, and IL-6) and inflammatory mediators (reactive oxygen and nitrogen species, E-selectin, and HMGB1) [81]. TH can also prevent leukocyte extravasation into neural tissue directly by reducing the endothelial expression of ICAM-1 [27, 48]. ICAM-1 is constitutively expressed by endothelial cells at very low levels, but the expression is precipitously increased following endothelial damage when it functions as an attachment point for the CD11/CD18 integrin of leukocytes (preceding extravasation

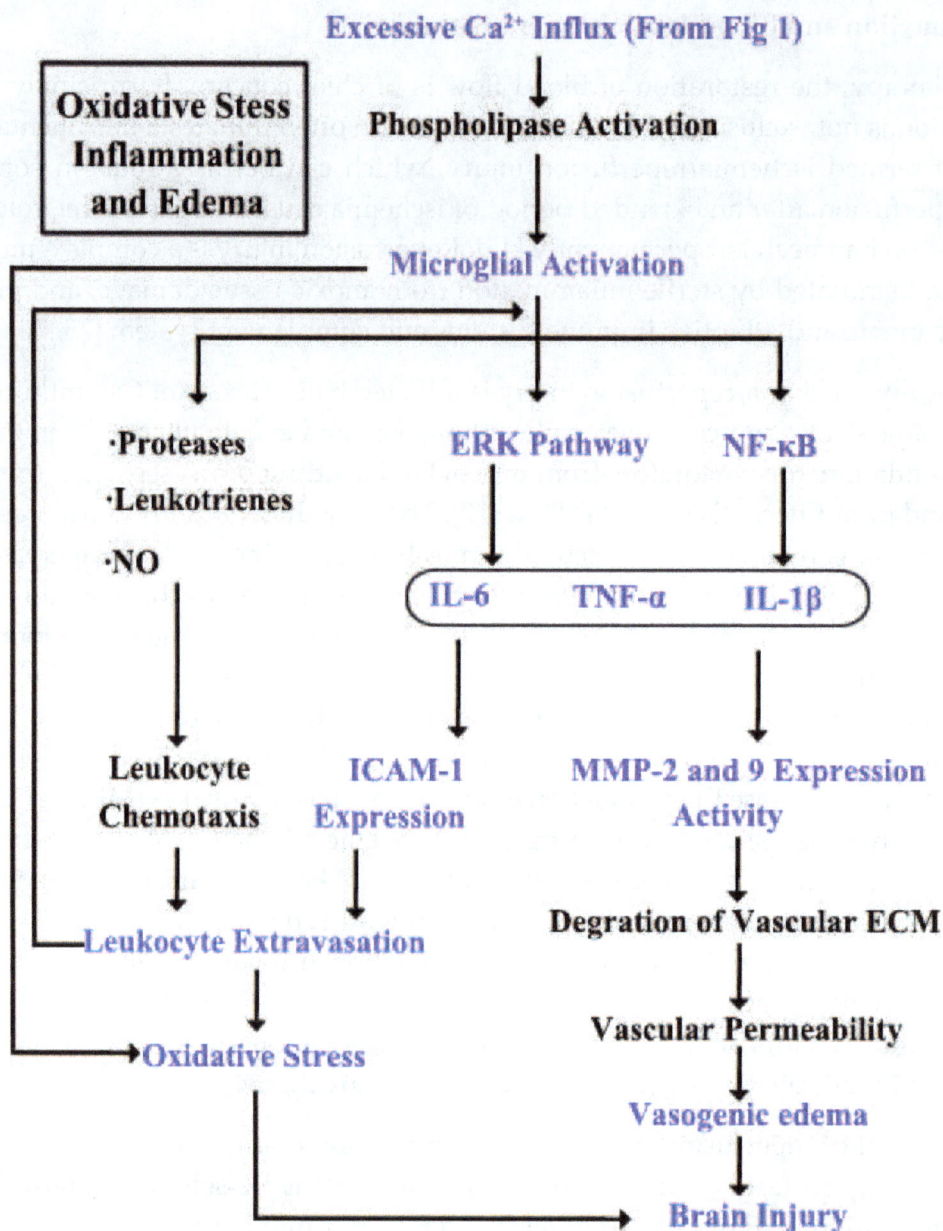

Figure 2. The figure describes the pathogenesis of stroke as it relates to ischemia-induced oxidative stress, inflammation, and edema. It is not known exactly where hypothermia exerts its neuroprotective effects. Studies have shown that TH attenuates a multitude of steps in the cascade of ischemia-induced brain damage compared to stroke without hypothermia, but whether the observed attenuations are direct effects of TH or byproducts of upstream attenuations has yet to be elucidated. As such, blue font indicates steps discussed in the present review that hypothermia has been shown to attenuate. Black font indicates steps that we have not discussed in the present review, but does not necessarily indicate that these steps are unaffected by hypothermia.

into damaged tissue) [82]. ICAM-1 knockout mice are resistant to cerebral ischemic injury [83], and antagonization of CD11/CD18 has been shown to substantially reduce leukocyte infiltration and subsequent cerebral edema (**Figure 2**) [82].

These effects seem to be associated with the inhibition of the extracellular signal-regulated kinase (ERK) pathway (**Figure 2**). ERK plays a significant role in the regulation of cell survival signals, and in the brain it is involved in responses to stress stimuli, including glutamate receptor stimulation and oxidative stress [84, 85]. ERK has been shown to contribute to NO and TNF-α secretion, and inhibition of the pathway prevents the release of excitotoxic amino acids following focal ischemia [86]. Transient hypothermia has been shown to reduce microglial activation, which translated to reduced phosphorylation (activation) of ERK and decreased IL-6 and TNF-α secretion [84]. However, induction of hypothermia in conjunction with U0216 (an ERK inhibitor) provided equal functional recovery to rats that did not receive U0216, implying that poststroke functional recovery progresses independently of ERK signaling [87]. Hypothermia has also been shown to reduce ICAM-1 expression in microglia in correlation with the ERK pathway, as administration of TH led to decreases in the activation of ERK as well as the inhibition of ICAM-1 expression [84].

Hypothermia-associated decreases in the expression of ICAM-1, IL-1β and TNF-α may also be due to attenuation of the NF-κB pathway (**Figure 2**). Therapeutic hypothermia has been shown to increase the expression of HSP70 in ischemic brains (but not in non-ischemic brains), and reports have suggested that HSP70 stabilizes NF-κB, thereby preventing its phosphorylation (activation) [73]. However, other NF-κB-associated proteins contribute as well. This pathway is puzzling, as the mechanism of NF-κB suppression varies depending on the type of ischemia. In models of focal ischemia, hypothermia suppresses NF-κB activity by inhibiting the activity of NF-κB kinase (IKK), a protein essential for degradation of the NF-κB inhibitor (IκB). In models of global ischemia, nuclear NF-κB levels in hypothermic subjects were still below normothermic levels, but IKK and IκB levels were unchanged [78]. These results are surprising, but emphasize the complexity of stroke pathogenesis and TH-associated neuroprotection. Moreover, regardless of the precise mechanism, therapeutic hypothermia seems to serve a beneficial role in NF-κB-associated neuroprotection.

Hypothermia can also prevent BBB breakdown directly. Nagel et al. recently found that TH increased functional recovery and reduced MMP-2 and -9 activities to the same degree as normothermic application of the MMP inhibitor minocycline, and that the application of TH in conjunction with minocycline was only marginally more effective than either by itself [88]. In addition to decreasing MMP activity, minocycline has been shown to decrease MMP production at the transcriptional level, and this report suggested that TH functions in the same way [88]. Other groups have found similar results, and this TH-induced MMP downregulation indeed translated to smaller infarct volumes and improved functional recovery [79, 89]. These data consistently show that TH is a powerful downregulator of MMP expression and activity, and that the modulation of MMP function leads to marked improvements in big-picture end goals of stroke therapy (decreased infarct volume, increased functional recovery, etc.) (**Figure 2**).

4.3. Apoptosis

Following the initial ischemia-induced insults (hours to days), long-term brain damage (days to weeks) is greatly influenced by cellular proapoptotic mechanisms. Hypothermia has been shown to affect several aspects of apoptotic cell death in both the intrinsic (intracellular-mediated) and extrinsic (receptor-mediated) cell death pathways, and ultimately prevent apoptosis after experimental stroke (**Figure 3**) [37].

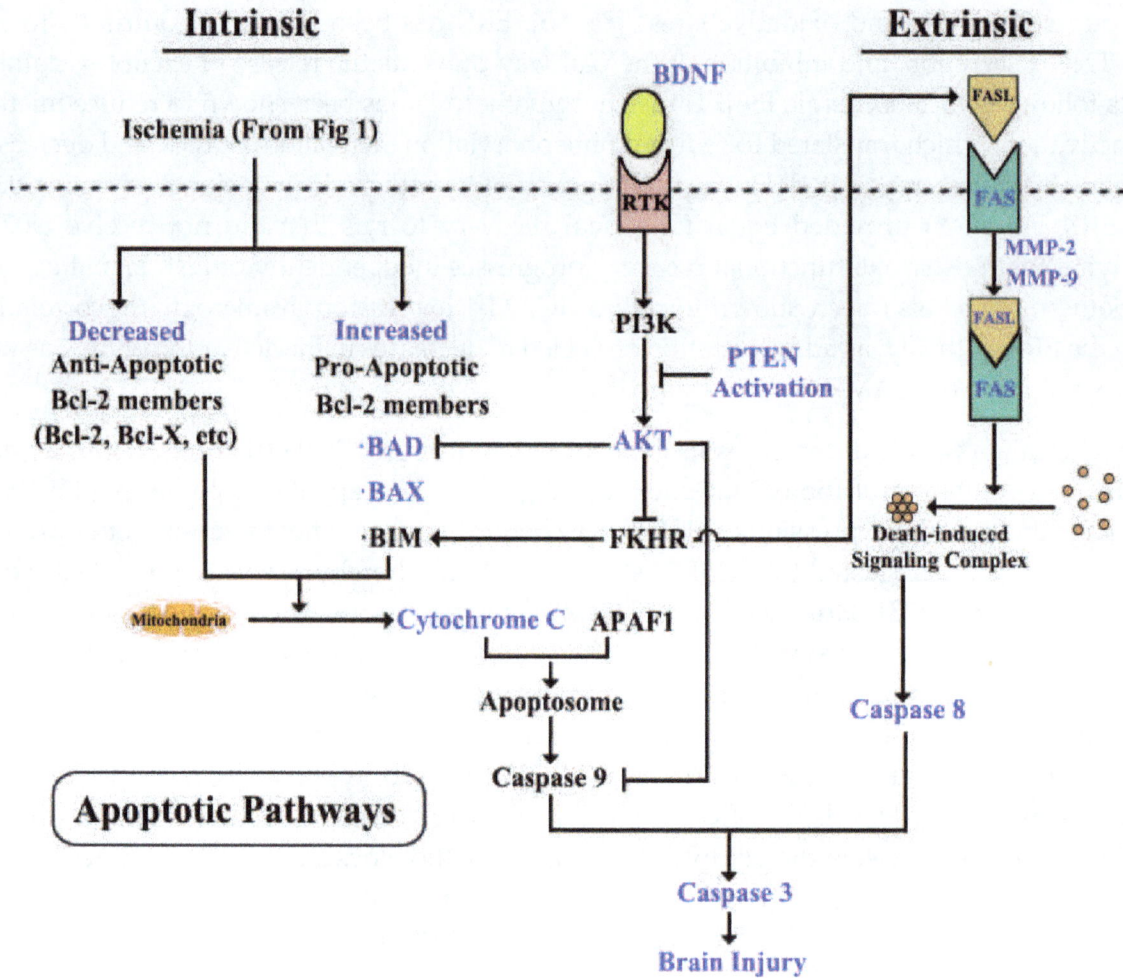

Figure 3. The figure describes the pathogenesis of stroke as it pertains to apoptotic pathways. It is not known exactly where hypothermia exerts its neuroprotective effects. Studies have shown that TH attenuates a multitude of steps in the cascade of ischemia-induced brain damage compared to stroke without hypothermia, but whether the observed attenuations are direct effects of TH or byproducts of upstream attenuations has yet to be elucidated. As such, blue font indicates steps discussed in the present review that hypothermia has been shown to attenuate. Black font indicates steps that we have not discussed in the present review, but does not necessarily indicate that these steps are unaffected by hypothermia. BDNF, brain-derived neurotropic factor; MMP, matrix metalloproteinase; RKT, receptor tyrosine kinase; PI3K, phosphoinositide-3 kinase; PTEN, phosphatase and tensin homologue; FKHR, forkhead transcription factor; APAF1, apoptotic protease-activating factor 1.

The extrinsic apoptotic pathway is initiated by ligand binding to cell death receptors; the best studied being the FAS-ligand (FASL) and its receptor, FAS. When FASL interacts with FAS, it triggers the intercellular assembly of death-induced-signaling complexes (DISCs), which leads to caspase 8 activation. Activated caspase 8 then triggers a caspase activation cascade resulting in the stimulation of apoptosis-inducing proteins such as caspase 3, thereby mediating cell death (**Figure 3**).

Hypothermia affects this pathway at multiple levels (**Figure 3**). Cooling has been shown to suppress the expression of caspase 8, caspase 3, FAS, and FASL [90]. Additionally, there is evidence that the FAS-FASL complex must be cleaved from the cell membrane by MMPs before becoming active [91]. TH has been shown to reduce levels of both MMPs and soluble

FASL in cooled rat brains [91], so is possible that the reduction in levels of these downstream effectors is simply the byproduct of inhibiting the FAS-FASL cleavage. While there are little available data to this end, the fact remains that, by one mechanism or another, hypothermia significantly reduces the production of a number of extrinsic apoptotic pathway intermediates, which translates to the preservation of penumbral tissue.

The intrinsic apoptotic pathway is triggered by intracellular cell stress signals including hypoxia, DNA damage, and cellular detachment from the extracellular matrix. These signals initiate apoptosis by disrupting the balance between proapoptotic Bcl-2 family members (BID, BAX, BAD, etc.) and anti-apoptotic Bcl-2 members (Bcl-2, Bcl-x, etc.) by a variety of mechanisms. Bcl-2 and Bcl-xL have both been found to be upregulated in neurons surviving hypoxia, while proapoptotic Bcl-2 members are highly expressed in neurons that will eventually die from hypoxic damage [37]. The imbalance between pro- and anti-apoptotic Bcl-2 members leads to the liberation of cytochrome C from the mitochondrial intermembrane space into the cytosol where it couples with APAF1 to form an apoptosome. The apoptosome activates caspase 9, which triggers a caspase activation cascade resulting in the activation of caspase 3 and apoptosis (**Figure 3**).

Hypothermia exerts its neuroprotective effects at several points along the intrinsic apoptotic pathway (**Figure 3**). TH has been found to inhibit BAX overexpression 4 h after 30 min of partial ischemia while having no effect on Bcl-2 expression [92]. TH has also been shown to diminish cytochrome C release without modifying BAX or Bcl-2 expression. This study did not observe caspase activity, which implied that TH endowed neuroprotection functions independently of caspases [93]. Interestingly, the same group found that hypothermia increased Bcl-2 expression in a global ischemia model [94], which underlines the importance of designing studies specific to local cooling in focal ischemia models. Additionally, mild hypothermia has been found to decrease cytochrome C translocation 5 h after reperfusion while leaving levels of caspase 9 and caspase 3 unchanged [74]. The conflicting nature of these findings leaves the point at which TH exerts its protective effects in question, but emphasizes the intricacy of TH-mediated neuroprotection.

Some of the anti-apoptotic effects of TH are mediated through the anti-apoptotic factor Akt/protein kinase B (**Figure 3**). Hypothermia attenuates decreases in Akt dephosphorylation (inactivation) after hypoxia [90]. In response to growth factors including BDNF (brain-derived neurotropic factor), membrane receptor tyrosine kinases activate PI3 kinase, which activates Akt via phosphorylation (p-Akt), thereby allowing it to phosphorylate (inhibit) numerous proapoptotic factors, including BAD, caspase 9, and forkhead transcription factor (FKHR) [90, 95]. Under normal physiological conditions, these proteins are phosphorylated by Akt, and their dephosphorylation can have severe repercussions. Dephosphorylation of BAD allows it to migrate into the mitochondria where it triggers the release of cytochrome C [91]. Dephosphorylated FKHR functions as a transcription factor to encourage overexpression of FASL and BIM [90]. Activation of caspase 9 activates a caspase cascade that results in apoptosis.

In normothermia, poststroke p-Akt levels fluctuate constantly; Zhao et al. found that, in normothermic rats, p-Akt levels decreased 30 min after stroke, increased at 1.5 and 5h, decreased at 9 and 24h, and increased again at 48h. Moderate hypothermia was found to stabilize these fluctuations at every time point except 24h, which translated to reduced infarct volumes and improved functional recovery up to 2 months after hypoxia. Interestingly, the reduction in infarct volumes was considerably less pronounced when TH was administered in conjunction with the PI3K inhibitor LY294002, although infarcts were still substantially smaller than in control animals [90]. It is very likely that this pathway provides a significant portion of TH-mediated neuroprotection. In line with this premise, mild hypothermia has also been found to inhibit the expression of caspase-3 and Fas after resolution of focal ischemia, which also translated to significantly decreased infarct volumes [96]. Hypothermia has also been shown to augment BDNF expression during cerebral ischemia [97], as well as attenuate the decrease in the Akt activity after stroke [90], so it is also possible that the effects of hypothermia on Akt activity are mediated at the level of BDNF.

While direct enhancement of the Akt pathway likely constitutes a portion of TH-mediated neuroprotection, cerebral cooling intervenes at other steps in the pathway as well. The PI3K/Akt pathway is inhibited by phosphatase and tensin homologue (PTEN), which de-phosphorylates upstream activators of Akt. PTEN is inhibited by phosphorylation (p-PTEN), and p-PTEN levels seem to play a crucial role in TH-mediated neuroprotection. Hypothermia has been found to stabilize p-PTEN levels more effectively than levels of p-Akt and other PI3K/Akt pathway participants (p-PDK1, p-GSK3β p-FKHR) [37]. A recent investigation from Lee et al. found that TH administered 15 min before reperfusion led to massive decreases in infarct volume while TH administered 15 min after reperfusion only had modest infarct reductions. Interestingly, while early and late TH had nearly identical effects on levels of p-Akt and other proteins, only early TH maintained high levels of p-PTEN [98]. Additionally, independent of hypothermia, PTEN inhibition was recently shown to confer a 75% reduction in infarct volume in rat models [95]. PTEN clearly plays a critical part in the story of neuroprotection, and should not be neglected in future investigations on the topic.

4.4. Long-term neuroprotection

There is compelling clinical evidence of neuroprotection with prolonged moderate cerebral hypothermia initiated within a few hours after hypoxia-ischemia and continued through the resolution of ischemia in term infants and adults [99–101]. The mechanisms underlying the neuroprotection are currently under investigation. Volser et al. showed that during the post-ischemic phase, the brain naturally activates restorative mechanisms to counteract the effects of the ischemic insult even without the induction of hypothermia [102]. This study, among others put forth the idea of long-term neuroprotection following an ischemic event in the brain. A study by Feng et al. went a step further and found that acute brain insult led to stimulation of neural stem cell proliferation, particularly in the subventricular and hippocampal subgranular zone, corroborating long-term neuroprotection [103]. However, evident from the lasting symptoms of acute ischemia, the brain is unable to completely regenerate and recover from the injury on its own. Thus, there is a dire need for the development of effective regenerative techniques and therapies to maximize patient recovery. This is where LEVI and hypothermia can be used to further the recovery of the brain.

Over the past decade, researchers have proposed the following mechanisms of long-term neuroprotection: neurogenesis, angiogenesis, gliogenesis, preservation of the integrity of neural networks, and inhibition of apoptosis [55]. These mechanisms will be discussed in detail below.

4.4.1. Neurogenesis

Contrary to prior belief, neurogenesis is a common event observed in the brain and while it is primarily limited to two neurogenic areas of the brain, the dentate gyrus of the hippocampus and the subventricular zone of the lateral ventricles, this process plays an important role in maintaining normal brain function [104, 105]. Two potential mechanisms can be attributed to neurogenesis: enhanced differentiation of neuroprogenitor cells into neurons and preferential differentiation of neuroprogenitor cells toward neurogenesis over gliogenesis.

The formation of new neural cells from neural progenitor cells has been identified as a major contributor to new populations of neurons, and TH seems to encourage this formation. An *in vivo* study by Silasi et al. found that when forebrain ischemia was induced in adult rodents, mild hypothermia following the ischemic event led to significantly increased neurogenesis in the dentate gyrus when compared to control groups with no hypothermia induction following an ischemic event [106]. Moreover, a very recent study in a neonatal hypoxic-ischemic injury mouse model showed that hypothermia provided partial protection for neural stem and progenitor cells (NSPCs) in the dentate gyrus subgranular zone, which may facilitate the recovery of function after injury and does not impair the proliferation of NSPCs during recovery [107]. This TH-mediated neurogenesis is thought to confer a more robust, long-term conservation of brain function than would be seen in normoxic stroke patients.

Preferential differentiation of neuroprogenitor cells into neurons also plays a major role in neuroprotection. Interestingly, an *in vivo* study found that cooling of rat brains to 33°C under hypoxic conditions led to an inhibition of hypoxia-induced apoptosis of proliferating neural stem cells and an increase in preferential maturation of neural progenitor cells into neural cells in the striatum [108]. Moreover, an *in vitro* study by Saito et al. found that moderate hypothermia to 32°C prevented apoptosis, preserved the naivety of neural stem cells, and led to lower expression of GFAP in neural stem cell culture, indicating less glial differentiation [109].

On the other hand, a study from early 2016 found that in aged rats, hypothermia induced by H_2S gas for 24 h after resolution of an MCAO only provided temporary therapeutic benefit and did not correlate with enhanced neurogenesis in the subventricular zone or infarcted area [110]. However, the duration of hypothermia induction in this study was shorter than the duration of hypothermia used in most clinical trials (24–48 h) and thus led to suboptimal hypothermia which is reflected in the temporary therapeutic effects [110]. Additionally, the use of hydrogen sulfide to induce hypothermia may not be representative of the conventional hypothermia-inducing agents used in other animal studies. H_2S is a weak and reversible inhibitor of oxidative phosphorylation, thus causing a suspended animation state with hypothermia [111]. It is quite possible that the mechanism of induction of hypothermia by H_2S may have interfered with various long-term protective mechanisms observed in other studies and in clinic using conventional hypothermia techniques.

4.4.2. Angiogenesis

Angiogenesis is a normal yet important biological process that is highly regulated and leads to the formation of new blood vessels during development, wound repair, and reproduction [111]. A study on rats by Xie et al. found that mild hypothermia enhanced angiogenesis in focal cerebral ischemia by increasing microvessel diameter, number of vascular branch points, and overall vessel surface area [112]. This was found to be a brain-derived neurotrophic factor (BDNF)-dependent process. Moreover, another study using a rat MCAO model showed that the injection of BDNF fused with a collagen-binding domain (CBD-BDNF) into the lateral ventricle specifically bound to collagen of the ventricular ependyma and consequently led to neural regeneration, angiogenesis, and reduced cell death [113]. This study further confirms the pro-angiogenic activity of BDNF in ischemic conditions. Vascular endothelial growth factor (VEGF) upregulation has also been found to correlate with acute cerebral ischemia [114, 115]. A very recent prospective cohort study observed increased brain perfusion over the first month in term-asphyxiated newborn babies treated with hypothermia during the first few days of life. This increase in brain perfusion came as a result of increased angiogenesis, which was found to be associated with VEGF expression in the injured brain of asphyxiated newborns treated with hypothermia [116]. VEGF has been consistently shown to increase angiogenesis, which translates to increased functional recovery in the months following an ischemic stroke [117–119].

4.4.3. Gliogenesis

While gliogenesis refers to the development of microglia, oligodendrocytes, and astrocytes in the brain, intriguingly, oligodendrocytes have been found to have a similar susceptibility to neurons for cell death. Early studies found that combined deprivation of oxygen and glucose led to selective death of mature oligodendrocytes over other glial cells *in vitro* [120–122]. *In vivo* studies have shown that cerebral white matter, specifically oligodendrocytes and astrocytes, are highly vulnerable to focal ischemia [123]. However, *in vitro* studies have shown that hypothermia increases the number of oligodendrocyte precursors in primary neural and glial cultures from mouse brains and maintains a cell population of oligodendrocyte progenitors in a less well-differentiated state [124]. Recent studies have found that susceptible oligodendrocyte progenitors and mature oligodendrocytes exposed to hypoxia could be protected by deep hypothermia [125]. Another study demonstrated that hypothermia promoted the differentiation and maturation of oligodendrocyte precursor cells (OPCs), and indicated that OPC death was significantly suppressed by hypothermia *in vitro*, alluding to the fact that hypothermia is protective of oligodendrogliogenesis [126]. More recent studies in fetal sheep have shown that cerebral ischemia is associated with significant loss in total numbers of oligodendrocytes, decreased myelin basic protein expression, and increased microglial activation [127, 128]. However, another study in fetal sheep countered these results by showing that delayed cerebral hypothermia partially protects white matter after global cerebral ischemia by stimulating oligodendrocyte proliferation, reducing microglial induction, and restoring the amount and pattern of expression of myelin basic protein, once again confirming the neuroprotective role of hypothermia toward oligodendrogenesis [129, 130]. Moreover, researchers have found that hypothermia attenuates demyelination, trauma-induced oligodendrocyte cell death, and overall circuit dysfunction [131, 132]. While a study in preterm fetal sheep found that TH was correlated with an overall reduction in the hypoxia-induced death of immature oligodendrocytes, hypothermia did not prevent the hypoxia-induced inhibition of oligodendrocyte proliferation in the periventricular white matter zone [133, 134]. Most importantly, a recent study in rats found that hypothermia reduced the extent of hypoxia-ischemia damage in axons and increased oligodendrocyte lineage proliferation, which was reflected in the increase in myelination of axons and decreases apoptosis and pre-oligodendrocyte lineage accumulation [134]. While an ischemic environment has been shown to be detrimental to oligodendrogenesis and oligodendrocyte survival, hypothermia has been shown to rescue these processes *in vivo* and *in vitro*, as discussed above.

Since astrocytes are the largest population of cells present in the ischemic core during the subacute to chronic period of stroke, astrogliogenesis is often considered to be therapeutic following insult to the brain [131, 135, 136]. However, we still lack much information and need more investigation in this area. Most of the current literature suggests astrogliogenesis as detrimental to the brain rather than neuroprotective. As we know, activated astrocytes form the glial scar in the brain following insult or injury [112, 137]. This brings about doubt on whether astrogliogenesis is therapeutic and may actually impede the postischemic healing process by forming a glial scar that could hinder neurite growth and synaptogenesis, and lead to leakage of proapoptotic factors from astrocyte gap junctions within the glial scar [138]. Moreover, a very recent study found that in mice, hypoxia diminished the protective function of astrocytes and activated them to initiate astrogliosis in the ischemic region [139]. In fact, many studies have shown that decreased astrogliosis correlates with decreased infarct size [140]. Intriguingly, a study conducted by Xiong et al. showed that postischemic hypothermia in rats for 24 h rescued hippocampal neurons by decreasing astrocyte activation and inflammatory cytokine release [141]. Such studies truly call into question the role of astrogliogenesis in neuroprotection. More investigation needs to be done in this area to better understand the role of astrogliogenesis in neuroprotection under hypothermic conditions.

4.4.4. Preservation of the integrity of neural networks

Neural networks are functional units representing the high complexity and processivity of the brain and thus repair and preservation of this circuitry is the key for recovery from brain injury. Some of the key processes involved in neural network maintenance are axonal and neurite growth, synaptogenesis, and maintenance of neuronal architecture. Studies have found that hypothermia of the brain by 17°C enhanced neurite and axonal outgrowth in brain slices [142, 143]. A recent study on spinal cord injury rat models found that regional hypothermia promoted neurite, axonal, and nerve fiber growth to the point that hind limb function was recovered in these rats, which emphasizes the plasticity and extent of recovery via hypothermia that the central nervous system is capable of [144]. However, deep hypothermia (20°C) followed by subsequent rewarming did not change the stability of dendritic spines or the presynaptic boutons in mouse somatosensory cortex [145]. Moreover, a gene profiling study on rat model of traumatic brain injury found that mild hypothermia had significant effects on gene expression for synapse organization and biogenesis; an analysis of the hippocampal gene expression profiles of these rats found that 133 genes showed statistically significant changes in expression compared to injured rat in normoxic conditions. Of the 133, 57 genes were upregulated and were responsible for synaptic organization and biogenesis [146]. An *in vitro* study showed that hypothermia to 33°C following *in* vitro ischemia decreased the neuronal actin polymerization that reduced spine calcium kinetics, disrupted detrimental cell signaling, and protected the neurons against damage [147]. While hypoxic conditions caused changes in F-actin architecture of dendritic spines, hypothermia decreased the actin modifications in dendritic spines preventing the neuronal death [148]. All of these studies support the notion of spine and synaptogenesis preservation by hypothermia treatment.

In a functional study on ischemic gerbils treated with moderate postischemic hypothermia, the untreated (normothermic) groups experienced a 95% reduction in CA1 cells, while cell counts in the TH group were equivalent to that of sham animals. Additionally, postischemic hypothermia preserved the electrophysiological properties of CA1 neurons, which reflects the functional preservation of neural networks [149]. Moreover, mice subjected to ischemia followed by hypothermia treatment showed neuroprotection against ischemia-induced long-term potentiation (LTP) impairment as well as synaptic plasticity [150]. While there are encouraging studies on mechanisms of neural network preservation by hypothermia treatment, further research is needed to better understand how neuronal networks are preserved in the ischemic and penumbra regions in response to hypothermia.

5. Future research directions

Between 1935 and 2010, cancer, heart disease, and stroke have consistently been in the top five causes of death in the United States [151]. While all three are complex, multifaceted diseases, stroke differs from cancer and heart disease in one critical way; a highly effective, easily administered, cost-effective therapy has already been devised. The main factor hindering significant progress on stroke therapy is not a lack of ideas, but rather a lack of research moving hypothermia toward clinical acceptance. Since TH is still predominately discussed in the context of cardiac arrest, the majority of studies on TH feature a global ischemia (cardiac arrest) model, which cannot always be extrapolated to studies on focal cerebral ischemia. Several papers in the present review alone have arrived at a finding using a global ischemia model that is directly opposed by results from a model of focal ischemia or vice versa [37, 93, 94]. In focal ischemia models, there is significant heterogeneity in experimental methods. Studies on TH in focal cerebral ischemia frequently differ in animal model, animal age, duration of ischemia, duration of hypothermia, depth of hypothermia, method of hypothermia induction, and rate of cooling, all of which have consistently been shown to play critical roles in the efficacy of TH treatments. It is also important to note that the vast majority of investigations on neuroprotective efficacy have used transient occlusion models, which produce much more uniform and encouraging results than those using a permanent occlusion model [37]. This is problematic, considering that an estimated 50% of ischemic stroke patients display vessel occlusion 3–4 days after symptom onset, which is considered a relatively permanent occlusion [152]. This heterogeneity is likely a large source of conflicting findings, and surely prevents investigators from coming to an agreement on TH mechanisms. Another issue with present research is the goal of hypotheses. While there have been innumerable studies on the mechanisms of hypothermia-mediated neuroprotection, these reports are usually correlative rather than causative, which makes it difficult to derive any concrete, widely applicable mechanisms from the literature. This overall lack of research has hindered publicization of the procedure; given that LEVI was only developed in 2002, many groups are simply unaware that such a procedure has been proposed. For instance, a highly cited 2012 review on the topic discussed numerous problems with global cooling, but failed to mention LEVI to any extent despite the fact that the procedure remedies every problem highlighted in the paper [58]. However, as the body of research on LEVI grows, so too will its clinical acceptance.

Overall, the picture of therapeutic hypothermia-mediated neuroprotection is favorable and encouraging. TH consistently decreases infarct volumes and facilitates short- and long-term preservation of function to an unprecedented degree. Although there is little widespread consensus as to how this is accomplished, a review of the literature is scarce with detrimental effects of TH. While many questions remain to be answered before TH can be consistently implemented in humans, such a promising therapy to such a ubiquitously disastrous disease warrants a significant time investment going forward.

Acknowledgements

This work was partially supported by the American Heart Association Grant-in-Aid (14GRNT20460246), Merit Review Award (I01RX-001964-01) from the US Department of Veterans Affairs Rehabilitation R&D Service, the National Natural Science Foundation of China (81501141), and the Beijing New-Star Plan of Science and Technology (xx2016061).

Author details

Mitchell Huber[1#], Hong Lian Duan[2#], Ankush Chandra[1], Fengwu Li[2], Longfei Wu[3], Longfei Guan[2], Xiaokun Geng[1,2]* and Yuchuan Ding[1,2]

*Address all correspondence to: xgeng@ccmu.edu.cn

1 Department of Neurological Surgery, Wayne State University School of Medicine, Detroit, MI, USA

2 Institute of Neuroscience, Beijing Luhe Hospital, Capital Medical University, Beijing, China

3 China-America Institute of Neuroscience, Xuanwu Hospital, Capital Medical University, Beijing, China

# These authors contributed equally for this work

References

[1] The National Institute of Neurological Disorders and Stroke rt-PA Stroke Study Group Tissue plasminogen activator for acute ischemic stroke. N Engl J Med, 1995. **333**(24): p. 1581–1588.

[2] Demaerschalk, B.M., et al., Scientific rationale for the inclusion and exclusion criteria for intravenous alteplase in acute ischemic stroke: a statement for healthcare professionals from the American Heart Association/American Stroke Association. Stroke, 2016. **47**(2): p. 581–641.

[3] O'Collins, V.E., et al., 1,026 experimental treatments in acute stroke. Ann Neurol, 2006. **59**(3): p. 467–477.

[4] Bernard, S.A., Gray, T.W., and Buist, M.D., Treatment of comatose survivors of out-of-hospital cardiac arrest with induced hypothermia. ACC Curr J Rev, 2002. **11**(4): p. 82–83.

[5] The Hypothermia After Cardiac Arrest Study Group Mild therapeutic hypothermia to improve the neurologic outcome after cardiac arrest. N Engl J Med, 2002. **346**(8): p. 549–556.

[6] van der Worp, H.B., et al., Hypothermia in animal models of acute ischaemic stroke: a systematic review and meta-analysis. Brain, 2007. **130**(12): p. 3063–3074.

[7] Hemmen, T.M. and Lyden, P.D., Hypothermia after acute ischemic stroke. J Neurotrauma, 2009. **26**(3): p. 5.

[8] Kollmar, R., et al., Different degrees of hypothermia after experimental stroke - Short- and long-term outcome. Stroke, 2007. **38**(5): p. 1585–1589.

[9] Gunn, A.J. and Thoresen, M., Animal studies of neonatal hypothermic neuroprotection have translated well in to practice. Resuscitation, 2015. **97**: p. 88–90.

[10] Gunn, A.J. and Bennet, L., Timing still key to treating hypoxic ischaemic brain injury. The Lancet Neurology. 2016. **15**(2): p. 126–127.

[11] Christian, E., et al., A review of selective hypothermia in the management of traumatic brain injury. Neurosurg Focus, 2008. **25**(4): p. 8.

[12] Ginsberg, M.D., et al., Therapeutic modulation of brain temperature: relevance to ischemic brain injury. Cerebrovasc Brain Metab Rev, 1992. **4**(3): p. 189–225.

[13] Krieger, D.W., et al., Cooling for acute ischemic brain damage (cool aid): an open pilot study of induced hypothermia in acute ischemic stroke. Stroke, 2001. **32**(8): p. 1847–1854.

[14] De Georgia, M.A., et al., Cooling for acute ischemic brain damage (COOL AID): a feasibility trial of endovascular cooling. Neurology, 2004. **63**(2): p. 312–317.

[15] Lyden, P.D., et al., Intravascular cooling in the treatment of stroke (ICTuS): early clinical experience. J Stroke Cerebrovasc Dis, 2005. **14**(3): p. 107–114.

[16] Pichon, N., et al., Efficacy of and tolerance to mild induced hypothermia after out-of-hospital cardiac arrest using an endovascular cooling system. Crit Care, 2007. **11**(3): p. R71.

[17] Simosa, H.F., et al., Increased risk of deep venous thrombosis with endovascular cooling in patients with traumatic head injury. Am Surg, 2007. **73**(5): p. 461–464.

[18] Hemmen, T.M., et al., Intravenous thrombolysis plus hypothermia for acute treatment of ischemic stroke (ICTuS-L): final results. Stroke, 2010. **41**(10): p. 2265–2270.

[19] Kammersgaard, L.P., et al., Feasibility and safety of inducing modest hypothermia in awake patients with acute stroke through surface cooling: a case-control study: The Copenhagen stroke study. Stroke, 2000. **31**(9): p. 2251–2256.

[20] Jeon, S.B., et al., Critical care for patients with massive ischemic stroke. J Stroke, 2014. **16**(3): p. 146–160.

[21] Polderman, K.H., Mechanisms of action, physiological effects, and complications of hypothermia. Crit Care Med, 2009. **37**(7 Suppl): p. S186–202.

[22] Zhang, J.N., et al., Effects of low temperature on shear-induced platelet aggregation and activation. J Trauma, 2004. **57**(2): p. 216–223.

[23] Connolly, J.E., Boyd, R.J., and Calvin, J.W., The protective effect of hypothermia in cerebral ischemia-experimental and clinical application by selective brain cooling in the human. Surgery, 1962. **52**(1): p. 15–24.

[24] Parkins, W.M., Jensen, J.M., and Vars, H.M., Brain cooling in the prevention of brain damage during periods of circulatory occlusion in dogs. AnnSurg, 1954. **140**(3): p. 284–289.

[25] Chen, J., et al., Endovascular hypothermia in acute ischemic stroke: pilot study of selective intra-arterial cold saline infusion. Stroke, 2016. **47**(7): p. 1933–1935.

[26] Ringer, A.J. and Tomsick, T.A., Developments in endovascular therapy for acute ischemic stroke. Neurol Res, 2002. **24(Suppl 1)**: p. S43–46.

[27] Ding, Y., Justin, C., Research progress of hypothermia: selective intra-arterial infusion and regional brain cooling in acute stroke therapy. Exp Stroke, 2012.

[28] Ding, Y., et al., Prereperfusion saline infusion into ischemic territory reduces inflammatory injury after transient middle cerebral artery occlusion in rats. Stroke, 2002. **33**(10): p. 2492–2498.

[29] Ding, Y., et al., Prereperfusion flushing of ischemic territory: a therapeutic study in which histological and behavioral assessments were used to measure ischemia-reperfusion injury in rats with stroke. J Neurosurg, 2002. **96**(2): p. 310–319.

[30] Ding, Y., et al., Local saline infusion into ischemic territory induces regional brain cooling and neuroprotection in rats with transient middle cerebral artery occlusion. Neurosurgery, 2004. **54**(4): p. 956–964; discussion 964-5.

[31] Ji, Y., et al., Therapeutic time window of hypothermia is broader than cerebral artery flushing in carotid saline infusion after transient focal ischemic stroke in rats. Neurol Res, 2012. **34**(7): p. 657–663.

[32] Ji, Y.-B., et al., Interrupted intracarotid artery cold saline infusion as an alternative method for neuroprotection after ischemic stroke. Neurosurg Focus, 2012. **33**(1): p. E10.

[33] Mattingly, T.K., et al., Catheter based selective hypothermia reduces stroke volume during focal cerebral ischemia in swine. J Neurointerv Surg, 2016. **8**(4): p. 418–422.

[34] Zhao, B., et al., A more consistent intraluminal rhesus monkey model of ischemic stroke. Neural Regener Res, 2014. **9**(23): p. 2087–2094.

[35] Wang, B., et. Al., Local cerebral hypothermia induced by selective infusion of cold lactated ringer's: a feasibility study in rhesus monkeys. 2016. Neurological Research. **38**(6): p. 545 - 552.

[36] Choi, J.H., et al., Selective brain cooling with endovascular intracarotid infusion of cold saline: a pilot feasibility study.Am J Neuroradiol, 2010. **31**(5): p. 928–934.

[37] Zhao, H., Steinberg, G.K., and Sapolsky, R.M., General versus specific actions of mild-moderate hypothermia in attenuating cerebral ischemic damage. J Cereb Blood Flow Metab, 2007. **27**(12): p. 1879–1894.

[38] van der Worp, H.B., et al., Can animal models of disease reliably inform human studies? PLoS Med., 2010. **7**(3): p. e1000245.

[39] Esposito, E., et al., In cold blood: intraarteral cold infusions for selective brain cooling in stroke. J Cereb Blood Flow Metab, 2014. **34**(5): p. 743–752.

[40] Roelfsema, V., et al., Window of opportunity of cerebral hypothermia for postischemic white matter injury in the near-term fetal sheep. J Cereb Blood Flow Metab, 2004. **24**(8): p. 877–886.

[41] Markarian, G.Z., et al., Mild hypothermia: therapeutic window after experimental cerebral ischemia. Neurosurgery, 1996. **38**(3): p. 542–550; discussion 551.

[42] Li, J., et al., Long-term neuroprotection induced by regional brain cooling with saline infusion into ischemic territory in rats: a behavioral analysis. Neurol Res, 2004. **26**(6): p. 677–683.

[43] Lassen, N.A., The luxury-perfusion syndrome and its possible relation to acute metabolic acidosis localised within the brain.Lancet, 1966. **288**(7473): p. 1113–1115.

[44] Heiss, W.D., et al., Repeat positron emission tomographic studies in transient middle cerebral artery occlusion in cats: residual perfusion and efficacy of postischemic reperfusion. J Cereb Blood Flow Metab, 1997. **17**(4): p. 388–400.

[45] Pan, J., et al., Reperfusion injury following cerebral ischemia: pathophysiology, MR imaging, and potential therapies. Neuroradiology, 2007. **49**(2): p. 93–102.

[46] Hsu, C.Y., et al., Arachidonic acid and its metabolites in cerebral ischemia. Ann N Y Acad Sci, 1989. **559**: p. 282–295.

[47] Chen, J., et al., The effect of a microcatheter-based selective intra-arterial hypothermia on hemodynamic changes following transient cerebral ischemia. Neurol Res, 2015. **37**(3): p. 263–268.

[48] Luan, X.D., et al., Regional brain cooling induced by vascular saline infusion into ischemic territory reduces brain inflammation in stroke. Acta Neuropathol, 2004. **107**(3): p. 227–234.

[49] Toyoda, T., et al., Intraischemic hypothermia attenuates neutrophil infiltration in the rat neocortex after focal ischemia-reperfusion injury. Neurosurgery, 1996. **39**(6): p. 1200–1205.

[50] Woitzik, J. and Schilling, L., A new method for superselective middle cerebral artery infusion in the rat. J Neurosurg, 2007. **106**(5): p. 872–878.

[51] Song, W., et al., Intra-carotid cold magnesium sulfate infusion induces selective cerebral hypothermia and neuroprotection in rats with transient middle cerebral artery occlusion. Neurol Sci, 2013. **34**(4): p. 479–486.

[52] Chen, J., et al., Enhanced neuroprotection by local intra-arterial infusion of human albumin solution and local hypothermia. Stroke, 2013. **44**(1): p. 260–262.

[53] Dang, S., et al., Neuroprotection by local intra-arterial infusion of erythropoietin after focal cerebral ischemia in rats. Neurol Res, 2011. **33**(5): p. 520–528.

[54] Pardridge, W.M., The blood-brain barrier: bottleneck in brain drug development. NeuroRx, 2005. **2**(1): p. 3–14.

[55] Lyden, P.D. and Lonzo, L., Combination therapy protects ischemic brain in rats. A glutamate antagonist plus a gamma-aminobutyric acid agonist. Stroke, 1994. **25**(1): p. 189–196.

[56] Huang, Z.G., et al., Biphasic opening of the blood-brain barrier following transient focal ischemia: effects of hypothermia. Can J Neurol Sci, 1999. **26**(4): p. 298–304.

[57] Polderman, K.H., Application of therapeutic hypothermia in the intensive care unit. Opportunities and pitfalls of a promising treatment modality-Part 2: Practical aspects and side effects. Intensive Care Med, 2004. **30**(5): p. 757–769.

[58] Yenari, M.A. and Han, H.S., Neuroprotective mechanisms of hypothermia in brain ischaemia. Nat Rev Neurosci, 2012. **13**(4): p. 267–278.

[59] Dong, X.-X., Wang, Y., and Qin, Z.-H., Molecular mechanisms of excitotoxicity and their relevance to pathogenesis of neurodegenerative diseases. Acta Pharmacol Sin, 2009. **30**(4): p. 379–387.

[60] Previch, L.M., L.; Wright, J.; Singh, S.; Geng, X.; Ding, Y., Progress in AQP research and new developments in therapeutic approaches to ischemic and hemorrhagic stroke. Int J Mol Sci, 2016. **17**(7).

[61] Yenari, M., et al., Metabolic downregulation: a key to successful neuroprotection? Stroke, 2008. **39**(10): p. 2910–2917.

[62] Erecinska, M., Thoresen, M., and Silver, I.A., Effects of hypothermia on energy metabolism in Mammalian central nervous system. J Cereb Blood Flow Metab, 2003. **23**(5): p. 513–530.

[63] Kimura, T., et al., Effect of mild hypothermia on energy state recovery following transient forebrain ischemia in the gerbil. Exp Brain Res, 2002. **145**(1): p. 83–90.

[64] Shimizu, H., et al., Effect of brain, body, and magnet bore temperatures on energy metabolism during global cerebral ischemia and reperfusion monitored by magnetic resonance spectroscopy in rats. Magn Reson Med, 1997. **37**(6): p. 833–839.

[65] Ooboshi, H., et al., Hypothermia inhibits ischemia-induced efflux of amino acids and neuronal damage in the hippocampus of aged rats. Brain Res, 2000. **884**(1–2): p. 23–30.

[66] Colbourne, F., et al., Hypothermia rescues hippocampal CA1 neurons and attenuates down-regulation of the AMPA receptor GluR2 subunit after forebrain ischemia. Proc Natl Acad Sci USA, 2003. **100**(5): p. 2906–2910.

[67] Kristian, T., Katsura, K., and Siesjo, B.K., The influence of moderate hypothermia on cellular calcium uptake in complete ischaemia: implications for the excitotoxic hypothesis. Acta Physiol Scand, 1992. **146**(4): p. 531–532.

[68] Papadopoulos, M.C., et al., Aquaporin-4 facilitates reabsorption of excess fluid in vasogenic brain edema. FASEB J, 2004. **18**(9): p. 1291-+.

[69] Zhao, H., et al., Molecular mechanisms of therapeutic hypothermia on neurological function in a swine model of cardiopulmonary resuscitation. Resuscitation, 2012. **83**(7): p. 913–920.

[70] Kurisu, K., et al., Transarterial regional brain hypothermia inhibits acute aquaporin-4 surge and sequential microvascular events in ischemia/reperfusion injury. Neurosurgery, 2016. **79**(1): p. 125–134.

[71] Morishima, T., et al., Lactic acid increases aquaporin 4 expression on the cell membrane of cultured rat astrocytes. Neurosci Res, 2008. **61**(1): p. 18–26.

[72] Vella, J., et al., The central role of aquaporins in the pathophysiology of ischemic stroke. Front Cell Neurosci, 2015. **9**: p. 108.

[73] Shintani, Y., Terao, Y., and Ohta, H., Molecular mechanisms underlying hypothermia-induced neuroprotection. Stroke Res Treat, 2010. **2011**: p. 809874.

[74] Xu, L., et al., Mild hypothermia reduces apoptosis of mouse neurons in vitro early in the cascade. J Cereb Blood Flow Metab, 2002. **22**(1): p. 21–28.

[75] Nour, M., Scalzo, F., and Liebeskind, D.S., Ischemia-reperfusion injury in stroke. Interv Neurol, 2013. **1**(3–4): p. 185–199.

[76] Eltzschig, H.K. and Eckle, T., Ischemia and reperfusion-from mechanism to translation. Nat Med, 2011. **17**(11): p. 1391–1401.

[77] Kim, J.Y., Kawabori, M., and Yenari, M.A., Innate inflammatory responses in stroke: mechanisms and potential therapeutic targets. Curr Med Chem, 2014. **21**(18): p. 2076–2097.

[78] Yenari, M.A. and Han, H.S., Influence of hypothermia on post-ischemic inflammation: role of nuclear factor kappa B (NFkappaB). Neurochem Int, 2006. **49**(2): p. 164–169.

[79] Truettner, J.S., Alonso, O.F., and Dalton Dietrich, W., Influence of therapeutic hypothermia on matrix metalloproteinase activity after traumatic brain injury in rats. Journal of cerebral blood flow and metabolism, 2005. **25**: p. 1516.

[80] Kahles, T. and Brandes, R.P., NADPH oxidases as therapeutic targets in ischemic stroke. Cell Mol Life Sci, 2012. **69**(14): p. 2345–2363.

[81] Ceulemans, A.-G., et al., The dual role of the neuroinflammatory response after ischemic stroke: modulatory effects of hypothermia. J Neuroinflamm, 2010. **7**: p. 74.

[82] Yenari, M.A., et al., Hu23F2G, an antibody recognizing the leukocyte CD11/CD18 integrin, reduces injury in a rabbit model of transient focal cerebral ischemia. Exp Neurol, 1998. **153**(2): p. 223–233.

[83] Connolly, E.S., Jr., et al., Cerebral protection in homozygous null ICAM-1 mice after middle cerebral artery occlusion. Role of neutrophil adhesion in the pathogenesis of stroke. J Clin Invest, 1996. **97**(1): p. 209–216.

[84] Schmitt, K.R., Hypothermia suppresses inflammation via ERK signaling pathway in stimulated microglial cells. Journal of neuroimmunology, 2007. **189**: p. 16.

[85] Aikawa, R., et al., Oxidative stress activates extracellular signal-regulated kinases through Src and Ras in cultured cardiac myocytes of neonatal rats. J Clin Invest, 1997. **100**(7): p. 1813–1821.

[86] Alessandrini, A., et al., MEK1 protein kinase inhibition protects against damage resulting from focal cerebral ischemia. Proc Natl Acad Sci U S A, 1999. **96**(22): p. 12866–12869.

[87] D'Cruz, B.J., et al., Hypothermia and ERK activation after cardiac arrest. Brain research, 2005. **1064**: p. 118.

[88] Nagel, S., Minocycline and hypothermia for reperfusion injury after focal cerebral ischemia in the rat: effects on BBB breakdown and MMP expression in the acute and subacute phase. Brain research, 2008. **1188**: p. 206.

[89] Burk, J., et al., Protection of cerebral microvasculature after moderate hypothermia following experimental focal cerebral ischemia in mice. Brain Res, 2008. **1226**: p. 248–255.

[90] Zhao, H., et al., Akt contributes to neuroprotection by hypothermia against cerebral ischemia in rats. J Neurosci, 2005. **25**(42): p. 9794–9806.

[91] Liu, L., et al., FasL shedding is reduced by hypothermia in experimental stroke. J. Neurochem, 2008. **106**(2): p. 541–550.

[92]   Eberspacher, E., et al., The effect of hypothermia on the expression of the apoptosis-regulating protein Bax after incomplete cerebral ischemia and reperfusion in rats. J Neurosurg Anesthesiol, 2003. **15**(3): p. 200–208.

[93]   Yenari, M.A., Mild hypothermia attenuates cytochrome c release but does not alter Bcl-2 expression or caspase activation after experimental stroke. 2002. **22**: p. 38.

[94]   Zhang, Z., et al., Mild hypothermia increases Bcl-2 protein expression following global cerebral ischemia. Brain research. Molecular brain research, 2001. **95**: p. 85.

[95]   Shi, G.D., et al., PTEN deletion prevents ischemic brain injury by activating the mTOR signaling pathway. Biochem Biophys Res Commun, 2011. **404**(4): p. 941–945.

[96]   Phanithi, P.B., et al., Mild hypothermia mitigates post-ischemic neuronal death following focal cerebral ischemia in rat brain: immunohistochemical study of Fas, caspase-3 and TUNEL. Neuropathology, 2000. **20**(4): p. 273–282.

[97]   Vosler, P.S., et al., Delayed hypothermia preferentially increases expression of brain-derived neurotrophic factor exon III in rat hippocampus after asphyxial cardiac arrest. Brain research. Molecular brain research, 2005. **135**: p. 29.

[98]   Lee, S.M., et al., The protective effect of early hypothermia on PTEN phosphorylation correlates with free radical inhibition in rat stroke. J Cereb Blood Flow Metab, 2009. **29**(9): p. 1589–1600.

[99]   Gunn, A.J. and Gluckman, P.D., Head cooling for neonatal encephalopathy: the state of the art. Clin Obstet Gynecol, 2007. **50**(3): p. 636–651.

[100] Hoehn, T., et al., Therapeutic hypothermia in neonates. Review of current clinical data, ILCOR recommendations and suggestions for implementation in neonatal intensive care units. Resuscitation, 2008. **78**(1): p. 7–12.

[101] Shah, P.S., Hypothermia: a systematic review and meta-analysis of clinical trials. Semin Fetal Neonatal Med, 2010. **15**(5): p. 238–246.

[102] Kernie, S.G. and Parent, J.M., Forebrain neurogenesis after focal Ischemic and traumatic brain injury. Neurobiol Dis, 2010. **37**(2): p. 267–274.

[103] Feng, J.F., et al., Effect of therapeutic mild hypothermia on the genomics of the hippocampus after moderate traumatic brain injury in rats. Neurosurgery, 2010. **67**(3): p. 730–742.

[104] Gage, F.H., Mammalian neural stem cells. Science, 2000. **287**(5457): p. 1433–1438.

[105] Ming, G.L. and Song, H., Adult neurogenesis in the mammalian brain: significant answers and significant questions. Neuron, 2011. **70**(4): p. 687–702.

[106] Silasi, G. and Colbourne, F., Therapeutic hypothermia influences cell genesis and survival in the rat hippocampus following global ischemia. J Cereb Blood Flow Metab, 2011. **31**(8): p. 1725–1735.

[107] Kwak, M., et al., Effects of neonatal hypoxic-ischemic injury and hypothermic neuro-protection on neural progenitor cells in the mouse hippocampus. Dev Neurosci, 2015. **37**(4–5): p. 428–439.

[108] Xiong, M., et al., Post-ischemic hypothermia promotes generation of neural cells and reduces apoptosis by Bcl-2 in the striatum of neonatal rat brain. Neurochem Int, 2011. **58**(6): p. 625–633.

[109] Saito, K., et al., Moderate low temperature preserves the stemness of neural stem cells and suppresses apoptosis of the cells via activation of the cold-inducible RNA binding protein. Brain Res, 2010. **1358**: p. 20–29.

[110] Sandu, R.E., et al., Twenty-four hours hypothermia has temporary efficacy in reducing brain infarction and inflammation in aged rats. Neurobiol Aging, 2016. **38**: p. 127–140.

[111] Otrock, Z.K., et al., Understanding the biology of angiogenesis: Review of the most important molecular mechanisms. Blood Cells Mol Dis, 2007. **39**(2): p. 212–220.

[112] Hawthorne, A.L., et al., The unusual response of serotonergic neurons after CNS Injury: lack of axonal dieback and enhanced sprouting within the inhibitory environment of the glial scar. J Neurosci, 2011. **31**(15): p. 5605–5616.

[113] Guan, J., et al., Neuronal regeneration and protection by collagen-binding BDNF in the rat middle cerebral artery occlusion model. Biomaterials, 2012. **33**(5): p. 1386–1395.

[114] Wang, Y., et al., VEGF overexpression induces post-ischaemic neuroprotection, but facilitates haemodynamic steal phenomena. Brain, 2005. **128**(Pt 1): p. 52–63.

[115] Margaritescu, O., Pirici, D., and Margaritescu, C., VEGF expression in human brain tissue after acute ischemic stroke. Rom J Morphol Embryol, 2011. **52**(4): p. 1283–1292.

[116] Shaikh, H., et al., Increased brain perfusion persists over the first month of life in term asphyxiated newborns treated with hypothermia: does it reflect activated angiogen-esis? Transl Stroke Res, 2015. **6**(3): p. 224–233.

[117] Dzietko, M., et al., Delayed VEGF treatment enhances angiogenesis and recovery after neonatal focal rodent stroke. Transl Stroke Res, 2013. **4**(2): p. 189–200.

[118] Sun, Y., et al., VEGF-induced neuroprotection, neurogenesis, and angiogenesis after focal cerebral ischemia. J Clin Invest, 2003. **111**(12): p. 1843–1851.

[119] Lee, H.J., et al., Human neural stem cells over-expressing VEGF provide neuroprotec-tion, angiogenesis and functional recovery in mouse stroke model. PLoS One, 2007. **2**(1): p. e156.

[120] McDonald, J.W., et al., Oligodendrocytes from forebrain are highly vulnerable to AMPA/kainate receptor-mediated excitotoxicity. Nat Med, 1998. **4**(3): p. 291–297.

[121] Lyons, S.A. and Kettenmann, H., Oligodendrocytes and microglia are selectively vul-nerable to combined hypoxia and hypoglycemia injury in vitro. J Cereb Blood Flow Metab, 1998. **18**(5): p. 521–530.

[122] Yoshioka, A., et al., Non-N-methyl-D-aspartate glutamate receptors mediate oxygen–glucose deprivation-induced oligodendroglial injury. Brain Res, 2000. **854**(1–2): p. 207–215.

[123] Pantoni, L., Garcia, J.H., and Gutierrez, J.A., Cerebral white matter is highly vulnerable to ischemia. Stroke, 1996. **27**(9): p. 1641–1647.

[124] Imada, S., et al., Hypothermia-induced increase of oligodendrocyte precursor cells: Possible involvement of plasmalemmal voltage-dependent anion channel 1. J Neurosci Res, 2010. **88**(16): p. 3457–3466.

[125] Agematsu, K., et al., Effects of preoperative hypoxia on white matter injury associated with cardiopulmonary bypass in a rodent hypoxic and brain slice model. Pediatr Res, 2014. **75**(5): p. 618–625.

[126] Xiong, M., et al., Effects of hypothermia on oligodendrocyte precursor cell proliferation, differentiation and maturation following hypoxia ischemia in vivo and in vitro. Exp Neurol, 2013. **247**: p. 720–729.

[127] Davidson, J.O., et al., Non-additive effects of delayed connexin hemichannel blockade and hypothermia after cerebral ischemia in near-term fetal sheep. J Cereb Blood Flow Metab, 2015. **35**(12): p. 2052–2061.

[128] Davidson, J.O., et al., Connexin hemichannel blockade improves outcomes in a model of fetal ischemia. Ann Neurol, 2012. **71**(1): p. 121–132.

[129] Davidson, J.O., et al., Extending the duration of hypothermia does not further improve white matter protection after ischemia in term-equivalent fetal sheep. Sci Rep, 2016. **6**: p. 25178.

[130] Davidson, J.O., et al., How long is too long for cerebral cooling after ischemia in fetal sheep? J Cereb Blood Flow Metab, 2015. **35**(5): p. 751–758.

[131] Lotocki, G., et al., Oligodendrocyte vulnerability following traumatic brain injury in rats: effect of moderate hypothermia. Ther Hypothermia Temp Manag, 2011. **1**(1): p. 43–51.

[132] Lotocki, G., et al., Oligodendrocyte vulnerability following traumatic brain injury in rats. Neurosci Lett, 2011. **499**(3): p. 143–148.

[133] Bennet, L., The effect of cerebral hypothermia on white and grey matter injury induced by severe hypoxia in preterm fetal sheep. Journal of Physiology, 2007. **578**: p. 506.

[134] Xiong, M., et al., Short-term effects of hypothermia on axonal injury, preoligodendrocyte accumulation and oligodendrocyte myelination after hypoxia-ischemia in the hippocampus of immature rat brain. Dev Neurosci, 2013. **35**(1): p. 17–27.

[135] Font, M.A., Arboix, A., and Krupinski, J., Angiogenesis, neurogenesis and neuroplasticity in ischemic stroke. Curr Cardiol Rev, 2010. **6**(3): p. 238–244.

[136] Gopurappilly, R., Stem cells in stroke repair: current success & future prospects. CNS & Neurological disorders drug targets, 2011. **10**: p. 756.

[137] Trendelenburg, G. and Dirnagl, U., Neuroprotective role of astrocytes in cerebral ischemia: focus on ischemic preconditioning, Glia, 2005. **50**: p. 320.

[138] Lin, J.H., et al., Gap-junction-mediated propagation and amplification of cell injury. Nat Neurosci, 1998. **1**(6): p. 494–500.

[139] Agematsu, K., et al., Hypoxia diminishes the protective function of white-matter astrocytes in the developing brain. J Thorac Cardiovasc Surg, 2016. **151**(1): p. 265–272 e1-3.

[140] Zhao, Y. and Rempe, D.A., Targeting astrocytes for stroke therapy. Neurotherapeutics, 2010. **7**(4): p. 439–451.

[141] Xiong, M., et al., Post-ischemic hypothermia for 24h in P7 rats rescues hippocampal neuron: association with decreased astrocyte activation and inflammatory cytokine expression. Brain Res Bull, 2009. **79**(6): p. 351–357.

[142] Schmitt, K.R.L., et al., Hypothermia-induced neurite outgrowth is mediated by tumor necrosis factor-alpha. Brain Pathol, 2010. **20**(4): p. 771–779.

[143] Schmitt, K.R., S100B modulates IL-6 release and cytotoxicity from hypothermic brain cells and inhibits hypothermia-induced axonal outgrowth. Neuroscience research, 2007. **59**: p. 173.

[144] Xu, X., et al., Beneficial effects of local profound hypothermia and the possible mechanism after experimental spinal cord injury in rats. J Spinal Cord Med, 2016. **39**(2): p. 220–228.

[145] Xie, Y., Chen, S., and Murphy, T., Dendritic spines and pre-synaptic boutons are stable despite local deep hypothermic challenge and re-warming in vivo. PLoS One, 2012. **7**(5): p. e36305.

[146] Feng, J.-F., et al., Effect of therapeutic mild hypothermia on the genomics of the hippocampus after moderate traumatic brain injury in rats. Neurosurgery, 2010. **67**(3): p. 730–742.

[147] Gisselsson, L.L., Matus, A., and Wieloch, T., Actin redistribution underlies the sparing effect of mild hypothermia on dendritic spine morphology after in vitro ischemia. J Cereb Blood Flow Metab, 2005. **25**(10): p. 1346–1355.

[148] Muniz, J., et al., Neuroprotective effects of hypothermia on synaptic actin cytoskeletal changes induced by perinatal asphyxia. Brain Res, 2014. **1563**: p. 81–90.

[149] Dong, H., et al., Electrophysiological properties of CA1 neurons protected by postischemic hypothermia in gerbils. Stroke, 2001. **32**(3): p. 788–795.

[150] Dietz, R.M., et al., Therapeutic hypothermia protects against ischemia-induced impairment of synaptic plasticity following juvenile cardiac arrest in sex-dependent manner. Neuroscience, 2016. **325**: p. 132–141.

[151] Hoyert, D.L., 75 years of mortality in the United States, 1935–2010. NCHS Data Brief, 2012(88): p. 1–8.

[152] Kassem-Moussa, H. and Graffagnino, C., Nonocclusion and spontaneous recanalization rates in acute ischemic stroke: a review of cerebral angiography studies. Arch Neurol, 2002. **59**(12): p. 1870–1873.

Permissions

All chapters in this book were first published in HHD, by InTech Open; hereby published with permission under the Creative Commons Attribution License or equivalent. Every chapter published in this book has been scrutinized by our experts. Their significance has been extensively debated. The topics covered herein carry significant findings which will fuel the growth of the discipline. They may even be implemented as practical applications or may be referred to as a beginning point for another development.

The contributors of this book come from diverse backgrounds, making this book a truly international effort. This book will bring forth new frontiers with its revolutionizing research information and detailed analysis of the nascent developments around the world.

We would like to thank all the contributing authors for lending their expertise to make the book truly unique. They have played a crucial role in the development of this book. Without their invaluable contributions this book wouldn't have been possible. They have made vital efforts to compile up to date information on the varied aspects of this subject to make this book a valuable addition to the collection of many professionals and students.

This book was conceptualized with the vision of imparting up-to-date information and advanced data in this field. To ensure the same, a matchless editorial board was set up. Every individual on the board went through rigorous rounds of assessment to prove their worth. After which they invested a large part of their time researching and compiling the most relevant data for our readers.

The editorial board has been involved in producing this book since its inception. They have spent rigorous hours researching and exploring the diverse topics which have resulted in the successful publishing of this book. They have passed on their knowledge of decades through this book. To expedite this challenging task, the publisher supported the team at every step. A small team of assistant editors was also appointed to further simplify the editing procedure and attain best results for the readers.

Apart from the editorial board, the designing team has also invested a significant amount of their time in understanding the subject and creating the most relevant covers. They scrutinized every image to scout for the most suitable representation of the subject and create an appropriate cover for the book.

The publishing team has been an ardent support to the editorial, designing and production team. Their endless efforts to recruit the best for this project, has resulted in the accomplishment of this book. They are a veteran in the field of academics and their pool of knowledge is as vast as their experience in printing. Their expertise and guidance has proved useful at every step. Their uncompromising quality standards have made this book an exceptional effort. Their encouragement from time to time has been an inspiration for everyone.

The publisher and the editorial board hope that this book will prove to be a valuable piece of knowledge for researchers, students, practitioners and scholars across the globe.

List of Contributors

Susana P. Gaytán and Rosario Pasaro
Department of Physiology, University of Seville, Sevilla, Spain

Shayna Sharma, Mona Alharbi, Andrew Lai and Miharu Kobayashi
Exosome Biology Laboratory, Centre for Clinical Diagnostics, University of Queensland Centre for Clinical Research, Royal Brisbane and Women's Hospital, The University of Queensland, Brisbane, QLD, Australia

Gregory E. Rice and Carlos Salomon
Exosome Biology Laboratory, Centre for Clinical Diagnostics, University of Queensland Centre for Clinical Research, Royal Brisbane and Women's Hospital, The University of Queensland, Brisbane, QLD, Australia
Department of Obstetrics and Gynecology, Maternal-Fetal Medicine, Ochsner Clinic Foundation, New Orleans, LA, USA

Richard Kline and Katrina Wade
Department of Obstetrics and Gynecology, Maternal-Fetal Medicine, Ochsner Clinic Foundation, New Orleans, LA, USA

Guomin Shen
Department of Medical Genetics, Medical College, Henan University of Science and Technology, Luoyang, Henan Province, China

Xiaobo Li
Department of Pathology & Translational Medicine Center, Harbin Medical University, Harbin, Heilongjiang Province, China

Kazuhiro Kaneko and Tomonori Yano
Division of Science and Technology for Endoscopy, National Cancer Center Hospital East, Chiba, Japan

Hiroshi Yamaguchi
Imaging Technology Center, FUJIFILM Corporation, Tokyo, Japan

Christopher B. Wolff and David J. Collier
William Harvey Heart Centre, Barts and the London School of Medicine and Dentistry, Queen Mary University of London, London, UK

Annabel H. Nickol
Oxford Centre, for Respiratory Medicine, Churchill Hospital, Oxford, UK

Nicoletta Charolidi and Veronica A. Carroll
Vascular Biology Research Centre, Molecular and Clinical Sciences Research Institute, St George's, University of London, London, UK

Wahyu Widowati
Faculty of Medicine, Maranatha Christian University, Bandung, Indonesia

Dwi Davidson Rihibiha and Khie Khiong
Biomolecular and Biomedical Research Center, Aretha Medika Utama, Bandung, Indonesia

M. Aris Widodo
Laboratory of Pharmacology, Faculty of Medicine, Brawijaya University, Malang, Indonesia

Sutiman B. Sumitro
Department of Biology, Faculty of Mathematics and Natural Sciences, Brawijaya University, Malang, Indonesia

Indra Bachtiar
Stem Cell and Cancer Institute, Jakarta, Indonesia

Nassera Aouali, Manon Bosseler, Delphine Sauvage, Kris Van Moer and Bassam Janji
Laboratory of Experimental Cancer Research, Department of Oncology, Luxembourg Institute of Health, Luxembourg City, Luxembourg

Guy Berchem
Laboratory of Experimental Cancer Research, Department of Oncology, Luxembourg Institute of Health, Luxembourg City, Luxembourg
Luxembourg Hospital Center, Department of Hemato-Oncology, Luxembourg City, Luxembourg

Yulia G. Birulina, Liudmila V. Smaglii and Svetlana V. Gusakova
Siberian State Medical University, Tomsk, Russia

Sergei N. Orlov
Siberian State Medical University, Tomsk, Russia
MV Lomonosov Moscow State University, Moscow, Russia

Mitchell Huber and Ankush Chandra
Department of Neurological Surgery, Wayne State University School of Medicine, Detroit, MI, USA

Xiaokun Geng and Yuchuan Ding
Department of Neurological Surgery, Wayne State University School of Medicine, Detroit, MI, USA
Institute of Neuroscience, Beijing Luhe Hospital, Capital Medical University, Beijing, China

Longfei Guan, Hong Lian Duan and Fengwu Li
Institute of Neuroscience, Beijing Luhe Hospital, Capital Medical University, Beijing, China

Longfei Wu
China-America Institute of Neuroscience, Xuanwu Hospital, Capital Medical University, Beijing, China

Index

www.ingramcontent.com/pod-product-compliance
Lightning Source LLC
Chambersburg PA
CBHW050442200326
41458CB00014B/5037